Hurst's
The Heart

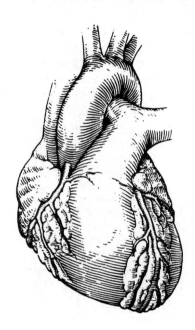

PreTest®
Self-Assessment
and Review

Hurst's The Heart

PreTest® Self-Assessment and Review

Eighth Edition

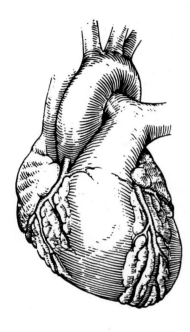

Edited by

Jerre Frederick Lutz, M.D.
Associate Professor of Medicine (Cardiology)
Emory University School of Medicine
Director, Coronary Care Unit
Emory Hospital
Atlanta, Georgia

John Willis Hurst, Jr., M.D.
Clinical Assistant Professor of Medicine (Cardiology)
Emory University School of Medicine
Atlanta, Georgia

J. Willis Hurst, M.D.
Consultant to the Division of Cardiology
(Professor and Chairman, Department of Medicine 1957–1986)
Emory University School of Medicine
Atlanta, Georgia

McGraw-Hill
Health Professions Division
PreTest® Series

New York   St. Louis   San Francisco   Auckland
Bogotá   Caracas   Lisbon   London   Madrid
Mexico City   Milan   Montreal   New Delhi
San Juan   Singapore   Sydney   Tokyo   Toronto

2 3 4 5 6 7 8 9 0   SEMSEM   9 9 8 7 6 5

ISBN 0-07-052011-9

The editors were Gail Gavert and Bruce MacGregor.
The production supervisor was Gyl A. Favours.
This book was set in Times Roman by Compset, Inc.
Quebecor/Semline was printer and binder.
Cover illustration reproduced with permission from S. B. King and J. S. Douglas,
    "Coronary Arteriography and Angioplasty." Copyright ©1985, McGraw-Hill, N.Y.
    Illustration by Michael Budowick, Medical Artist, Emory University School of
    Medicine, Office of Medical Illustration.
This book is printed on acid-free paper.

Library of Congress Cataloging-in-Publication Data

The heart : PreTest self-assessment and review / edited by Jerre
    Frederick Lutz, John W. Hurst, Jr., J. Willis Hurst. — 8th ed.
        p.   cm.
    Includes bibliographical references.
    ISBN 0-07-052011-9
        1. Cardiovascular system—Diseases—Examinations, questions, etc.
    I. Lutz, Jerre F.   II. Hurst, John Willis, III. Hurst, J.
    (John Willis).
        [DNLM: 1. Cardiovascular Diseases—examination questions.   WG 18
    H4365   1996]
    RC669.2.H43   1996
    616.1'0076—dc20
    DNLM/DLC
    for Library of Congress   94-3584

McGraw-Hill, a Division of *The McGraw-Hill Companies*.

• •

Dedicated to

Those who test their knowledge in order to
improve the care of their patients

• •

Contents

CONTENTS

Contributors

Michael Balk, M.D.

Assistant Professor of Medicine (Cardiology)
Emory University School of Medicine
Atlanta, Georgia

Ziyad Ghazzal, M.D.

Assistant Professor of Medicine (Cardiology)
Emory University School of Medicine
Atlanta, Georgia

J. Willis Hurst, M.D.

Consultant to the Division of Cardiology
Professor and Chairman, Department of Medicine
  (1957–1986)
Emory University School of Medicine
Atlanta, Georgia

John Willis Hurst, Jr., M.D.

Clinical Assistant Professor of Medicine (Cardiology)
Emory University School of Medicine
Atlanta, Georgia

Thomas S. Johnston, M.D.

Assistant Professor of Medicine (Cardiology)
Emory University School of Medicine
Atlanta, Georgia

Michael E. Kutcher, M.D.

Associate Professor of Medicine
Director, Interventional Cardiology
Bowman Gray School of Medicine
Winston-Salem, North Carolina

Jerre Frederick Lutz, M.D.

Associate Professor of Medicine (Cardiology)
Emory University School of Medicine
Director, Coronary Care Unit
Emory Hospital
Atlanta, Georgia

Steven V. Manoukian, M.D.

Assistant Professor of Medicine (Cardiology)
Emory University School of Medicine
Atlanta, Georgia

Jeffrey Marshall, M.D.

Assistant Professor of Medicine (Cardiology)
Emory University School of Medicine
Chief of Cardiology and Director of the Cardiac
Catheterization Laboratory
Atlanta VA Medical Center
Atlanta, Georgia

J. David Talley, M.D.

Professor of Internal Medicine
Chief of Cardiology
John L. McClellan Memorial Veterans Hospital
Associate Director, Division of Cardiology
University of Arkansas
Little Rock, Arkansas

Preface

For three decades, Dr. J. Willis Hurst, then Chairman of the Department of Medicine at Emory University, emphasized the importance of learning and teaching medicine. He has also emphasized that the more physicians teach, the more they learn. We as physicians learn from the literature, we learn from each other, and we especially learn from our patients. The end product of the learning process is the delivery of quality care to the patient.

In recognition of the emphasis on self-directed learning in continuing medical education, this review book presents a total of 655 multiple-choice questions. Each answer is discussed and referenced to the appropriate page or pages in *Hurst's The Heart.* The editors carefully reviewed and edited questions, some of which went through many drafts until they were right.

One of the dangers of a self-assessment exercise is the idea that a good score implies expertise. The editors of this book believe that good doctoring consists not only of basic knowledge but of the ability to gather the appropriate medical data from the patient, to create a list of health problems, to act with the best possible clinical judgment, and to be properly involved in the humane effort of caring for the patient. This book will assist the reader in the first step of this sequence—assessing one's basic medical knowledge.

We wish to thank Myrna Esbrandt and Kelly Pinkston for their help in preparing the manuscript—a task that is more difficult than one might think—and Gail Gavert, Bruce MacGregor, and Gyl A. Favours at McGraw-Hill for their expertise in shepherding the manuscript through to completion.

Jerre F. Lutz, M.D.
John W. Hurst, Jr., M.D.
J. Willis Hurst, M.D.

Introduction

Hurst's The Heart: PreTest® Self-Assessment and Review, 8th ed., has been designed to provide physicians with a comprehensive, relevant, and convenient instrument for self-evaluation and review of topics within the field of cardiology. Although it should be particularly helpful for fellows preparing for the American Board of Internal Medicine Subspecialty Examination in Cardiovascular Disease, it should also be useful for internists, family practitioners, and other physicians in practice who are simply interested in maintaining a high level of competence in cardiology. Study of this self-assessment and review book should help readers to (1) identify areas of relative weakness, (2) confirm areas of expertise, (3) assess knowledge of the sciences fundamental to cardiology, (4) assess clinical judgment and problem-solving skills, and (5) review recent developments in cardiology.

This book consists of 655 multiple-choice questions that (1) are representative of the major areas covered in *Hurst's The Heart,* 8th ed., and (2) parallel the degree of difficulty of the questions on the above-mentioned board examinations. Each question is accompanied by an answer, a paragraph-length explanation, and a reference to a specific page or pages in *Hurst's The Heart,* as well as in some cases references to more specialized textbooks and current journal articles. A list of all the sources used for the questions can be found in the Bibliography. All figures are taken from *Hurst's The Heart.*

We have assumed that the time available to the reader is limited; as a result, this book can be used profitably a part at a time. By allowing no more than two and a half minutes to answer each question, you can simulate the time constraints of the actual board examinations. When you finish answering all the questions in a part, spend as much time as necessary verifying answers and carefully reading the accompanying explanations. If after reading the explanations for a given part, you feel a need for a more extensive and definitive discussion, consult the pages in *Hurst's The Heart* or any of the other references listed.

Considerable editorial time has been spent trying to ensure that each question is clearly stated and discriminates between those physicians who are well-prepared in the subject and those who are less knowledgeable. This book is a teaching device that provides readers with the opportunity to objectively evaluate and update their clinical expertise, their ability to interpret data, and their ability to diagnose and solve clinical problems. We hope that you will find this book interesting, relevant, and challenging. The authors, as well as the McGraw-Hill Health Professions staff, would be very happy to receive your comments and suggestions.

Hurst's
The Heart

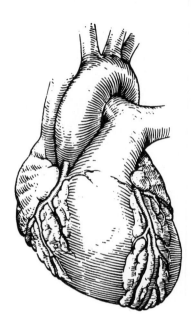

PreTest®
Self-Assessment
and Review

I. Basic Foundations of Cardiology

DIRECTIONS: Each question below contains five suggested responses. Select the **one best** response to each question.

1. All the following statements regarding cardiac myocytes are true EXCEPT

   (A) cardiac myocytes are large cells
   (B) the working unit of contraction is the T tubule
   (C) myosin and actin are the primary proteins in the sarcomere
   (D) sarcomeres compose about 50 percent of the cardiac myocytes
   (E) sarcomeres are joined in a series via the Z lines

2. Which of the following statements best describes the polymerase chain reaction?

   (A) This reaction is easier than cloning and can provide a million copies of a DNA fragment in 3 to 4 hours
   (B) Messenger RNA (mRNA) can be amplified without being converted to complementary DNA (cDNA) first
   (C) The DNA must not be denatured
   (D) Viral RNA cannot be amplified by this process even after it is converted to cDNA
   (E) Many copies (greater than 50,000) of RNA or DNA must be present, or the polymerase chain reaction will fail

3. Smooth muscle contraction can be stimulated by a variety of hormones and molecules including all the following EXCEPT

   (A) norepinephrine
   (B) vasopressin
   (C) angiotensin II
   (D) endothelin
   (E) prostacyclin

4. All the following statements concerning ion channels are correct EXCEPT

   (A) ion channels regulate the flow of ions across the cell membrane, thus modulating the electric potential of the cell
   (B) adenosine triphosphate (ATP) is not expended during ion movement
   (C) channels open and close in response to stimuli to maintain an electrical potential
   (D) proteins regulate the opening of pores in the cell membrane to facilitate movement of specific ions across the membrane
   (E) the potassium (K^+)-selective channel is the most important and diverse of the inward current channels

5. The inward current channels of the myocyte membrane are described by all the following statements EXCEPT

(A) the two main channels are the sodium (Na^+) and calcium (Ca^{2+}) channels
(B) the three major classes of voltage-dependent Ca^{2+} channels (L, N, and T types) can be differentiated by their sensitivity to dehydropyridines, by the membrane potential at which they are activated, and by their gating and permeation characteristics
(C) The Ca^{2+} channel can be opened by β-adrenergic receptors activating via the G_s protein
(D) the Na^+ channel leads to the rapid inward movement of Na^+, moving the resting potential from 0 mV to +80 mV
(E) to increase intracellular Ca^{2+} concentration, leading to muscle contraction, Ca^{2+} and Na^+ channels are needed

6. All the following statements concerning the constituents of the cell membrane are correct EXCEPT

(A) fatty acid chains, which are unsaturated (i.e., have double bonds between carbons), lead to greater mobility within the membrane
(B) cholesterol in the membrane promotes rigidity not fluidity
(C) glycolipids, which are found on the intracellular face, contain lipids and oligosaccharides
(D) glycolipids probably promote cell-cell interaction and act as cell-surface receptors
(E) the hydrophobic core of the lipid bilayer prevents the passage of charged molecules

7. Increased levels of the G_s protein have been found in patients with

(A) insulin-dependent diabetes mellitus
(B) non–insulin-dependent diabetes mellitus
(C) hyperthyroidism
(D) hypothyroidism
(E) idiopathic dilated cardiomyopathy

8. Structures visible within the right atrium include all the following EXCEPT the

(A) thebesian valve
(B) eustachian valve
(C) sulcus terminalis
(D) moderator band
(E) coronary sinus orifice

9. Correct statements concerning the right ventricle include all the following EXCEPT

(A) the right ventricle is a crescent-shaped chamber compared to the left ventricle, which is an ellipsoidal sphere
(B) the right ventricle is 4 to 5 mm thick compared to the left ventricle, which is 8 to 15 mm thick
(C) the trabecular muscles in the right ventricle are more coarse than in the left ventricle with trabeculae carneae forming ridges along the inner surface found in the right ventricle
(D) the moderator band is a muscle that carries the right bundle branch from the ventricular septum to the right ventricular endocardium
(E) the right ventricle lies anteriorly and provides most of the inferior heart border on a frontal view of the cardiac silhouette

10. Correct statements about cardiac valves include all the following EXCEPT

(A) the fibrous tissue of the annular rings forms the fibrous skeleton of the heart
(B) the valves consist of a central collagenous core covered by loose fibroelastic tissue and then with endothelium
(C) both atrioventricular (AV) valves and the semilunar valves are avascular structures
(D) all the valves normally have three cusps except the mitral valve, which has two cusps
(E) the annulus of the tricuspid valve is larger than that of the mitral valve

11. The cardiac structure least innervated by the vagus nerve is the

    (A) sinoatrial (SA) node
    (B) atrioventricular (AV) node
    (C) atrial myocardium
    (D) ventricular myocardium
    (E) His-Purkinje system

12. Which of the following branches most consistently arises from the right coronary artery?

    (A) Atrioventricular (AV) node artery
    (B) Sinoatrial (SA) node artery
    (C) Right ventricular branches
    (D) Posterior descending artery
    (E) Conus branch

13. The epicardial blood supply to the anterolateral papillary muscle is the

    (A) left anterior descending coronary artery
    (B) circumflex artery
    (C) right coronary artery
    (D) left anterior descending coronary artery and circumflex artery
    (E) left anterior descending and right ventricular branches of the right coronary artery

14. With total occlusion of the proximal right or circumflex artery, flow to the distal posterior descending artery may be provided through the atrioventricular (AV) node by

    (A) the bridging collaterals
    (B) the circle of Vieussens
    (C) the circle of Willis
    (D) the oblique vein of Marshall
    (E) Kugel's artery

15. Coronary veins that drain into the right atrium via the coronary sinus include all the following EXCEPT the

    (A) great cardiac vein
    (B) middle cardiac vein
    (C) small cardiac vein
    (D) oblique vein of Marshall
    (E) thebesian vein

16. A major determinant of myocardial oxygen consumption in the beating heart is

    (A) external work (load × shortening)
    (B) intramyocardial wall tension (pressure × volume)
    (C) basal oxygen requirements
    (D) coronary blood flow
    (E) activation energy

17. The heart preferentially uses which of the following substrates for oxidative energy production?

    (A) Proteins
    (B) Fatty acids
    (C) Carbohydrates
    (D) Ketones
    (E) Glucose

18. Uptake of glucose by the heart is controlled by the glucose transporter in the sarcolemmal membrane. The glucose transporter is stimulated by all the following EXCEPT

    (A) hypoxia
    (B) the actions of insulin
    (C) high plasma glucose concentrations
    (D) increased work performance
    (E) fasting conditions

19. Factors affecting protein synthesis and degradation of heart muscle include all the following EXCEPT

    (A) availability of amino acids
    (B) supply of oxidative substrates
    (C) availability of hormones
    (D) presence of histamine in mast cells
    (E) level of aortic pressure

20. All the following statements concerning protein degradation are correct EXCEPT

(A) lysosomes and cytoplasmic proteases appear to be involved with protein degradation to free amino acids

(B) lysosomes contain hydrolytic enzymes, which degrade proteins to free amino acids

(C) lysosomal proteases have an optimal pH of 7 to 9

(D) energy is required in protein degradation to maintain a low intralysosomal pH

(E) lysosomes often appear in the perinuclear region of myocardial cells and in rows of mitochondria

21. Correct statements concerning the regulation of protein degradation and the efficiency of protein synthesis include all the following EXCEPT

(A) in cardiomyocytes, global protein synthesis required for hypertrophy is regulated by the cytoplasmic concentration of messenger RNA (mRNA)

(B) hypertrophy and reduction in cardiac mass depend on relative rates of synthesis and degradation of heart proteins

(C) the half-time for turnover of heart protein and RNA varies from 1 hour to several days

(D) enzymatic components of the heart can change in quantity or type of isozyme over short periods of time

(E) decreased availability of hormones, growth factors, oxidative substrates, and oxygen disturb the protein balance of the heart

22. Concentrations of amino acids within the intracellular pool are determined by all the following EXCEPT the

(A) rate of entry from the extracellular space

(B) rate of exit from the cell

(C) rate of formation or destruction of the compound by transamination, oxidation, or other metabolic processes

(D) levels of calcium ion (Ca^{2+})–calmodulin-dependent kinase

(E) rates of protein synthesis and degradation

23. Which of the following statements regarding antiplatelet therapy is true?

(A) Dipyridamole provides additional benefit when coadministered with aspirin for the treatment of cerebral vascular disease

(B) Dipyridamole decreases cyclic adenosine monophosphate (cAMP)

(C) Ticlopidine inhibits phosphodiesterase

(D) Ticlopidine is effective in preventing the occurrence of nonfatal stroke and death in patients with transient ischemic attacks (TIAs)

(E) Aspirin increases platelet production of thromboxane A_2 (TXA_2) and endothelial cell synthesis of prostacyclin (PGI_2)

24. All the following statements regarding anticoagulation are true EXCEPT

(A) low-molecular-weight heparin inhibits activated factor X

(B) dermatan sulfate catalyzes heparin cofactor II–thrombin interaction

(C) heparin catalyzes complex formation between plasma antithrombin III and serine protease

(D) warfarin is effective through inhibition of clotting factors II, VII, IX, and X and proteins C and S

(E) an international normalized ratio (INR) of 1.0 to 2.0 is recommended for anticoagulation of patients with mechanical heart valves

25. Thrombosis is accurately described by which of the following statements?

(A) Arterial thrombosis is due to slow flow
(B) Thrombosis after hip surgery may be due to injury of the femoral vein
(C) An increase in endogenous tissue plasminogen activator (tPA) activity results in venous thrombosis
(D) A decrease in plasminogen activator inhibitor 1 (PAI-1) results in arterial thrombosis
(E) The use of fibrin-specific agents is not recommended for venous thrombosis

26. Each of the following statements regarding the incidence or mortality of cardiovascular disease is true EXCEPT

(A) coronary heart disease accounts for slightly more than one-fourth of all deaths in persons over the age of 35
(B) the recent decline in cardiovascular mortality extends to both sexes, all races, every age group, and all geographic areas in the United States
(C) 1 in every 3 men in the United States can expect to develop major cardiovascular disease before reaching the age of 60
(D) cardiovascular disease declines as a cause of death to less than 50 percent of patients beyond the age of 75
(E) cardiovascular diseases, although on the decline, still account for approximately 45 percent of all deaths in the United States

27. True statements regarding the differences between men and women in the incidence, prevalence, and mortality of cardiovascular diseases include all the following EXCEPT

(A) the average age of occurrence of cardiovascular disease, excluding stroke, is 10 years later in females
(B) death rates from cardiovascular disease are highest in black males followed in descending order by white males, white females, and black females
(C) the first clinical symptom in women with coronary heart disease is likely to be angina, whereas in men it is more likely to be myocardial infarction
(D) surgical menopause carries the same risk as natural menopause regarding the incidence of coronary heart disease in women
(E) after surviving acute myocardial infarction, men are twice as likely as women to have sudden cardiac death

28. Blood pressure is accurately described by all the following statements EXCEPT

(A) hypertension is the most prevalent of all the cardiovascular diseases
(B) in the United States, about 15 percent of all people ages 18 to 74 have a blood pressure greater than or equal to 140/90 mmHg
(C) the prevalence of hypertension is higher among blacks than whites
(D) in general, between the ages of 30 and 60, systolic blood pressure increases approximately 20 mmHg and diastolic blood pressure increases 10 mmHg
(E) the treatment of isolated systolic hypertension in the elderly reduces the risk of stroke and coronary artery disease

29. All the following statements regarding heart failure are true EXCEPT

   (A) hypertension or hypertension accompanied by coronary artery disease accounts for the majority of all causes of heart failure

   (B) after the age of 65, the annual occurrence of congestive heart failure approaches 1 percent of the population

   (C) adjusting for age, there has been a marked improvement in the prognosis of patients with congestive heart failure over the last 4 decades

   (D) 5-year survival rates for congestive heart failure are approximately 25 percent in men and 40 percent in women

   (E) the increasing number of patients with heart failure is probably due to the improved survival of patients with coronary heart disease who ultimately develop heart failure

30. All the following statements regarding the prevalence, incidence, and mortality of stroke are true EXCEPT

   (A) atherothrombotic brain infarction accounts for more than 50 percent of all strokes in the United States

   (B) the reduction in death rates from all causes of stroke has exceeded the rate of decline in all other causes of cardiovascular death

   (C) even though the age-adjusted death rate for stroke has decreased by 55 percent over the last 2 decades, it is still the third leading cause of death in the United States

   (D) the chances of having a stroke before age 70 is approximately 1 in 20 in men and 1 in 40 in women

   (E) long-term survival following stroke is worse in men than in women

DIRECTIONS: Each question below contains four suggested responses of which **one or more** is correct. Select

A	if	**1, 2, and 3**	are correct
B	if	**1 and 3**	are correct
C	if	**2 and 4**	are correct
D	if	**4**	is correct
E	if	**1, 2, 3, and 4**	are correct

31. The proposed mechanism by which actin filaments slide over myosin filaments to induce muscle contraction and relaxation includes which of the following steps?

(1) Release of calcium ions (Ca^{2+}) by the sarcoplasmic calcium adenosine triphosphatase (ATPase)

(2) Decrease in cytosolic Ca^{2+} after the muscle is stimulated

(3) Hydrolysis of adenosine triphosphate (ATP)

(4) Myosin binding of actin, which is potentiated by the presence of troponin and tropomyosin in the relaxed state

32. Correct statements regarding contractile proteins include which of the following?

(1) Myosin is present in nonmuscle and muscle cells

(2) Actin is a necessary component of the cytoskeleton of most cells

(3) Muscle contraction involves the occupation by calcium ions (Ca^{2+}) at all the Ca^{2+}-binding sites of troponin C

(4) There is only one type of actin expressed in adult mammals

33. The endothelial cells play a major role in the homeostasis of the vascular system. Normal functions of the endothelium include

(1) secretion of vasoactive substances into the lumen and into the vessel wall

(2) prevention of platelet aggregation and thrombosis

(3) regulation of the influx of plasma macromolecules into the arterial wall

(4) regulation of smooth muscle cell proliferation by various growth factors

34. Correct statements regarding the structure of the arterial wall include which of the following?

(1) Arteries consist of three layers, including the intima, the media, and the adventitia

(2) The intima is composed primarily of smooth muscle cells

(3) Large conduit arteries tend to have a high ratio of elastic laminae to smooth muscle cells

(4) Veins do not contain smooth muscle cells

35. The response of the arterial wall to the injury induced by angioplasty involves several distinct events including

(1) removal of endothelium, which exposes a thrombogenic surface to which platelets can adhere

(2) infiltration of macrophages into the vessel wall

(3) formation of a neointima over a period of weeks to months (restenosis)

(4) stimulation of endothelium-derived growth factors

36. Conditions known to regulate receptor signaling on cardiovascular membranes include

(1) changes in steroid levels

(2) myocardial ischemia

(3) diabetes mellitus

(4) congestive heart failure (CHF)

37. Cell types involved in the system of impulse formation and rapid conduction include

(1) P cells

(2) transitional cells

(3) ameboid cells

(4) Purkinje cells

SUMMARY OF DIRECTIONS

A	B	C	D	E
1, 2, 3 only	1, 3 only	2, 4 only	4 only	All are correct

---

38. In the left ventricular function curve depicted below, if *curve A* represents normal function, then *curve B* could represent

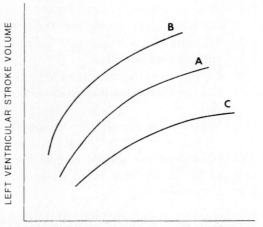

(1) extensive myocardial ischemia
(2) a response to digitalis
(3) a result of excessive doxorubicin
(4) a response to an infusion of epinephrine

39. Mechanisms of cardiac reserve that the heart may use to meet increased demands on the normal heart or to maintain cardiac function in the presence of disease include

    (1) increased heart rate
    (2) cardiac hypertrophy
    (3) anaerobic metabolism
    (4) cardiac dilatation

40. The major physical factors of the cardiac cycle that may result in an increase of coronary blood flow to the left ventricle include an increase in the

    (1) time spent in the first half of systole
    (2) arterial pressure gradient (aortic pressure − left ventricular diastolic pressure)
    (3) time spent in the second half of systole
    (4) time spent in diastole

41. At the cellular level of myocardial contraction, depolarization of the sarcolemma and transverse T-tubular system by an action potential initiates sequential calcium ion (Ca^{2+}) dynamics, which include

    (1) transsarcolemmal influx of Ca^{2+}
    (2) active uptake of Ca^{2+} by the sarcoplasmic reticulum
    (3) increased binding of Ca^{2+} to troponin C
    (4) direct Ca^{2+} activation of actin-myosin contraction

42. The physiological events of the normal cardiac cycle of the left ventricle may be correlated with which of the following valvular events?

    (1) Isovolumic contraction is associated with mitral valve closure
    (2) The beginning of the rapid ventricular ejection phase is indicated by the opening of the mitral valve
    (3) Isovolumic relaxation is signified by closure of the aortic valve
    (4) The rapid ventricular filling phase coincides with the closure of the mitral valve

43. Correct statements regarding oxidative metabolism in the heart include which of the following?

    (1) Forty percent of the heart's energy production is derived from the oxidation of carbon-based fuels
    (2) The oxidation of fatty acids leads to much higher yields of adenosine triphosphate (ATP) per molecule than the oxidation of glucose
    (3) Oxidative metabolism occurs in the cytosol of the myocyte
    (4) The availability of substrate to the heart and substrate preference by the heart can influence the bioenergetic balance and respiratory efficiency at a given level of cardiac performance

44. Correct statements regarding thrombosis include which of the following?

(1) Fibrinolysis is the process by which fibrin is broken down to fibrin fragments

(2) Thrombolytic agents are plasminogen activators

(3) Fibrin-selective plasminogen activators result in a higher recanalization rate than do nonfibrin-selective agents

(4) Repeat administration of either streptokinase (SK) or anisoylated plasminogen-streptokinase activator complex (APSAC) has been shown to be effective in the treatment of arterial thrombosis

45. Which of the following technologies can provide information regarding the metabolic support of the heart?

(1) NMR spectroscopy

(2) Echocardiography

(3) Positron emission tomography (PET)

(4) Cardiac catheterization

DIRECTIONS: Each question below contains five suggested responses. For **each** of the **five** responses listed with every question, you are to respond either YES (Y) or NO (N). In a given item **all, some, or none of the alternatives may be correct.**

46. Correct statements regarding molecular biology include which of the following?

    (A) A single gene may give rise to several messenger RNAs (mRNAs)
    (B) Gene expression is regulated only in response to signals from within the cell
    (C) Any tissue can be used to obtain a DNA sample for use in recombinant technology
    (D) Southern and northern blotting are used to detect proteins, and a western blot is used to detect DNA and RNA
    (E) It is necessary to isolate the DNA fragment of interest prior to the DNA cloning process

47. Correct statements regarding endothelial-cell dysfunction, an important concept in vascular biology, include which of the following?

    (A) Normal endothelium is generally in an inhibitory mode, preventing thrombosis, contraction, white-cell adhesion, and vascular smooth muscle growth
    (B) Endothelial dysfunction in atherosclerosis accounts for the relative tendency of diseased arteries to relax inappropriately
    (C) Endothelial-dependent vasodilator dysfunction only occurs in patients with angiographically demonstrable coronary disease
    (D) Hypercholesterolemic endothelium produces increased amounts of nitric oxide (NO), but NO is rapidly degraded into inactive metabolites
    (E) Cholesterol-fed animals have high levels of vascular cell adhesion molecule 1 (VCAM-1) expression, which leads to recruitment of monocytes and macrophages into the vessel wall

48. Correct statements regarding the interaction of endothelium and smooth muscle cells include which of the following?

    (A) Normal endothelium inhibits proliferation of smooth muscle cells
    (B) Experimental removal of the endothelium allows initiation of the mitogenic response of smooth muscle cells
    (C) Smooth muscle cells are relatively immature cells that are constantly reproducing
    (D) Cultured vascular smooth muscle cells exposed to sodium nitroprusside, which mimics the effect of nitric oxide (NO) on vascular smooth muscle, can inhibit mitogenesis
    (E) NO plays a large role in the control of vascular tone of large arteries

49. Correct statements concerning the coronary circulation include which of the following?

    (A) The conus artery originates within the right sinus of Valsalva as a separate ostium from the right coronary artery in 50 percent of hearts
    (B) The ostium of the left coronary artery is slightly inferior and anterior to that of the right coronary artery
    (C) In 40 to 50 percent of hearts, the atrioventricular (AV) node is supplied by the left circumflex artery
    (D) The circle of Vieussens is an important collateral from the circumflex artery to the AV node and the posterior circulation
    (E) The thebesian veins drain directly into the cardiac chambers, primarily the right atrium and right ventricle

50. Which of the following general processes occur during the contraction cascade of vascular smooth muscle?

    (A) Phosphorylation of actomyosin
    (B) Cross-bridge formation
    (C) Attachment of myosin to cytoplasmic enzymes
    (D) Phosphorylation of the myosin light chain
    (E) Decrease in intracellular calcium ion (Ca^{2+}) concentration in response to a vasoconstrictor hormone

51. Correct statements regarding the valves of the heart include which of the following?

    (A) Small perforations are found normally in the aortic cusps
    (B) The mitral orifice is larger than the tricuspid orifice
    (C) The anterior leaflet of the mitral valve provides an important boundary of the left ventricular outflow tract
    (D) The tricuspid valve is in close proximity to the coronary sinus and the atrioventricular (AV) node
    (E) The largest papillary muscle in the right ventricle is the septal papillary muscle

52. Correct statements regarding the gross anatomy of the right side of the heart include which of the following?

    (A) The right ventricle lies directly below the sternum and is normally the most anterior cardiac chamber
    (B) In normal subjects, the interventricular septum contributes predominantly to right ventricular function
    (C) The moderator band is a muscle that joins the lower ventricular septum and the anterior papillary muscle in the right ventricle
    (D) The right atrium is in close proximity to the aortic root
    (E) The coronary sinus opens into the anteromedial aspect of the right atrium

53. Correct statements concerning the ultrastructure of the myocardium include which of the following?

    (A) P cells are special cells involved in the generation and rapid conduction of the electrical impulse and are located in the Purkinje system
    (B) According to the "sliding filament hypothesis," the actin and myosin filaments slide by each other causing the muscle fiber to shorten
    (C) Free intracellular calcium (Ca^{2+}) increases following the release of the actin-myosin inhibition
    (D) The A band consists of thin actin filaments attached to either side of the dark Z band
    (E) The length of each sarcomere varies from 1.5 to 2.2 μm

54. True statements about the gross anatomy of the left side of the heart include which of the following?

    (A) The relative thinness of the apex of the left ventricle is in part responsible for the tendency toward formation of aneurysms
    (B) The presence of true valves at the junction of the pulmonary veins and the left atrium prevents the reflux of blood during atrial systole or mitral regurgitation
    (C) The trabecular muscles in the left ventricle are much more coarse than those in the right ventricle
    (D) Enlargement of the left atrial appendage may directly compress the esophagus and lead to esophageal obstruction or achalasia
    (E) A patent foramen ovale can be found in 15 percent of hearts

DIRECTIONS: Each group of questions below consists of lettered headings followed by a set of numbered items. For each numbered item select the **one** lettered heading with which it is **most** closely associated. Each lettered heading may be used **once, more than once, or not at all.**

Questions 55–58

Vessel tone is dependent on the balance between different vasoconstrictor and vasorelaxing factors. For each description that follows, select the vasoconstrictor or vasorelaxing factor that it most aptly describes.

(A) Prostacyclin
(B) Adenosine
(C) Endothelin
(D) Endothelium-derived relaxing factor
(E) Angiotensin-converting enzyme (ACE)

55. Peptides made and secreted by the endothelial cells in some vascular beds; it is an extremely potent vasoconstrictor and produces a slow, sustained contraction in smooth muscle

56. Protein that degrades and inactivates bradykinin; when this enzyme is associated with the endothelial cell membrane, it modifies both locally produced and circulating bradykinin and angiotensin I and contributes to the regulation of vasomotor tone

57. A nucleoside released by the endothelium in response to thrombin and flow

58. A prostanoid derived from the action of cyclooxygenase on arachidonic acid; it is released by the endothelium and relaxes vascular smooth muscle

Questions 59–61

For each statement or definition listed below, select the physiological principle that it best represents.

(A) Bowditch effect
(B) Poiseuille's equation
(C) Laplace's law
(D) Anrep effect
(E) Woodworth phenomenon

59. The tension tending to expand the wall of a blood vessel is greater if the radius of the vessel is greater or if the blood vessel wall is thinner

60. The predominant influence on flow is the radius of the vessel raised to the fourth power

61. An increase in heart rate may in itself increase myocardial contractility

I. Basic Foundations of Cardiology

Answers

1. **The answer is B.** *(pp 16–17)* Cardiac myocytes are large cells (i.e., up to 120 μm in length). The working unit of contraction is the sarcomere, which is composed primarily of myosin and actin, also known as the thick and thin filaments, respectively. There are several other proteins that attach to the actin filament, including tropomyosin and troponins C, T, and I. The sarcomeres are joined together in a series via the Z lines and comprise about 50 percent of the cardiac myocytes.

2. **The answer is A.** *(pp 15–16)* The polymerase chain reaction was developed in 1985. This procedure can provide a billion copies of DNA within 24 hours by taking advantage of the natural DNA replication process. Prior to amplification, messenger RNA (mRNA) must be converted to complementary DNA (cDNA), using the enzyme reverse transcriptase. The process requires the DNA to be thermally denatured by increasing the temperature; then the temperature is decreased so that primers can reanneal to the native DNA strands. Any type of viral RNA or DNA for which primers can be made can be used in this process. The polymerase chain reaction is, therefore, a helpful tool when diagnosing viral myocarditis. It can be used to amplify a specific viral RNA from a myocardial biopsy. Compared to conventional techniques, the polymerase chain reaction is much more sensitive, and only one copy of RNA or DNA is needed for it to amplify accurately and generate a million copies of the RNA or DNA.

3. **The answer is E.** *(pp 32–55)* Vascular endothelial cells secrete the peptide endothelin, an endothelial-derived contracting factor, which acts as a vasoconstrictor. Angiotensin II induces a transient constriction of many vessels, whereas norepinephrine and vasopressin nearly always cause a sustained contraction. Prostacyclin (PGI_2) is a potent vasodilator and potent inhibitor of platelet aggregation that is produced by vascular endothelial cells.

4. **The answer is E.** *(p 49)* Ion channels regulate the flow of specific ions across the cell membrane, thus modulating the electrical potential at all times. Ion channels act as passive conduits, allowing ions to move down a concentration gradient. Thus, adenosine triphosphate (ATP) is not expended during ion movement. Channels must have the ability to open and close in response to stimuli or no ionic gradient could be maintained and cell death would ensue. Proteins regulate channel opening and closing. Pores are opened, allowing specific ions to enter and traverse the pore. The potassium (K^+)-selective channel is the most important and diverse in terms of the outward current channels.

5. **The answer is D.** *(p 50)* The calcium (Ca^{2+}) and sodium (Na^+) channels are the two main inward current channels of the myocyte membrane. The Na^+ channel leads to the rapid inward movement of Na^+, which changes the resting potential of -80 mV to -100 mV in a positive direction. The ensuing inward Ca^{2+} flux leads to increased intracellular Ca^{2+} and muscle contraction. There are three major voltage-depen-

dent Ca²⁺ channels (L, N, and T types), which can be differentiated by their sensitivity to the dehydropyridine class of calcium antagonists, by the membrane potential at which they are activated, and by gating and permeation characteristics. The opening of Ca²⁺ channels can be promoted by β-adrenergic receptors acting via the G_s protein.

6. The answer is C. *(p 48)*   Constituents of the cell membrane are illustrated in the figure below. Fatty acid chains are unsaturated (i.e., have double bonds between carbon atoms), which leads to a kinking of the chain. Since the molecules cannot be packed together as tightly, there is greater mobility or fluidity within membranes. Cholesterol promotes rigidity rather than fluidity by decreasing the ability of the fatty acid tails to move. Glycolipids are formed on the extracellular surface when the glycan component is exposed to the extracellular space. Their function is cell-cell interaction with the moiety acting as a class of specific cell-surface receptors. The lipid bilayer has a hydrophobic core that prevents the passage of charged molecules. Thus, a water molecule is 10 billion times more likely to cross the lipid bilayer than a sodium (Na⁺) molecule.

Extracellular Space

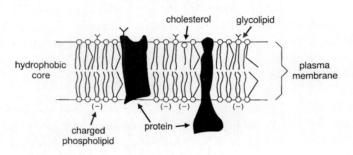

Intracellular Space

7. The answer is C. *(p 56)*   Cell-surface receptors regulate intracellular function with extracellular substances. The G-protein coupled receptors use G proteins to act as intermediaries between the cell-membrane receptor and the inhibition or activation of an intracellular process. Hyperthyroidism has been associated with an increased level of G_s, while hypothyroidism is associated with low G_s levels.

8. The answer is D. *(pp 62–63)*   Venous blood from the head and upper extremities returns to the right atrium via the superior vena cava while blood returns from the lower extremities to the right atrium via the inferior vena cava. There is no valve at the ostium of the superior vena cava, but a rudimentary valve called the eustachian valve guards the inferior vena cava. The coronary venous return enters the right atrium via the coronary sinus, which is guarded by the thebesian valve. On the posterior external surface of the right atrium a ridge, the sulcus terminalis, extends from the superior to inferior vena cava. The moderator band joins the lower ventricular septum to the anterior papillary muscle in the right ventricle.

9. The answer is C. *(pp 63–65)*   The right ventricle has a crescent-shaped cavity and is 4 to 5 mm thick since it is designed to pump against low-resistance pulmonary arteries. The left ventricle is smooth and 8 to 15 mm thick as it is designed to pump against high resistance, but it still contains the ridgelike trabeculae carneae like the right ventricle. The right bundle does course through the moderator muscle band to the right ventricular endocardium. The right ventricle is an anterior structure, which comprises most of the inferior surface of the heart on a frontal roentgenogram, while the right atrium makes up most of the right heart border on the frontal cardiac silhouette.

10. The answer is C. *(pp 66–70)*   The fibrous tissue of the annular rings of the two semilunar and the two atrioventricular (AV) valves form the fibrous skeleton of the heart. The mitral valve annulus is indeed smaller than the tricuspid annulus. Normal mitral valve orifice size is 3 to 4 cm² while normal tricuspid valve orifice size is 5 to 7 cm². All the valves normally have three cusps except the mitral valve, which has two cusps. The valve leaflet consists of a central collagenous core covered by loose fibroelastic tissue and then with endothelium. The semilunar valves are avascular. Smooth and striated muscles extend onto the proximal third of the atrial endothelium, which often contains blood vessels. The remainder of the normal AV valve is avascular.

11. The answer is E. *(pp 82–83)*   The sinoatrial (SA) node, the atrioventricular (AV) node, and the lower conduction system all possess intrinsic pacemaker capabilities; however, the autonomic nervous system also influences the rate of impulse spread, the rate of depolarization and repolarization, and the contractility of both the atria and the ventricles. Parasympathetic innervation arises from the medulla and passes through the right and left vagus nerves. The superior cardiac nerves and the inferior cardiac nerves arise from either the vagi or the recurrent branches of the vagi. Both sympathetic and parasympathetic fibers influence the SA node, AV node, and both atrial and ventricular muscles. The vagal fibers to the ventricles are sparse, and vagal fibers directly to the His-Purkinje system are not described.

12. The answer is C. *(pp 84–87)*   In about 50 percent of humans, the conus artery arises separately in the right sinus of Valsalva rather than as a right coronary branch. The sinoatrial (SA) node artery arises from the proximal right coronary in 50 to 60 percent of cases. The posterior descending and atrioventricular (AV) node arteries arise from the circumflex artery in 10 to 15 percent of cases. The right coronary gives rise to arteriographically identified right ventricular branches.

13. The answer is D. *(p 74)*   The left anterior descending coronary artery provides most of the blood supply to the anterolateral papillary muscle while the right coronary artery supplies the posteromedial papillary muscle. The left circumflex artery provides blood to both papillary muscles.

14. The answer is E. *(p 89)*   Kogel's artery arises from the proximal right coronary artery or left circumflex artery; it courses through the posterior atrial septum to join the atrioventricular (AV) artery and retrograde fills the posterior descending artery. This vessel is usually seen with a total proximal occlusion of the right coronary artey or the circumflex artery. Occlusion is accompanied by excellent collateral flow to the posterior descending via the above communication. Bridging collaterals connote a total occlusion with ipsilateral local collateralization around the focal occlusion. Occlusion of the proximal right coronary artery may be accompanied by excellent collateralization of the right ventricular branch from a large wraparound left anterior descending vessel (circle of Vieussens).

15. The answer is E. *(p 91)*   The coronary sinus is the major venous drainage of the left ventricle. The coronary sinus receives its blood supply from the great, middle, and small cardiac veins; the posterior veins of the left ventricle; and the oblique vein of Marshall. Thebesian veins are tiny venous channels that drain the myocardium directly into either the right atrium or right ventricle.

16. The answer is B. *(p 134, Table 5-2)*   The four major determinants of myocardial oxygen consumption are myocardial mass, intramyocardial tension or wall stress (pressure × volume), inotropic state (contractility), and heart rate. Of the major determinants of myocardial oxygen consumption, wall tension and heart rate are the most important. Three minor determinants of myocardial oxygen consumption are external work (load × shortening), basal oxygen requirements, and activation energy. The oxygen cost of electrical activation is less than 1 percent of the total myocardial oxygen consumption, and the costs for contractile-state activation and deactivation and for the maintenance of the active state are small. Coronary flow and pressure affect oxygen consumption in the nonworking heart but have variable effects in the beating heart.

17. **The answer is B.**   *(pp 158–159)*   The normal heart preferentially uses fatty acids as the substrate for oxidative energy production, although nutritional, metabolic, and hormonal influences can induce a greater contribution from carbohydrates. Less used fuels include amino acids and ketones.

18. **The answer is E.**   *(pp 154–155)*   The first step of regulation in the utilization of glucose within the myocyte occurs at the level of the sarcolemmal membrane. Uptake of glucose is controlled by a glucose transporter in the sarcolemmal membrane. Glucose uptake is stimulated by increased demands for anaerobic glycolysis as in hypoxia, increased work, high plasma glucose concentration, and the actions of insulin. Reduced activity of the transporter occurs in situations of decreased cardiac work, fasting conditions, and uncontrolled diabetes.

19. **The answer is D.**   *(p 168)*   Factors that affect protein synthesis or degradation in heart muscle include the availability of amino acids, especially leucine, the supply of oxidative substrates, the availability of hormones, such as insulin, which accelerates synthesis and inhibits degradation, the adequacy of oxygen delivery, and the level of aortic pressure.

20. **The answer is C.**   *(p 168)*   Lysosymes appear usually in the mitochondria and in the perinuclear region of myocardial cells. These organelles contain hydrolytic enzymes, which include acid proteases capable of degrading protein to free amino acids. These acid proteases function optimally in the pH range of 2 to 4. Energy is then expended in the protein degradation process to maintain this low pH.

21. **The answer is A.**   *(p 166)*   In cardiomyocytes, the cytoplasmic concentration of messenger RNA (mRNA) regulates specific protein synthesis, but global protein synthesis required for hypertrophy is not dependent on mRNA concentration. Rapid protein turnover rates lead to the ability to change myofibrillar or enzymatic components in quantity or type of isozyme in short periods of time. The half-time for turnover of cardiac proteins or mRNA is brief, varying from 1 hour to several days. Hypertrophy and reduction in cardiac mass are dependent on the relative rate of protein synthesis and degradation. Protein turnover in the heart is dependent on mechanical activity and the availability of growth factors, hormones, oxidative substrates, and oxygen.

22. **The answer is D.**   *(p 167)*   Concentrations of amino acids within the intracellular pool are determined by the rate of amino acid entry from the extracellular space, the rate of amino acid exit from the cell, the rate of destruction or amino acid formation by oxidation, transamination, or other metabolic processes, and the rates of protein synthesis and degradation.

23. **The answer is D.**   *(p 178)*   Antiplatelet drugs work by a variety of mechanisms. Aspirin inhibits platelet production of thromboxane A_2 (TXA_2) and endothelial cell synthesis of prostacyclin (PGI_2). Dipyridamole increases cyclic adenosine monophosphate (cAMP) by inhibiting phosphodiesterase activity. The mechanism by which ticlopidine works is unknown. It does not affect phosphodiesterase. Ticlopidine has been shown to prevent the occurrence of nonfatal stroke and death in patients with transient ischemic attacks (TIAs). Dipyridamole is ineffective by itself and provides no additional effect when coadministered with aspirin for the prevention of thrombosis of saphenous vein bypass grafts or for the treatment of cerebral vascular disease.

24. **The answer is E.**   *(pp 179–180)*   Low-molecular-weight heparin has an antithrombotic effect without considerable bleeding due to its ability to inhibit activated factor X with a relative decrease in levels of thrombin. A new anticoagulant, dermatan sulfate, catalyzes the heparin cofactor II–thrombin interaction; however, it has no effect on the formation of antithrombin III and serine protease. Vitamin K is necessary for gamma carboxylation of clotting factors II, VII, IX, and X and proteins C and S, and warfarin is the most widely used vitamin K antagonist. Heparin catalyzes the interaction between plasma antithrombin III and serine protease, thus inhibiting thrombin. Recently introduced is the international normalized ratio

(INR), which is used to monitor the anticoagulant activity of vitamin K antagonists. An INR of 2.0 to 3.0 is recommended for treatment of patients with venous thrombus, atrial fibrillation, or acute myocardial infarction. Higher levels of anticoagulation (INR of 2.5 to 3.5) are recommended for patients with evidence of thromboembolism despite adequate anticoagulation and for patients with mechanical heart valves.

25. The answer is B.   *(pp 173–175)*   Arterial thrombosis is usually due to vascular injury; venous thrombosis is usually due to static blood flow. Venous thrombosis after hip surgery is due to a combination of events that includes injury to the femoral vein and prolonged immobilization. Increased venous thrombosis is also seen in "acquired" prothrombotic states such as pregnancy, malignancy, and hypofibrinolytic states, including conditions that result in a decrease in activity of endogenous tissue plasminogen activator (tPA) or an increase in activity of plasminogen activator inhibitor 1 (PAI-1). Finally, a patient with massive venous thrombosis, such as one with large, deep venous thrombosis, may gain benefit from the use of fibrinolytic agents.

26. The answer is D.   *(pp 185–187)*   Cardiovascular diseases are the major cause of death in the United States. In 1991, they accounted for 43 percent of the total deaths in the United States. These cardiovascular diseases include hypertension, coronary artery disease, cerebral vascular disease, and occlusive peripheral vascular disease. Cardiovascular disease is the leading cause of death in men after the age of 40 and in women after the age of 65. In addition, coronary heart disease accounts for slightly more than one-fourth of all deaths in persons over the age of 35. Since 1940 there has been a downward trend in mortality from cardiovascular diseases, and these declines have been universal: death rates have declined in both sexes, all races, all age groups, and in every geographic area in the United States. The greatest declines have been seen in young adults and in higher socioeconomic subgroups. Cardiovascular diseases cause approximately 70 percent of all deaths in patients beyond the age of 75.

27. The answer is B.   *(pp 185–197)*   Coronary heart disease is the leading or one of the leading causes of death in men and women in every racial and ethnic group. However, extensive differences are found between men and women regarding the incidence, prevalence, and mortality of coronary heart disease. For instance, the death rate for coronary heart disease is approximately 5 times higher in men than women from the ages of 25 to 34. However, that ratio declines to 1.5 by age 75 to 84. Men usually have the first occurrence of coronary heart disease 10 years earlier. Premenopausal women are generally protected from clinical coronary heart disease. However, following menopause the incidence of coronary heart disease increases rapidly. Indeed, the rates of coronary heart disease in postmenopausal women are 2 to 3 times that of women the same age who remain premenopausal. This finding applies whether the menopause is surgical or natural. In addition to the differences in incidence and prevalence, the clinical presentation and prognosis of coronary heart disease also vary between men and women. Women are more likely to have angina as their first coronary presentation, whereas men are more likely to have a myocardial infarction. Following a myocardial infarction, sudden cardiac death is almost twice as prevalent in men as in women.

28. The answer is B.   *(pp 185–197)*   Hypertension is the most prevalent of all cardiovascular diseases and one of the most powerful contributors to mortality and morbidity from cardiovascular causes. It is estimated that approximately 30 percent of the U.S. population between the ages of 18 and 74 have a blood pressure greater than or equal to 140/90 mmHg. The number of people in the United States with mild hypertension, defined as a diastolic pressure of 90 to 104 mmHg, was approximately 25 million in 1989. The number of patients in the United States with isolated systolic hypertension, defined as a systolic blood pressure greater than 160 mmHg and a diastolic blood pressure less than 95 mmHg, was approximately 4 million. The prevalence of hypertension increases with age and is highest in the black population. Although in some populations around the world, blood pressure does not increase with age, in most affluent populations there is a rise. In general, between the third and the sixth decades, the systolic pressure rises 20 mmHg and the diastolic pressure rises approximately 10 mmHg. Treatment of systolic hypertension in the elderly was efficacious against the incidence of stroke and coronary heart disease in the Systemic Hypertension in the Elderly Program (SHEP).

29. **The answer is C.** *(pp 185–197)*   Despite improvement in the overall survival of patients with cardiovascular diseases, there has been no significant change in the prognosis of patients with congestive heart failure over the last 4 decades. This dismal fact remains despite dramatic improvements in the clinical armamentarium used for this condition. Hypertension remains the dominant cause of congestive heart failure and alone or in combination with coronary heart disease accounts for the vast majority of patients with congestive heart failure. The National Heart, Lung, and Blood Institute estimates that 2 to 3 million Americans have heart failure. The incidence increases with age and the annual occurrence rate may approach 1 percent of the population for those greater than age 65. The overall 5-year survival rates are approximately 25 percent for men and 40 percent for women. It is postulated that the lack of improvement in survival of patients with congestive heart failure may be due to improved survival among patients with angina and subsequent myocardial infarction that eventually progresses to heart failure. This increases the prevalence of heart failure in the population and inflates the absolute numbers of patients dying from heart failure.

30. **The answer is D.** *(p 192)*   Cerebrovascular disease is the third leading cause of death in the United States, accounting for 147,000 deaths in 1989. As with other causes of cardiovascular death, the death rate from stroke has dramatically decreased over the last 40 years. In fact, over the last 20 years the death rate has declined approximately 55 percent. Indeed, the rate of decline of death from strokes has exceeded the rate of decline of death from other cardiovascular diseases. Unlike other cardiovascular diseases, the risk of having a stroke before age 70 is equivalent in men and women (approximately 1 in 20). The most common types of strokes are atherothrombotic brain infarction followed by cerebral embolism, subarachnoid hemorrhage, and finally intracerebral hemorrhage. Even though the risk of stroke is similar in men and women, the prognosis following stroke is markedly poorer in men. Marked ethnic differences regarding mortality from stroke also exist. The death rate from stroke is approximately 3 times greater in the black population than in the white population. This is felt to be due, in part, to the increased prevalence and severity of hypertension in the black population.

31. **The answer is B (1, 3).** *(p 20)*   Calcium ions (Ca^{2+}) play an integral role in the contraction and relaxation of cardiac muscle. The sarcoplasmic calcium adenosine triphosphatase (ATPase) releases Ca^{2+} which leads to contraction; when Ca^{2+} is sequestered, the muscle relaxes. Systolic contraction is induced when Ca^{2+} binds to troponin C. This induces a slight motion of the tropomyosin, which exposes the receptor site on actin for myosin. The increase in cytosolic Ca^{2+} and tropomyosin movement follows muscle stimulation by 17 ms. As the actin binds to myosin, the ATPase activity is increased by 200-fold, and adenosine triphosphate (ATP) is hydrolyzed to adenosine diphosphate (ADP). This causes the myosin head to flex from a 90° to a 45° angle, bringing the actin filaments closer together. The reverse process relaxes the sarcomere. Tropomyosin and troponin block the receptor site for myosin and inhibit binding in the relaxed state.

32. **The answer is A (1, 2, 3).** *(pp 19–20)*   There are six actin proteins expressed in the adult mammal; each is the product of a separate gene. Different actins are expressed in skeletal muscle, heart muscle, smooth muscle, and nonmuscle cells. Calcium ions (Ca^{2+}) are an integral part of muscle contraction. When Ca^{2+} binds to troponin C, the tropomyosin–troponin I inhibition of actin-myosin adenosine triphosphatase (ATPase) activity is released, and muscle contraction is activated. Myosin is present in muscle and nonmuscle cells.

33. **The answer is E (all).** *(pp 32–33, 40)*   The endothelium has three major functions: these include a metabolically active secretory function in which vasoconstrictors and vasodilators are secreted. Plasma lipids are also metabolized in various ways by enzymes, including lipoprotein lipase. Normal endothelial cells present an antithrombotic surface; however, when stimulated with cytokines and other inflammatory

agents, they are capable of secreting prothrombotic factors. The endothelium also contains intracellular tight junctions, vesicles, and transendothelial channels that enable the intact endothelium to serve as a barrier to prevent vasoactive and thrombotic substances from coming into contact with the underlying vascular smooth muscle. Both growth-promoting and growth-inhibiting factors are secreted by endothelial cells, which are involved in normal angiogenesis and abnormal growth of smooth muscle during disease.

34. The answer is B (1, 3). *(p 31)* Arteries consist of three layers: the intima, media, and adventitia. The intima is a single layer of endothelial cells embedded in an extracellular matrix. The adventitial layer varies, depending upon the type of artery. Large conduit arteries tend to have a high ratio of elastic laminae to smooth muscle cells, whereas muscular arteries are generally smaller and have a prevalence of smooth muscle cells. Veins have a similar architecture to that of the arterial system but differ in the orientation of the smooth muscle cells within the wall.

35. The answer is A (1, 2, 3). *(p 42)* It is theorized that one of the most important causes of restenosis after angioplasty is the loss of endothelium-derived growth inhibitory factors. Experimental removal of endothelium allows the initiation of the mitogenic response, and regrowth of normal endothelium inhibits further proliferation. During angioplasty, the stretching of the vessel wall and injury lead to several distinct events, including an altered hormonal environment in which the vascular smooth muscle cells exist, thrombus formation, and induction of growth factors from the underlying smooth muscle, which may have mitogenic effects on the remaining smooth muscle cells. The normal endothelium seems to be in an inhibitory mode, and loss of the normal endothelium plays a crucial role in the response of the vessel wall to injury.

36. The answer is E (all). *(p 55)* Cell-surface receptors interact with proteins, such as the G protein, to influence intracellular processes in either an agonistic or antagonistic fashion. Conditions now known to modulate receptor signaling on cardiovascular membranes include agonist-induced desensitization, antagonist-induced sensitization, changes in steroid and thyroid hormone levels, cyclic adenosine monophosphate (cAMP) changes, congestive heart failure (CHF), diabetes, and ischemia. Down-regulation denotes a condition in which there is a decrease in the total cellular pool of receptors and decreased agonist responsiveness.

37. The answer is E (all). *(p 105)* P cells, transitional cells, ameboid cells, and Purkinje cells are all involved in the system of impulse formation and rapid conduction. P cells are pale in appearance and are thought to be the site of pacemaker impulse origin; they are numerous in the sinoatrial node (SA), atrioventricular (AV) node, and internodal pathways. Transitional cells are a group of cells with an appearance between P cells and more complex working cardiac cells. They are found in the SA node, AV node, internodal pathways, and atrial tissue. Ameboid cells are recognized on electron microscopy by the presence of a eustachian ridge. These cells have multilobar nuclei and many mitochondria and myofibrils. They may act as an auxiliary pacemaker or may serve as a source of atrial natriuretic factor. Purkinje cells are recognized on the basis of their ultrastructure, being broader and shorter than working cells. Purkinje cells are found in the SA node, AV node, His bundle, and bundle branches.

38. The answer is C (2, 4). *(pp 121–122)* A left ventricular function curve in which left ventricular stroke volume is plotted as a function of left ventricular end-diastolic pressure is a curvilinear relationship. *Curve A* represents a normal functioning left ventricle. In *curve B,* the shift to the left is a reflection of increased contractility such as may result from sympathetic stimulation or the infusion of epinephrine or norepinephrine. In addition, inotropic agents can cause a shift to the left. *Curve C* is a shift to the right of the original curve and occurs with decreased contractility such as may result from ventricular failure due to ischemia or myocardial depressant drugs. The chemotherapeutic agent doxorubicin hydrochloride, in cumulative toxic quantities, produces cardiomyopathy and a failing heart. In congestive heart failure (CHF), the action of digitalis or other inotropic agents will shift *curve C* to the left to resemble the original normal *curve A.*

39. **The answer is E (all).** *(pp 128–130, Table 5-1)* Mechanisms of cardiac reserve that the heart may use to meet increased demands in the normal or diseased circulatory system include increased heart rate, increased stroke volume, increased oxygen extraction, redistribution of blood flow, anaerobic metabolism, cardiac dilatation, and cardiac hypertrophy. The two basic mechanisms that the heart may use to increase its minute output in the face of increased demand are change in rate and change in stroke volume. Anaerobic metabolism has a limited value as cardiac reserve but may account for about 5 percent of the energy used in a normal person during moderate exercise and up to 30 percent in patients with heart failure. Both dilatation and hypertrophy are forms of compensatory reserve with their own inherent consequences.

40. **The answer is C (2, 4).** *(p 135)* The arterial pressure gradient (aortic pressure − left ventricular diastolic pressure) and the time spent in diastole are the major determinants of coronary blood flow. Essentially, the left ventricle receives the most coronary blood flow during diastole. During ventricular systole, the left ventricular intramyocardial pressure exceeds the left ventricular cavitary pressure or aortic systolic pressure; thus, the penetrating coronary vessels in the wall of the left ventricle are exposed to marked compression, which prevents forward coronary blood flow and may even produce retrograde flow.

41. **The answer is B (1, 3).** *(pp 113–116; Figure 5-3)* The action potential of the cardiac cell membranes is initiated by a depolarization related to a sudden influx of sodium ions (Na^+), followed by a slower influx of calcium ions (Ca^{2+}). The initial transsarcolemmal influx of Ca^{2+} triggers and release of Ca^{2+} from the sarcoplasmic reticulum. Actually, the transsarcolemmal Ca^{2+} current has both a fast and a slow component. The fast component triggers the release of Ca^{2+} from the sarcoplasmic reticulum, whereas the slow component may cause the sarcoplasmic reticulum to accumulate Ca^{2+}. Ca^{2+} release is predominant in contraction. The active uptake of Ca^{2+} by the sarcoplasmic reticulum by an unknown stimulus is an event that initiates relaxation. The higher concentration of Ca^{2+} in the sarcoplasm binds to the troponin C subunit. This produces a conformational change in the whole troponin complex (troponin I-troponin C-troponin T). This conformational change then relieves a troponin I interaction with actin, which allows tropomyosin to roll back into the groves of the F-actin superhelix. This release of the baseline inhibition of actin and myosin results in actin-myosin contraction and overall myocardial contraction.

42. **The answer is B (1, 3).** *(pp 138–139, Color Plate II)* The classic Wiggers' diagram divides the cardiac cycle into two periods, systole and diastole, with each period subdivided into phases of cardiac activity. The following phases of left ventricular systole correlate with valvular events: isovolumic contraction–mitral closure; rapid ventricular ejection–opening of the aortic valve; and reduced ventricular ejection, which occurs when the shape of the ventricular volume curve indicates a significant decrease in the rate of ejection. The following phases of left ventricular diastole correlate with valvular events: protodiastole (the very brief initial phase of diastole) precedes the incisura of the aortic pressure tracing; isovolumic relaxation–closure of the aortic valve; rapid ventricular filling–opening of the mitral valve; and slow ventricular filling–*a* wave with left atrial contraction.

43. **The answer is C (2, 4).** *(p 159)* The heart derives 90 percent of its energy production from the oxidation of carbon-based fuels. Oxidative metabolism occurs in the mitochondria. The oxidative breakdown of 1 molecule of glucose by the heart produces 38 molecules of adenosine triphosphate (ATP). Other substrates such as fatty acids can yield much greater amounts of ATP per molecule that is oxidized. Substrate oxidation is an efficient source of energy for the heart, and the availability of substrate to the heart and substrate preference by the heart can influence the bioenergetic balance and respiratory efficiency at a given level of cardiac performance.

44. **The answer is A (1, 2, 3).** *(pp 175–177)* The conversion of fibrinogen to fibrin is the final result of the coagulation cascade. Fibrinolysis is the process by which insoluble fibrin is catalyzed to soluble fibrin fragments. This reaction is catalyzed by the conversion of plasminogen to plasmin. Currently available fibrinolytic or thrombolytic agents involve the activation of plasminogen to plasmin. Fibrin-specific agents including tissue plasminogen activator (tPA) and single-chain urokinase-type plasminogen activator (scuPA) have a 1000-fold increase in activity when bound to fibrin and have a higher recanalization rate than non-fibrin-selective agents. The repeat administration of streptokinase (SK) or anisoylated plasminogen-streptokinase activator complex (APSAC) to a patient who had already received such an agent is not advised. The initial use of these agents results in anti-SK antibodies, and therefore, repeat administration can result in an anaphylactic reaction or neutralization of the thrombotic agent. This interaction can usually be prevented with the preadministration of intravenous corticosteroids.

45. The answer is B (1, 3). *(p 163)* Traditional methods to study metabolism are not well suited to concurrent measurements of physiological functions because of the requirements of tissue sampling and difficulties with the enzyme assays. The invasive nature of metabolic analyses limits our understanding of the basic physiology of the heart in normal and diseased states. New technologies such as positron emission tomography (PET) and nuclear magnetic resonance (NMR) spectroscopy can provide nondestructive, kinetic information regarding metabolic support of the heart.

46. The answers are: A-Y, B-N, C-Y, D-N, E-Y. *(pp 8–14)* A single gene can give rise to several different messenger RNAs (mRNAs) with rearrangement of the exons. This will, therefore, translate into several unique polypeptides. Thus, the primary transcript, or initial mRNA, can undergo different splicing processes by which introns are removed and exons are properly respliced to provide different mRNAs.

The local environment as well as signals from within the cell regulate the process of gene expression, a situation that has great potential for therapeutic intervention; for example, altering the way a cell responds to an external stimuli may affect gene expression and cell growth.

Although all cells contain the same DNA and the same genes, the phenotype of each cell is determined by the genes that are expressed. This complicated process of selective gene expression is the basis of cell differentiation. If recombinant DNA technology is used on specific DNA that is expressed, then the mRNA is isolated using the enzyme reverse transcriptase to derive complimentary DNA (cDNA) from the mRNA.

Northern and southern blotting are used to electrophoretically separate different sized molecules of mRNA and DNA, respectively. When this procedure is used for the detection of proteins, it is referred to as western blotting.

DNA cloning techniques can produce a million copies of a DNA fragment rapidly. During this process, a DNA fragment is inserted into the DNA of a vector or extrachromosomal segment of DNA that is able to propagate independently of the host DNA. It is, therefore, necessary to isolate the DNA of interest prior to the cloning process.

47. The answers are: A-Y, B-N, C-N, D-Y, E-Y. *(p 40)* Atherosclerosis is frequently viewed as a disease of endothelial dysfunction. The primary impairment lies with endothelial-dependent relaxation, which accounts for the tendency of diseased arteries to have a vasospastic tendency, possibly due to defective generation or delivery of nitric oxide (NO). In fact, impairment in coronary endothelial-dependent vasodilator function occurs in patients with high cholesterol prior to angiographically demonstrable coronary disease. In hypercholesterolemic animals, enhanced NO production is rapidly degraded to inactive metabolites, which leads to less of a vasodilator effect in the vessel wall. This vasodilator defect can be corrected by the administration of superoxide dysmutase, which led to the theory that excessive oxygen-free radicals produced by the endothelium degrade NO and account for the decreased vasodilator activity. Vascular cell adhesion molecule 1 (VCAM-1) induction leads to recruitment of monocytes and macrophages into the vessel wall and may be secondary to inflammatory cytokines produced by the endothelium.

48. The answers are: A-Y, B-Y, C-N, D-Y, E-N. *(p 38)* Smooth muscle cells are relatively quiescent, well-differentiated cells that are prevented from proliferation by normal endothelium. Removal of endothelium in experimental conditions allows the initiation of smooth muscle proliferation. There is much experimental evidence supporting the theory that endothelial-derived inhibitors play a large role in preventing smooth muscle cell growth. Cultured vascular smooth muscle cells exposed to sodium nitroprusside, which mimics the effect of nitric oxide (NO), can inhibit mitogenesis. This suggests that NO may have an important role in maintaining the normal artery in a state refractory to mitogenesis. NO is usually associated with vascular relaxation, but it seems to play a less important role in the control of vascular tone of large arteries. It is theorized that NO may have an additional function in these vessels, and multiple studies have shown that a variety of factors, such as heparin and transforming growth factor β (TGF-β), can inhibit smooth muscle cell growth.

49. The answers are: A-Y, B-N, C-N, D-N, E-Y. *(pp 84–89)* The conus branch of the right coronary artery may indeed arise as a separate ostium from the right sinus of Valsalva in 40 to 50 percent of hearts. The origin of the left coronary artery is slightly superior and posterior to that of the right coronary artery. The left circumflex artery supplies the atrioventricular (AV) node in only 10 to 15 percent of hearts, most arising from the right coronary artery. The artery to the sinoatrial (SA) node, however, may originate in 40 to 50 percent of hearts from the circumflex artery rather than the right coronary artery. Kugel's artery is an important collateral from the base of the atrial septum to the AV node and the posterior circulation and may arise from either the proximal right or left coronary artery. The circle of Vieussens provides collateral circulation from the left anterior descending artery to the anterior right ventricle. Three venous drainages are present in the heart: the coronary sinus and its tributaries, the anterior right ventricular veins, and the thebesian veins. The coronary sinus drains blood mostly from the left ventricle via conduits in parallel with the coronary arteries. The anterior cardiac veins drain the anterior right ventricular wall via conduits to the right atrium. Thebesian veins are tiny venous channels, most of which drain directly into the right atrium and right ventricle.

50. The answers are: A-Y, B-Y, C-N, D-Y, E-N. *(pp 34–35)* In general, smooth muscle vessel vasoconstriction occurs in response to a vasoconstrictor agonist hormone. These hormones interact with specific receptors on the vascular smooth muscle and are linked to a G protein. This leads to production of inositol triphosphate (IP_3), which releases calcium ion (Ca^{2+}) from intracellular stores and activates calmodulin. This, in turn, activates myosin light chain kinase, which phosphorylates the myosin light chain and allows it to interact with actin, resulting in cross-bridge formation and force generation. When the intracellular Ca^{2+} concentration drops, the Ca^{2+} dissociates from calmodulin, and the process is reversed. The myosin then becomes dephosphorylated and cross-bridge cycling ceases.

51. The answers are: A-Y, B-N, C-Y, D-Y, E-N. *(pp 66–75)* Small perforations or fenestrations are found in normally functioning aortic and pulmonary valves. Tearing of a fenestration may lead to gross valvular insufficiency. The tricuspid valve orifice is larger than the mitral valve orifice. The three tricuspid leaflets are thinner and less well defined as compared with the two mitral leaflets. In hypertrophic cardiomyopathy, systolic anterior movement of the anterior (aortic) mitral leaflet into the left ventricular outflow tract coincides with maximal left ventricular outflow obstruction. The atrioventricular (AV) node lies within the triangle of Koch, the base of which is defined by the annulus of the tricuspid valve and the os of the coronary sinus. These landmarks are all important as guides to the surgeon during surgery for AV nodal reentrant tachycardia. The largest of the three papillary muscles in the right ventricle is the anterior papillary muscle. The septal papillary muscle is not infrequently absent.

52. The answers are: A-Y, B-N, C-Y, D-Y, E-N. *(pp 62–64, 91)* Palpation of the sternum and lower left sternal border is important in evaluating the right ventricle since the right ventricle lies beneath the sternum and is the most anterior cardiac chamber. Although the ventricular septum provides the medial wave for both ventricular chambers, the ventricular septum contributes predominantly to left ventricular rather than right ventricular function in normal persons. The right bundle courses through the moderator band on its path from the interventricular septum to the anterior papillary muscle prior to reaching the endocardium of the right ventricle. Since the right atrium is in close proximity to the aortic root, an aneurysm of the sinus of Valsalva may rupture into the right atrium and cause a continuous murmur. The coronary sinus opens into the inferior-posterior medial aspect of the right atrium. Retrograde cannulation of the coronary sinus is best approached from the left arm.

53. **The answers are: A-N, B-Y, C-N, D-N, E-Y.** *(pp 104–107)* P cells constitute one of four types of cells involved in impulse formation and rapid conduction. They are present in the sinoatrial (SA) node, atrioventricular (AV) node, and internodal pathways. Purkinje cells are found in both the His bundle and the bundle branches. Huxley and Hanson proposed the "sliding filament hypothesis," which applies to both myocardial and skeletal cells. According to this theory, the actin and myosin fibers slide past each other causing shortening of the muscle fiber. Although the length of each sarcomere varies from 1.5 to 2.2 μm, optimal overlap between the thin actin and the thick myosin filaments resulting in maximal shortening of the muscle fiber occurs at sarcomere lengths of 2.2 μm. Periodicity between the actin and myosin filaments results in A, I, and Z bands. The A bands contain both actin and myosin filaments. Release of the actin-myosin inhibition follows the increase in free intracellular calcium (Ca^{2+}) and its binding to troponin.

54. **The answers are: A-Y, B-N, C-N, D-N, E-Y.** *(pp 65–66)* Ventricular muscle at the apex of the left ventricle sometimes measures 2 mm or less. This may partially account for the fact that 85 percent of left ventricular aneurysms following acute myocardial infarction involve the apex. Although muscular sleeves may enter from the left atrium onto the pulmonary veins for 1 to 2 cm and may have a sphincterlike effect on retrograde flow, no true valves occur at the junction of the pulmonary veins and the left atrium. The right ventricular endocardium is much more trabeculated than the left ventricular as can be easily seen during constant ventriculography. Dilatation of the left atrium may compress the posteriorly located esophagus and can result in dysphagia. The left atrial appendage forms the anterolateral border of the left atrium and, thus, does not impinge on the esophagus. A patent foramen ovale, found in 15 percent of hearts, may account for some cases of paradoxical thromboembolism, especially those occurring during periods of elevated right atrial pressure.

55–58. **The answers are: 55-C, 56-E, 57-B, 58-A.** *(pp 36–37)* Smooth muscle tone is dependent on a balance between vasoconstrictor and vasorelaxing factors. The endothelium, which is responsible for this function, secretes both relaxing and constricting factors.

The endothelins are peptides that are secreted by endothelial cells, which activate the phosphoinositide protein kinase C signaling pathway and lead to a slow, sustained contraction of smooth muscle.

Angiotensin-converting enzyme (ACE) is a protein that converts angiotensin I to the potent vasoconstrictor angiotensin II. It also degrades and inactivates bradykinin.

Adenosine, a nucleoside released by the endothelium in response to thrombin and flow, can bond to purinergic receptors and activate cyclic adenosine monophosphate (cAMP), leading to relaxation.

Prostacyclin (PGI_2) also increases the intracellular content of cAMP. Because it is derived from the arachidonic acid pathway, there has been some debate about the ideal dose of aspirin that should be used in ischemic coronary syndromes—that is, a dose that will inhibit platelet function without inhibiting endothelial PGI_2 synthesis.

Nitric oxide (NO) is an endothelium-derived relaxing factor that is rapidly oxidized to form nitrite and nitrate. It enhances the formation of cyclic guanosine monophosphate (cGMP), which reduces intracellular calcium ion (Ca^{2+}) concentrations, leading to dephosphorylation of the myosin light chain and causing vascular smooth muscle relaxation. Nitroglycerin causes vascular relaxation by being converted to NO.

59–61. The answers are: 59-C, 60-B, 61-A. *(pp 124–126, 130–131)*   Important relations between the distending pressure and the tension in the wall of a blood vessel are expressed in Laplace's law:

$$\text{wall tension} = \text{distending pressure} \times \frac{\text{vessel radius}}{2 \times \text{wall thickness}}$$

The relation of the various factors affecting the resistance to fluid flow in rigid tubing is expressed by Poiseuille's equation:

$$\text{fluid flow} = \frac{\pi \, (\text{pressure difference}) \, \text{radius}^4}{8 \, (\text{vessel length}) \, (\text{fluid viscosity})}$$

The Bowditch effect (staircase phenomenon) is a force-frequency relationship in which an increase in pulse rate may also increase myocardial contractility. The "recuperative effect of a long pause" upon the strength of contraction is known as the Woodworth phenomenon (negative or reverse staircase).

The Anrep effect describes an additional influence in afterload changes, whereby there is an increase in ventricular performance several beats after the aortic pressure is raised. This may be due to recovery from transient subendocardial ischemia caused by the sudden change in arterial pressure.

II. General Evaluation of the Patient

DIRECTIONS: Each question below contains five suggested responses. Select the **one best** response to each question.

62. Which of the following statements regarding statistical terminology is true?

    (A) Sensitivity is defined as the frequency of a negative test result in a population of patients without a certain disease
    (B) Bayes' theorem states that the predictive value of the test result is determined by the pretest probability of the disease in the population being tested
    (C) Specificity indicates the frequency of a positive test result in a population of patients with a certain disease
    (D) The efficiency of a test is defined as the percentage of patients correctly classified
    (E) The prevalence of a disease is defined as a number of clinical events that are present in the general population

63. Angina pectoris due to myocardial ischemia is associated with all the following characteristics EXCEPT

    (A) symptoms may be effort-related or experienced at rest
    (B) the discomfort is described as retrosternal in location but may be referred elsewhere
    (C) it can be associated with electrocardiographic abnormalities
    (D) it persists for 30 to 60 min
    (E) it is promptly relieved by nitroglycerin

64. Anxiety frequently produces symptoms referable to the cardiovascular system such as

    (A) chest pain located along the right costosternal junction
    (B) chest pain that typically occurs on exertion
    (C) dyspnea with effort but not with rest
    (D) dyspnea associated with perioral and peripheral dysesthesia
    (E) periodic fatigue that occurs primarily with effort

65. Which of the following statements about the classification of heart disease is true?

    (A) The new New York Heart Association classification has the following categories: etiology, anatomy, physiology, functional capacity, and therapy
    (B) Heart failure is classified according to the Canadian Cardiovascular Society
    (C) Angina is graded according to the Canadian Cardiovascular Society
    (D) Class III heart failure indicates the presence of symptoms at rest
    (E) Grade I angina pectoris indicates absolute absence of symptoms regardless of activity

66. In the right panel below, which of the following conditions is most likely?

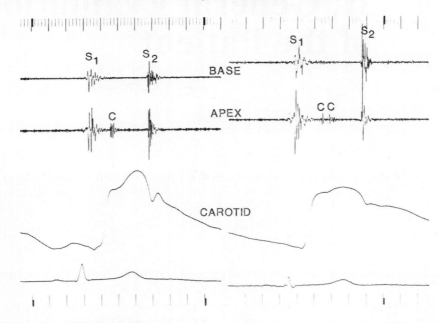

(From Shaver JA: Current uses of phonocardiography in clinical practice. In Rapaport E (ed): *Cardiology Update—Reviews for Physicians.* New York, Elsevier, 1981, p 370.)

(A) Mitral stenosis
(B) Mitral valve prolapse
(C) Bicuspid aortic valve
(D) Valvular pulmonary stenosis
(E) Ebstein's anomaly

---

67. Symptoms related to the cardiovascular system have which of the following characteristics?

(A) There is a direct correlation between the severity of symptoms and the seriousness of the disease process
(B) The magnitude of symptoms is inversely related to the severity of the disease
(C) Decreased physical activity may obscure the apparent severity of the disease process
(D) Sudden cardiac death is usually preceded by prodromal symptoms
(E) In approximately 70 percent of cardiac patients, assessment of the patient's history without additional diagnostic testing can provide a diagnosis

68. Which of the following is a correct description of an abnormal pulse?

(A) A dicrotic arterial pulse is characterized by two peaks in systole and is seen in patients with left ventricular dysfunction
(B) A hypokinetic pulse is a small, weak pulse seen in patients with an increased stroke volume
(C) A hyperkinetic pulse is a bounding pulse seen in patients with increased stroke volume
(D) A bisferiens pulse is characterized as having two peaks, one in systole and the other in diastole, and is seen in patients with hypertrophic obstructive cardiomyopathy
(E) A parvus et tardus pulse is a hypokinetic pulse with a slow upstroke and is seen in patients with aortic insufficiency

69. The phonocardiogram below represents which of the following conditions?

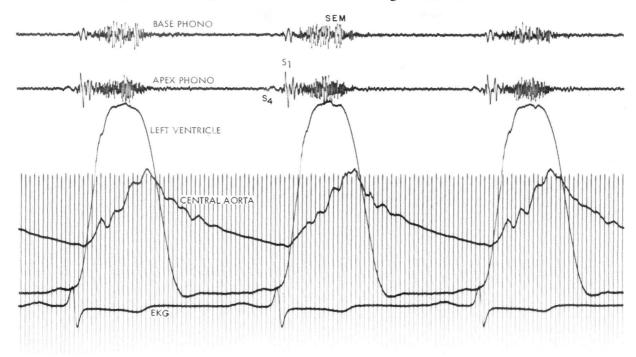

(A) Congenital valvular aortic stenosis
(B) Congenital subvalvular aortic stenosis
(C) Congenital supravalvular aortic stenosis
(D) Acquired aortic stenosis
(E) Hypertrophic obstructive cardiomyopathy

---

70. All the following statements regarding the first heart sound (S_1) in a healthy person are true EXCEPT

(A) auscultation reveals a widely split S_1
(B) on phonocardiography, four sequential components of S_1 can be identified
(C) a large high-frequency vibration is related to mitral valve closure
(D) a second high-frequency vibration is related to tricuspid valve closure
(E) low-frequency vibrations indicate that movement of aortic blood into the great vessel has already occurred

71. Which of the following statements regarding the first heart sound (S_1) is true?

(A) Paradoxical splitting of S_1 is seen with a right bundle branch block (RBBB)
(B) There is decreased intensity of S_1 with mitral valve prolapse
(C) There is increased intensity of S_1 in patients with Lown-Ganong-Levine syndrome
(D) There is increased intensity of S_1 in patients with mitral valve calcification and severe mitral stenosis
(E) S_1 is increased in intensity in patients with left bundle branch block (LBBB)

72. What is the abnormal retinal finding illustrated in the figure below?

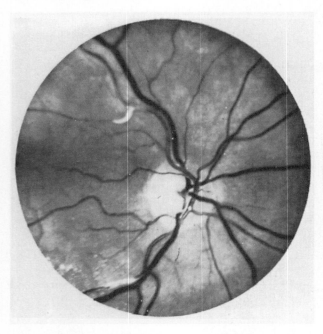

- (A) Platelet embolus
- (B) Roth's spot
- (C) Fat embolus
- (D) Hollenhorst plaque
- (E) Calcium plaque

73. Which of the following statements concerning auscultatory events and prosthetic valves is true?

- (A) The Bjork-Shiley valve has a prominent opening and soft closing sound
- (B) The Starr-Edwards valve has a closing but no opening sound
- (C) A tissue prosthetic valve in the aortic position usually has an opening sound
- (D) A central disk occluding valve has an opening and closing sound
- (E) A tissue prosthetic valve has neither a closing sound nor an opening sound

74. Which of the following statements concerning retinal changes in systemic disease is true?

- (A) Arteriovenous compression (nicking) is commonly seen in patients with isolated systemic arterial hypertension
- (B) Microaneurysms are seen in patients with increased intracranial pressure
- (C) Neovascularization is seen in conditions that predispose patients to the development of microaneurysms
- (D) Hard exudates are a sign of retinal ischemia due to a systemic illness
- (E) Cotton-wool spots result from prior edema due to systemic illnesses such as diabetes mellitus or systemic arterial hypertension

75. Which of the following statements concerning ventricular depolarization and repolarization is correct?

- (A) The sequence of ventricular repolarization is from epicardium to endocardium with positive charges in front of the negative charges
- (B) The sequence of ventricular repolarization is from endocardium to epicardium with positive charges in front of the negative charges
- (C) The sequence of ventricular depolarization is from epicardium to endocardium with negative charges in front of the positive charges
- (D) The sequence of ventricular depolarization is from endocardium to epicardium with positive charges in front of the negative charges
- (E) The sequence of ventricular depolarization both begins and terminates in the endocardium with positive charges leading negative charges

76. The figure below is consistent with which of the clinical presentations?

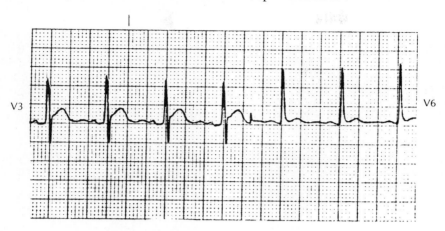

(A) A deaf child who has experienced sudden cardiac death
(B) A 76-year-old man with multiple myeloma and a calcium of 14.4 mg/dL
(C) A 45-year-old woman with glomerulonephritis, end-stage renal disease, and a potassium level of 7.6 meq/L
(D) A 52-year-old man with ventricular tachycardia who has been on a maintenance dose of amiodarone
(E) A 30-year-old alcoholic man with acute pancreatitis and a serum calcium of 7.0 mg/dL

77. The figure below represents which of the following electrocardiographic abnormalities?

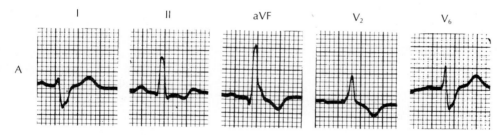

(A) Right bundle branch block (RBBB)
(B) Left bundle branch block (LBBB)
(C) LBBB with right axis deviation
(D) RBBB with left posterior hemiblock
(E) LBBB with left axis deviation

78. The chest roentgenogram below is most compatible with which of the following entities?

79. The chest roentgenogram below represents which of the following entities?

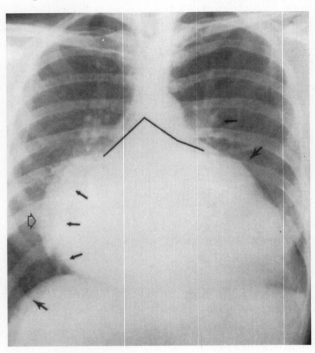

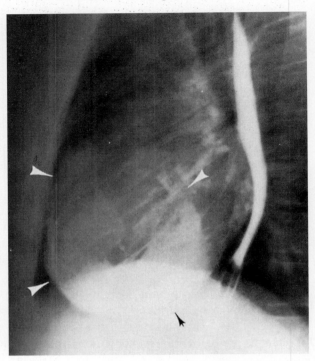

(A) Tricuspid stenosis
(B) Pulmonary stenosis
(C) Mitral regurgitation (severe)
(D) Aortic stenosis
(E) Tracheal stenosis

(A) Restrictive cardiomyopathy
(B) Calcific aortic stenosis
(C) Mitral annular calcification
(D) Calcific constrictive pericarditis
(E) Severe mitral stenosis

80. A 52-year-old man who smokes three packs of cigarettes per day and has a long-standing history of systemic arterial hypertension, type I diabetes mellitus, and hypercholesterolemia is admitted to the hospital with exertional chest discomfort that is relieved with rest and nitroglycerin. A lateral chest roentgenogram is obtained. Based on the history and roentgenographic findings shown below, what is the likelihood that this patient's chest discomfort is the result of myocardial ischemia?

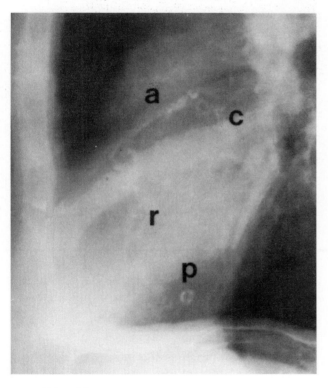

(A) 25 percent
(B) 40 percent
(C) 60 percent
(D) 75 percent
(E) 90 percent

81. The radiograph below identifies which of the following cardiac valves?

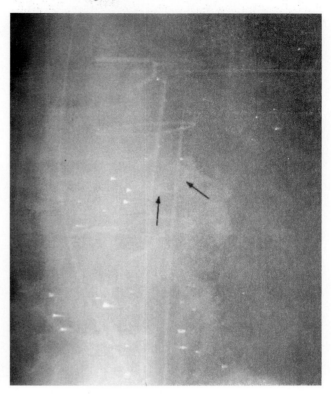

(A) Bjork-Shiley valve
(B) St. Jude prosthesis
(C) Tissue bioprosthetic valve
(D) Starr-Edwards valve
(E) Bovine pericardial valve

82. Which of the following abnormalities is compatible with the chest roentgenograms below?

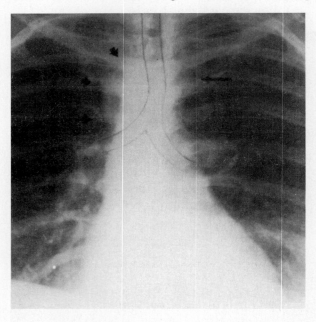 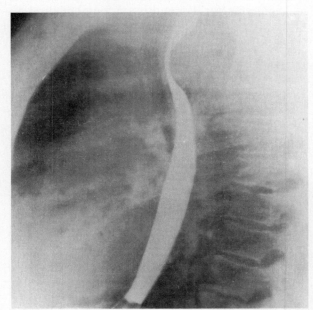

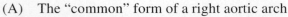

    (A)   The "common" form of a right aortic arch
    (B)   An enlarged left atrium
    (C)   The "avian" right-sided aortic arch
    (D)   Tetralogy of Fallot
    (E)   Holt-Oram syndrome

---

83. The advantages of echocardiography over other noninvasive diagnostic tests include all the following EXCEPT

    (A)   delineation of complete cardiac anatomic information is possible
    (B)   it provides both anatomic (from two-dimensional imaging) as well as physiological (from Doppler) information about cardiac structure, function, and great vessel anatomy
    (C)   the equipment is mobile and, therefore, can be moved to the patient's bedside, an advantage in the critical care setting
    (D)   it is useful for following serial changes over an extended period of time
    (E)   it is a relatively quick and inexpensive test

84. Echocardiographic criteria for the diagnosis of hypertrophic obstructive cardiomyopathy include all the following EXCEPT

    (A)   asymmetric septal hypertrophy
    (B)   left ventricular dilation
    (C)   systolic anterior motion of the mitral valve
    (D)   midsystolic notching or closure of the aortic valve
    (E)   left atrial dilation

85. Amyloidosis is characterized by all the following echocardiographic signs EXCEPT

    (A)   concentric left ventricular hypertrophy
    (B)   abnormal left ventricular function both in systole and diastole
    (C)   thinning of the interatrial septum
    (D)   thickening of the valves
    (E)   a glittering, ground-glass appearance of the left ventricular walls

86. The chest roentgenogram below represents which type of heart failure?

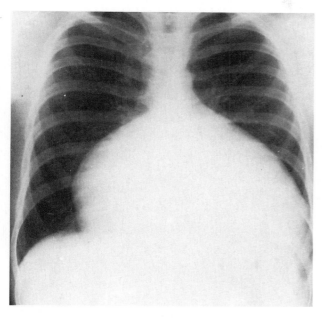

(A) Acute right-sided heart failure
(B) Acute left-sided heart failure
(C) Chronic right-sided heart failure
(D) Chronic left-sided heart failure
(E) Chronic biventricular failure

87. In mitral valve prolapse, which echocardiographic view should be used when determining leaflet displacement above the plane of the mitral annulus?

(A) Apical four-chamber view
(B) Apical two-chamber view
(C) Subcostal view
(D) Parasternal long axis view
(E) Parasternal short axis view

88. Echocardiographic features of aortic valve stenosis include all the following EXCEPT

(A) aortic stenosis is usually associated with concentric left ventricular hypertrophy and a dilated aortic root
(B) in aortic stenosis, the aortic valve areas can be calculated accurately by planimeter
(C) severe aortic stenosis can usually be excluded when the aortic cusps are separated by more than 12 mm
(D) aortic cusp separation of less than 7 mm is only suggestive of severe stenosis
(E) the Doppler modality accurately measures the peak and mean pressure gradients across the aortic valve

89. A 60-year-old man with a history of well-controlled hypertension on angiotensin-converting enzyme (ACE) inhibitors undergoes exercise testing to evaluate exertional chest discomfort that has been present for 6 months. The physician is surprised to find that there was no ischemic ST-segment depression. The most probable reason for the normal treadmill response is

(A) the ACE mediates bradykinin responses and limits the exercise-induced spasm that usually occurs
(B) exercise testing on the treadmill is not very sensitive for diagnosing single-vessel coronary disease
(C) the prevalence of coronary artery disease in this age-group is too low for exercise testing to be useful
(D) the cardiologist performing the test misread the test
(E) the patient exercised for only 12 min on a Bruce protocol, and this is an unlikely level of exercise to precipitate ischemia

90. The hemodynamic tracing below illustrates which of the following conditions?

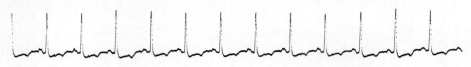

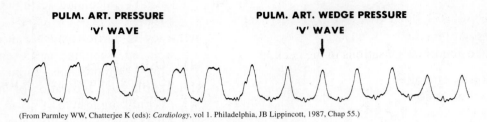

PULM. ART. PRESSURE   PULM. ART. WEDGE PRESSURE
'V' WAVE   'V' WAVE

(From Parmley WW, Chatterjee K (eds): *Cardiology*, vol 1. Philadelphia, JB Lippincott, 1987, Chap 55.)

(A) Acute mitral regurgitation
(B) Acute aortic insufficiency
(C) Chronic mitral regurgitation
(D) Chronic aortic insufficiency
(E) Chronic aortic stenosis

---

91. Echocardiographic features of endocarditis include all the following EXCEPT

(A) the absence of a vegetation on echocardiography rules out infective endocarditis
(B) vegetations are mobile, irregular, echodense structures attached to the leaflets
(C) the size of the vegetation is not an indication for surgery
(D) leaflet destruction is readily visualized
(E) valve ring abscesses may be diagnosed

92. Lung volume measurements in patients with congestive heart failure (CHF) due to cardiomyopathy but no pulmonary disease are characterized by

(A) normal lung volume measurements
(B) low lung volume measurements
(C) decreased total lung capacity, normal functional residual capacity, and normal or increased residual volume
(D) decreased inspiratory capacity and normal residual volume
(E) normal lung volume measurements except for decreased expiratory volume

DIRECTIONS: Each question below contains four suggested responses of which **one or more** is correct. Select

A	if	**1, 2, and 3**	are correct
B	if	**1 and 3**	are correct
C	if	**2 and 4**	are correct
D	if	**4**	is correct
E	if	**1, 2, 3, and 4**	are correct

93. In which of the following conditions may disease processes involving the cardiovascular system lead to abnormal sensations in the neck?

    (1) Pulmonary emboli
    (2) Acute pericarditis
    (3) Dissecting aneurysm of the aorta
    (4) Severe tricuspid regurgitation

94. Symptoms associated with severe pulmonary hypertension include

    (1) hemoptysis
    (2) anterior exertional chest discomfort
    (3) peripheral edema
    (4) Cheyne-Stokes respiratory pattern

95. True statements regarding abnormal skin color include which of the following?

    (1) A bluish tint to the skin is seen in patients with a left-to-right intracardiac shunt
    (2) A bronze hue to the skin may be caused by cardiomyopathy due to hemochromatosis
    (3) Sudden flushing of the skin, occasionally precipitated by the use of alcohol, is seen in patients with hepatic congestion due to congestive heart failure (CHF)
    (4) A slatelike tint to the skin occasionally is seen as a side effect in patients taking amiodarone

96. A ventricular septal defect is a common manifestation of which of the following congenital cardiovascular abnormalities?

    (1) Cardiofacial syndrome
    (2) Ellis–van Creveld syndrome
    (3) Cornelia de Lange syndrome
    (4) Rubella syndrome

97. Bacterial endocarditis may have which of the following peripheral manifestations?

    (1) Osler's nodes
    (2) Splinter hemorrhages of the nails
    (3) Janeway's lesions
    (4) Jaccoud's arthritis

98. Congenital cardiac abnormalities associated with ocular manifestations are found in which of the following conditions?

    (1) Down's syndrome
    (2) Wilson's disease
    (3) Osteogenesis imperfecta
    (4) Kawasaki's disease

99. Conduction disturbances have been linked to

    (1) neonates born to mothers with systemic lupus erythematosus
    (2) congenitally deaf children
    (3) patients with sarcoidosis
    (4) adults with Emery-Dreifuss muscular dystrophy

100. True statements regarding abnormal arterial pressure include which of the following?

    (1) Pulsus paradoxus is seen in patients with severe congestive heart failure
    (2) Pulsus alternans is seen in patients with cardiac tamponade
    (3) An increased pulse pressure is seen in patients with severe aortic stenosis
    (4) Unequal pulse pressure between the right and left arms is seen in infants with supravalvular aortic stenosis and adults with subclavian steal syndrome

SUMMARY OF DIRECTIONS

A	B	C	D	E
1, 2, 3 only	1, 3 only	2, 4 only	4 only	All are correct

101. A patient with a hemodynamically significant atrial septal defect and normal pulmonary artery pressures will present with which of the following auscultatory findings?

    (1) Increased intensity of the first heart sound (S_1)
    (2) Fixed splitting of the second heart sound (S_2)
    (3) A pulmonary vascular ejection sound
    (4) An aortic vascular ejection sound

102. Cardiac noise that may be audible to the patient includes which of the following?

    (1) Hamman's sign or mediastinal crunch
    (2) The "cooing dove" murmur of a ruptured or retroverted aortic cusp
    (3) The systolic murmur of a large ventricular septal defect
    (4) The systolic "honk" of mitral valve prolapse

103. Correct statements concerning the normal second heart sound (S_2) include

    (1) normal physiological splitting with inspiration is due to an early aortic closure sound (A_2)
    (2) a pulmonic closure sound (P_2) occurs simultaneously with the anacrotic notch of the pulmonary artery pressure tracing
    (3) normal physiological splitting with inspiration is due to a delay in P_2
    (4) when P_2 is audible at the apex, it indicates normal physiological splitting

104. Reversed splitting of the second heart sound (S_2) indicates significant cardiovascular disease such as

    (1) left bundle branch block (LBBB)
    (2) hypertrophic cardiomyopathy with significant outflow tract gradient
    (3) right ventricular premature contractions
    (4) severe pulmonic stenosis

105. Acute severe aortic regurgitation is characterized by which of the following auscultatory findings?

    (1) An Austin Flint rumble
    (2) Decreased intensity of the first heart sound (S_1)
    (3) A third heart sound (S_3)
    (4) A fourth heart sound (S_4)

106. Correct statements regarding pharmacological and positional changes that can discriminate murmurs of similar quality include which of the following?

    (1) Isometric handgrip decreases the murmur of mitral regurgitation
    (2) Phase II of the Valsalva maneuver increases the murmur of hypertrophic obstructive cardiomyopathy
    (3) Nitroglycerin increases the murmur of aortic regurgitation
    (4) Squatting increases the murmur of subvalvular pulmonary stenosis in a patient with tetralogy of Fallot

107. A 45-year-old male with severe chronic bronchitis presents with an acute exacerbation of cor pulmonale. Which of the following optical signs will most likely be observed?

    (1) A darkening of the blood column
    (2) Retinal edema
    (3) Disk edema
    (4) Arterial venous compression (nicking)

108. In the phonocardiograms below, the *left panel* illustrates the sound and pressure correlates of the second heart sound (S_2) of a patient with normal artery pressure. The *two right panels* illustrate the sound and pressure correlates of two patients with pulmonary hypertension. Choose the statements below that reflect the underlying physiological events of at least one of the patients represented by the *two right panels*.

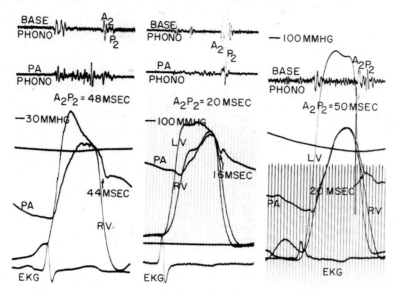

(From Shaver JA: Clinical implications of the hangout interval. *Int J Cardiol* 5:396, 1984.)

(1)   The hangout interval is decreased
(2)   There is narrow physiological splitting of S_2
(3)   There is wide physiological splitting of S_2
(4)   The hangout time is increased

109. The phonocardiogram below is from a patient with an abnormal heart sound, the genesis of which may be explained by the

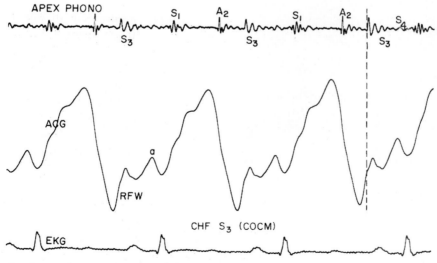

(From Shaver JA, et al: Early diastolic events associated with the physiologic and pathologic S_3. *J Cardiogr* 14 (Suppl 5): 30, 1984.)

(1)   root theory
(2)   impact theory
(3)   valvular theory
(4)   ventricular theory

SUMMARY OF DIRECTIONS

A	B	C	D	E
1, 2, 3 only	1, 3 only	2, 4 only	4 only	All are correct

110. Conditions in which Q waves may be seen on electrocardiographic studies include

    (1)   unstable angina pectoris
    (2)   hypertrophic cardiomyopathy
    (3)   coronary artery spasm
    (4)   transmural myocardial infarction

111. The cardiac size illustrated in the radiograph below is consistent with which of the following conditions?

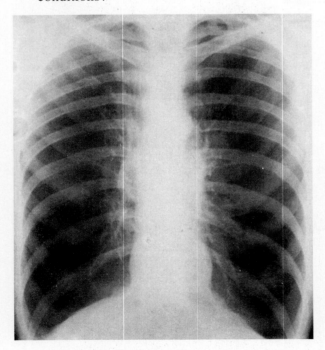

    (1)   Chronic obstructive pulmonary disease (COPD)
    (2)   Addison's disease
    (3)   Anorexia nervosa
    (4)   Hemochromatosis

112. An atrial infarction is suggested by which of the following electrocardiographic characteristics?

    (1)   PR-segment elevation in the left chest leads
    (2)   PR-segment depression in the right chest leads
    (3)   PR-segment elevation in lead I
    (4)   PR-segment depression in lead III

113. Correct statements concerning exercise testing in patients with cardiac disease include which of the following?

    (1)   Maximal oxygen uptake ($\dot{V}_{O_2}$ max) is below normal
    (2)   The anaerobic threshold is not reached
    (3)   Oxygen saturation is maintained
    (4)   The highest minute ventilation is near maximum voluntary ventilation (MVV)

114. Complications of hemodynamic monitoring include

    (1)   septicemia
    (2)   pneumothorax
    (3)   pulmonary infarction
    (4)   pulmonary artery rupture

115. Indications for pulmonary artery monitoring include

    (1)   assessment of inotropic and vasopressor intervention
    (2)   monitoring patients with noncardiogenic pulmonary edema
    (3)   determination of volume status in a hypotensive patient who has received appropriate volume
    (4)   routine placement in patients with acute myocardial infarction

116. The 12-lead electrocardiogram below is diagnostic of which of the following cardiac presentations?

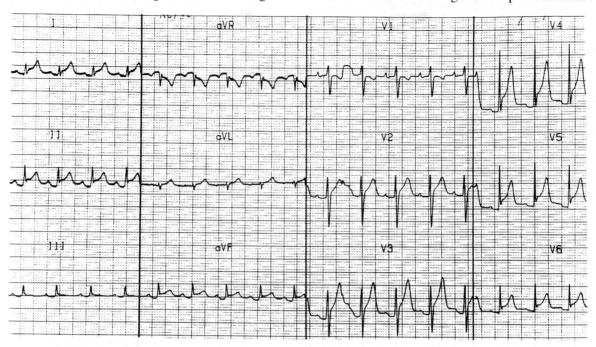

(1) Inferior myocardial infarction
(2) Pulmonary embolism
(3) Lateral myocardial infarction
(4) Pericarditis

117. The figure below illustrates which of the following entities?

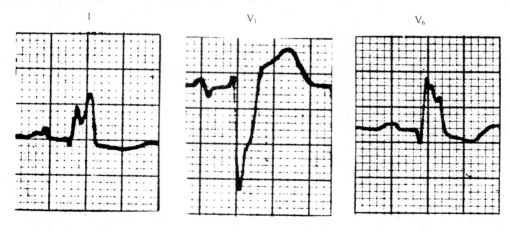

(1) Left bundle branch block (LBBB)
(2) Cabrera's sign
(3) Anteroseptal myocardial infarction
(4) Concealed right bundle branch block (RBBB)

118. The differential diagnosis of "rib notching" includes

    (1)   superior vena cava syndrome
    (2)   neurofibromatosis
    (3)   coarctation of the aorta
    (4)   osteodysplasia

119. The 12-lead electrocardiogram reproduced below illustrates a particular electrocardiographic abnormality that has which of the following characteristics?

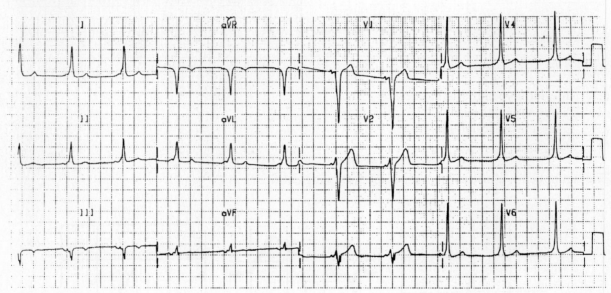

    (1)   A delta wave
    (2)   A narrow QRS complex
    (3)   A short PR interval
    (4)   Secondary repolarization abnormalities due to Mahaim (nodal-ventricular) fibers

DIRECTIONS: Each question below contains five suggested responses. For **each** of the **five** responses listed with every question, you are to respond either YES (Y) or NO (N). In a given item **all, some, or none of the alternatives may be correct.**

120. Dyspnea has many clinical presentations. Indicate the following correct relationships.

   (A) "Two-pillow" orthopnea may be seen with both chronic heart failure and severe pulmonary disease
   (B) Paroxysmal nocturnal dyspnea is pathognomonic of severe left ventricular dysfunction
   (C) Dyspnea may be secondary to nitroglycerin toxicity
   (D) Cheyne-Stokes breathing may be seen in a normal newborn
   (E) Thyrotoxicosis is associated with dyspnea caused by a low metabolic rate

121. True statements include which of the following?

   (A) Kussmaul's sign is an inspiratory decrease in venous pressure
   (B) Tietze's syndrome is characterized by tenderness of the costochondral, chondrosternal, and xiphisternal joints
   (C) Mondor's disease is characterized by tender superficial veins on the anterior abdomen
   (D) A "CV" wave is seen in patients with tricuspid regurgitation
   (E) Pulsations in the epigastrium may be secondary to an abdominal aortic aneurysm or right ventricular hypertrophy

122. All the following murmurs are correctly paired with the physiological anomalies most likely to cause them EXCEPT

   (A) a Graham Steel murmur and low-pressure pulmonary valve regurgitation
   (B) an Austin Flint murmur and mitral valve regurgitation
   (C) a Duroziez's murmur and tricuspid stenosis
   (D) a Carey Coombs murmur and mitral stenosis
   (E) Still's murmur and insignificant aortic stenosis

123. Acute right-sided heart failure can be associated with which of the following radiographic hallmarks?

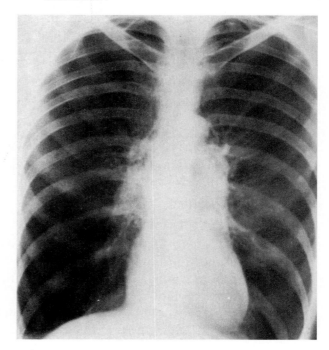

   (A) "Butterfly pattern"
   (B) Lateralized oligemia
   (C) Normal right atrial and ventricular size
   (D) Pulmonary parenchymal calcifications
   (E) Bilateral pulmonary opacification

124. Correct statements regarding the M-mode pattern of the anterior mitral valve leaflet include which of the following?

   (A) The point of maximum excursion of the anterior leaflet is designated the E point
   (B) The nadir of the initial diastolic closing of the valve is designated the F point
   (C) The middiastolic closing motion, referred to as EF slope, represents the velocity of blood moving from the left atrium into the left ventricle
   (D) The peak of the leaflet opening during atrial systole is the X point
   (E) Complete closure of the leaflet during ventricular systole marks the J point

125. The opening snap illustrated below has been assosiated with

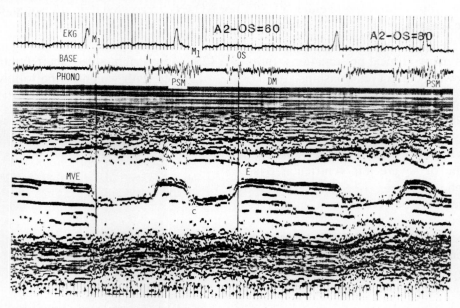

(From Reddy PS, et al: Normal and abnormal heart sounds in cardiac diagnosis. Part 2. Diastolic sounds in cardiac diagnosis. *Curr Probl Cardiol* 10 (3):12, 1985.)

(A)   severe calcific mitral stenosis with immobile leaflets
(B)   tricuspid stenosis
(C)   a large atrial septal defect and increased flow across the tricuspid valve
(D)   thyrotoxicosis
(E)   tricuspid atresia and a large atrial septal defect

126. Correct statements regarding the pattern of aortic leaflet motion include which of the following?

(A)   Late closure of the aortic valve is evidence for hypertrophic obstructive cardiomyopathy
(B)   Very early systolic closure of the aortic valve is seen with outflow tract obstruction secondary to discrete membranous subvalvular aortic stenosis
(C)   Severe aortic regurgitation may cause late opening of the aortic valve
(D)   The opening pattern of the aortic valve and pattern of leaflet motion provide information about left ventricular stroke volume
(E)   In low-output states, the aortic leaflets tend to open abruptly but close gradually throughout systole

127. Criteria suggestive of the diagnosis of cardiac tamponade by two-dimensional echocardiography include

(A)   systolic collapse of the right atrium
(B)   diastolic collapse of the right ventricle
(C)   a massive pericardial effusion with 4 cm of fluid separating the layers of pericardium, anteriorly
(D)   plethora of the inferior vena cava with blunted respiratory variation
(E)   a dilated right ventricle

128. Which of the following exercise test parameters are associated with poor prognosis and increased severity of coronary disease?

(A) Failure to complete stage IV of a Bruce protocol or an equivalent work load
(B) Development of limiting symptoms before reaching a heart rate of 120 beats per minute in the absence of beta blockers
(C) Prolonged duration of ST depression into the recovery stage
(D) Exercise-induced U-wave inversion
(E) a hypertensive response to exercise

DIRECTIONS: The group of questions below consists of four lettered headings followed by a set of numbered items. For each numbered item select

A	if the item is associated with	(A) **only**
B	if the item is associated with	(B) **only**
C	if the item is associated with	**both** (A) and (B)
D	if the item is associated with	**neither** (A) nor (B)

Each lettered heading may be used **once, more than once, or not at all.**

Questions 129–131

    (A)   Right pleural effusion
    (B)   Left pleural effusion
    (C)   Both
    (D)   Neither

129. Acute left-sided heart failure

130. Acute right-sided heart failure

131. Chronic right-sided heart failure

DIRECTIONS: Each group of questions below consists of lettered headings followed by a set of numbered items. For each numbered item select the **one** lettered heading with which it is **most** closely associated. Each lettered heading may be used **once, more than once, or not at all.**

Questions 132–135

Match each disorder listed below with its characteristic presentation. Answer E if none of the figures apply.

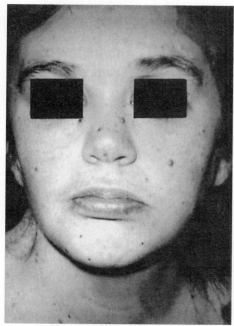

A

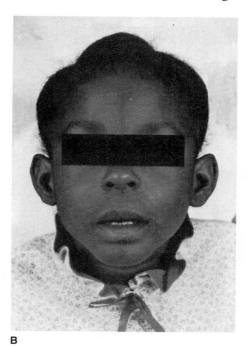

B

(From Silverman ME: Visual clues to diagnosis. *Primary Cardiol* August 1987.)

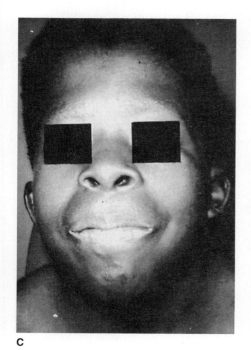

C

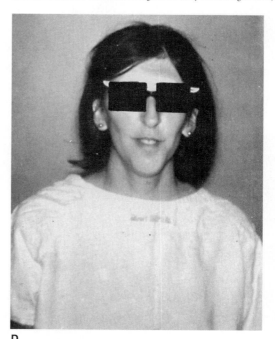

D

132. Fetal alcohol syndrome

133. Noonan's syndrome

134. Marfan's syndrome

135. Turner's syndrome

Questions 136–140

Match each pathologic finding with the appropriate radiograph.

136. Localization

137. Lateralization

138. Cephalization

139. Collateralization

140. Centralization

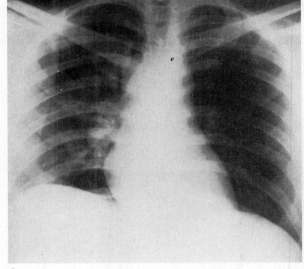

C

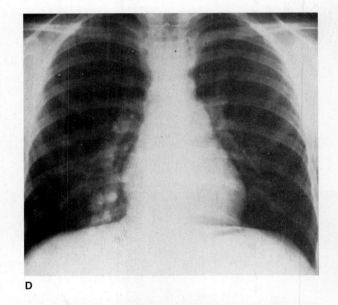

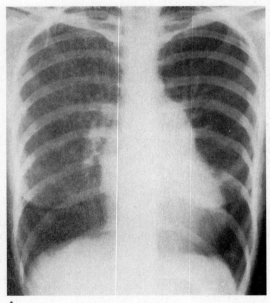

A

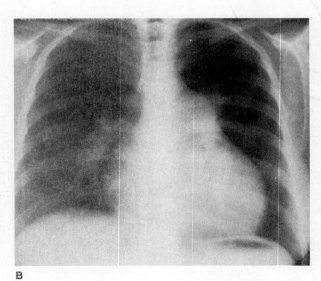

B

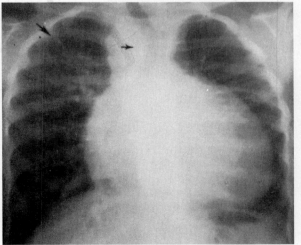

D

E

Questions 141–145

Match each proper finding with the radiograph.

141. Acute myocardial infarction

142. Pulmonary emboli

143. Tetralogy of Fallot

144. Coarctation of the aorta

145. Left ventricular aneurysm

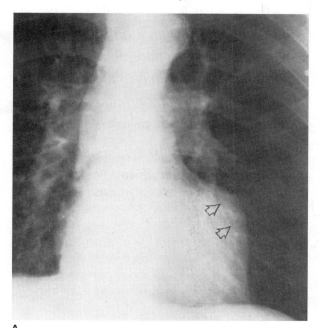

A

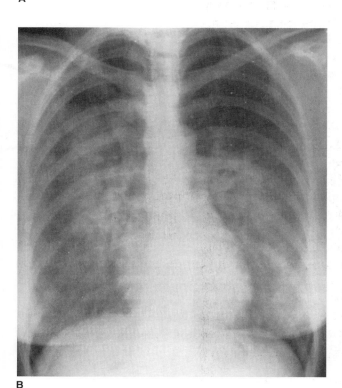

B

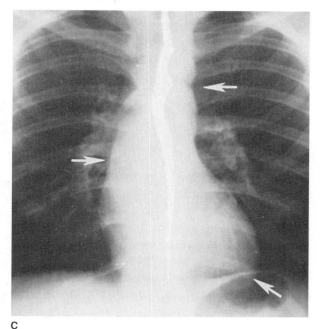

C

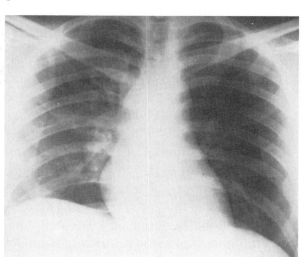

D

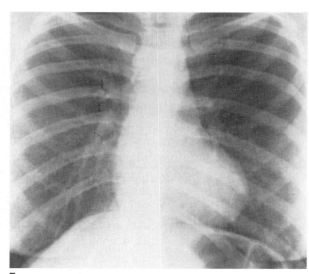

E

II. General Evaluation of the Patient

Answers

---

62. The answer is B. *(pp 201–203)* Physicians practicing today must have a thorough understanding of analytic medicine. This includes knowledge of the terminology used in determining the accuracy of diagnostic tests. Test results can be characterized as true positive (TP), true negative (TN), false positive (FP), or false negative (FN). The sensitivity of a test is defined as the proportion of total patients with the disease who have a positive test. It is defined as

$$\frac{TP}{TP + FN}.$$

The *specificity* of a test is defined as the proportion of total patients without a disease who have a negative test. Its arithmetic relationship is defined as

$$\frac{TN}{FP + TN}.$$

Thomas Bayes, an English theologian and mathematician, was among the first to use probability inductively. *Bayes' theorem* states that the predictive value of a test is determined by the pretest probability of that test result in the patient population being studied. It should be remembered that the *prevalence* of a disease state is defined as the incidence of a number of events applied to the general population. The efficacy of a test is defined as the percentage of patients correctly identified and is indicated by the following formula:

$$\frac{TP + TN}{TP + TN + FP + FN \times 100}.$$

63. The answer is D. *(pp 205–215)* Angina pectoris due to myocardial ischemia is transient, usually effort-related, and promptly relieved by nitroglycerin. It does not last longer than 20 min; pain of longer duration represents a prodrome to acute myocardial infarction. Angina pectoris due to myocardial ischemia is usually, but not always, associated with electrocardiographic abnormalities. The discomfort due to angina is usually retrosternal in location but may be referred widely. It is not unusual for a patient to describe symptoms as being more severe in the jaw, arm, or neck. The discomfort is often described as a "pressure-squeezing" sensation rather than as "pain." Symptoms are usually effort-related; however, with the Prinzmetal's variety of angina pectoris, which is associated with enhanced vasomotor activity of the coronary artery, symptoms may occur at rest.

64. The answer is D. *(pp 209–211)* Anxiety produces a variety of cardiovascular symptoms. The chest discomfort typically associated with anxiety is along the left precordium. Other symptoms occur both at rest and following exertion. The presence of persistent fatigue or dyspnea predominantly at rest is an important discriminating feature. The dyspnea associated with anxiety may be due to hyperventilation and is associated with numbness of the arms and hands as well as lips. If hyperventilation is prolonged, an episode of tetany may result.

65. The answer is C. *(pp 201–203)* The new (after 1973) New York Heart Association classification identifies specific cardiac status and prognosis, relying on a complete assessment of etiology, anatomy, and altered physiological states. A thorough understanding of prognosis indicates how medical and surgical techniques can alter the natural history of the disease. The old (prior to 1973) New York Heart Association classification indicates the functional capacity of a patient with congestive heart failure (CHF). The Canadian Cardiovascular Society's classification indicates the grade of angina pectoris. Class III heart failure indicates the presence of symptoms with minimal activity and marked limitation of normal exertion. Grade I angina pectoris indicates that ordinary activity does not produce angina; however, strenuous activity may produce symptoms of myocardial ischemia.

66. The answer is B. *(pp 259–261)* The *left panel* of the phonocardiograms that accompany the question represents a nonejection click, and the *right panel* represents two close clicks due to mitral valve prolapse. These single or multiple clicks are due to prolapse of the redundant leaflets into the left atrium. A nonejection click is not seen in patients with mitral stenosis. The sound associated with this condition occurs in early diastole and is termed a loud "opening snap." Ejection clicks are seen in patients with a bicuspid aortic valve or with valvular pulmonary stenosis. These conditions are associated with an early ejection sound. The timing of the clicks associated with mitral valve prolapse can be varied according to left ventricular volume. With increased filling, as with sudden squatting, the anterior and posterior mitral leaflets coapt better, and the click occurs later. When volume in the left ventricle is diminished, as with sudden standing, there is poor coaptation of the leaflets, and the click occurs early in systole.

67. The answer is C. *(pp 205–215)* Analysis of the history of a patient's symptoms is extremely important in the cardiovascular examination. Physicians must be familiar with the concepts of analytic medicine, including sensitivity, specificity, and predictive value as they apply to laboratory tests as well as to historical details. The severity of symptoms may not reflect the severity or accurately predict the prognosis of the disease process, nor does the absence of symptoms negate the presence of severe disease. The patient may voluntarily restrict activity that would unmask the underlying cardiovascular abnormality. Sudden cardiac death is usually not preceded by symptoms. A diagnosis of cardiac disease is commonly made with a complete history and physical and laboratory examinations. Reliance on a single historical detail usually will not provide an accurate diagnosis.

68. The answer is C. *(pp 235–237)* A dicrotic pulse is seen in patients with left ventricular systolic dysfunction. Left ventricular dysfunction, however, is characterized as having two beats, one in systole and one in diastole. A low-amplitude hypokinetic pulse is seen in patients with a decreased stroke volume such as that due to hypovolemia, left ventricular dysfunction, or mitral and aortic valve stenosis. A hyperkinetic pulse is a bounding pulse seen in patients with an increased stroke volume due to aortic insufficiency and other conditions associated with decreased peripheral vascular resistance. A bisferiens pulse, in which both peaks occur in systole, can be seen in some patients with aortic insufficiency. Patients with hypertrophic obstructive cardiomyopathy may exhibit the "dart and dome" pattern in the arterial pulse. Patients with severe aortic stenosis may occasionally exhibit a hypokinetic pulse with a delayed upstroke, parvus et tardus pulse. The parvus et tardus pulse may have a "notch" on the ascending limb, occasionally referred to as an anacrotic shoulder.

69. The answer is D. *(pp 285–305)* The phonocardiograms that accompany the question have a crescendo-decrescendo murmur, an absent second heart sound (S$_2$), and a low-frequency fourth heart sound (S$_4$). The murmur is of maximal intensity on the apex phonocardiogram. These characteristics correctly identify a patient with severe acquired calcific aortic stenosis. In patients with congenital valvular or subvalvular aortic stenosis, the maximal intensity of the systolic ejection murmur is at the first or second right intercostal space. In patients with congenital supravalvular aortic stenosis, the maximal intensity of the murmur is at the first right intercostal space or over the right carotid. Hypertrophic obstructive cardiomyopathy is characterized by a murmur of maximal intensity at the apex; however, S$_2$ is audible as either a single or paradoxically split S$_2$.

70. The answer is A. *(pp 255–256)* The first heart sound (S$_1$) is heard best between the left lower sternal border and the apex. S$_1$ is usually single, but when split, the mitral and tricuspid valve closure sounds are separated by only 20 to 30 ms and are usually heard as a single sound in the healthy patient. As demonstrated by phonocardiography, S$_1$ consists of four components. The first component represents the beginning of left ventricular contraction, is muscular in origin, and is not audible to the human ear. The second and third components reflect mitral and tricuspid valve closures, respectively. The fourth component consists of low-frequency vibrations, reflecting ejection of the blood into the aortic root.

71. The answer is C. *(pp 256–261)* The intensity of the first heart sound (S$_1$) is determined by six factors: (1) the integrity of valve closure, (2) mobility of the valve, (3) velocity of valve closure, (4) status of ventricular contraction, (5) transmission characteristics of the thoracic cavity and thorax, and (6) physical characteristics of the vibrating structures. Patients with mitral valve prolapse have increased mobility of the valve and, therefore, an increase in intensity of S$_1$. The converse is seen in patients with severe long-standing mitral stenosis and valvular calcification. In this circumstance, S$_1$ is diminished or absent. Lown-Ganong-Levine syndrome is characterized by short PR intervals; the ventricle has a short time to fill, and the leaflets are separated maximally at the beginning of ventricular systole, resulting in a loud S$_1$. With left bundle branch block (LBBB), there is electrical delay of left ventricular systole, and therefore, S$_1$ is decreased in intensity and delayed. Delay in onset of right ventricular contraction with right bundle branch block (RBBB) can lead to side splitting of S$_1$. Thus, S$_1$ is widely split, rather than paradoxically split with RBBB.

72. The answer is D. *(p 318)* The figure that accompanies the question represents retinal embolization of an atheroma, which has classically been called a Hollenhorst plaque. It is typically a glistening yellow-orange and occurs at bifurcations ofthe retinal vessels. At times, the plaque looks larger than the vessel it obstructs. A platelet embolus is dull pink to gray and often has associated fibrin. It can be seen in patients with endocarditis and mural thrombi. Roth's spot, once thought to be pathognomonic of endocarditis may also be seen in blood dyscrasias; it appears as a hemorrhage with a gray-white center. A fat embolus appears as a fuzzy bordered, gray-white spot without hemorrhage and occurs as a result of long-bone fractures. Its appearance connotes a grave prognosis. A calcium plaque appears as a glistening white plaque and is seen with embolization from severe aortic stenosis.

73. The answer is D. *(pp 282–283)* A caged-ball valve such as a Starr-Edwards valve or central disk occluder valve such as the Beall valve produces opening and closing sounds. The tilting disk Bjork-Shiley valve produces a prominent closing sound. A soft opening sound can occasionally be demonstrated with phonocardiography. The porcine valves function like normal valves, although an opening sound in the mitral position may be recorded in 50 percent of patients with phonocardiography.

74. The answer is C. *(pp 316–317)* Arteriovenous compression or "nicking" is due to arteriosclerotic thickening that compresses the underlying venous channel where these vessels intersect at right angles. It is not commonly seen in patients with isolated systemic arterial hypertension. Microaneurysms and neovascularization are changes seen in conditions which produce both retinal hypoxia and viable capillary endothelial cells. They are both seen in a variety of conditions, including diabetes mellitus, sickle cell disease, the dysproteinemias, Behçet's disease, sarcoidosis, uveitis, and retinal venous obstructive disease. A microaneurysm, however, is not a feature of increased intracranial pressure. Hard exudates are residues of prior edema. They are associated with systemic arterial hypertension, diabetes mellitus, venous outflow obstruction, and retinal angiomas. Cotton-wool spots are not exudates, but rather a sign of serious systemic disease and are due to ischemia, which occurs secondary to occlusion of peripapillary capillaries, occlusion of small arteries, or hypoxia.

75. The answer is D. *(pp 321–322)* The correct sequence of ventricular depolarization is from endocardium to epicardium. Depolarization consists of a moving wave of positive charges in front of negative charges. The sequence of ventricular repolarization occurs from epicardium to endocardium with negative charges in front of positive charges.

76. The answer is B. *(pp 342–346)* The figure that accompanies the question represents hypercalcemia. The QT interval is short despite the relative slow rate. A short QT interval can also be noted with hyperkalemia, digitalis, and right or left ventricular hypertrophy; however, other electrocardiographic features differentiate these abnormalities. Patients with the Jervell and Lange-Nielsen syndrome have congenital prolongation of the QT interval associated with deafness. These individuals are predisposed to sudden cardiac death. The electrocardiographic manifestations of hyperkalemia include a tall, peaked T wave with a narrow base. With more advanced levels of potassium elevation, the PR and the QRS intervals are prolonged and the T wave flattens. Amiodarone prolongs the QT interval. Additional effects include mild-to-moderate prolongation of the PR interval and the QRS complex.

77. The answer is D. *(pp 330–341)* The electrocardiogram that accompanies the question represents a right bundle branch block (RBBB) with the characteristic findings of a QRS duration greater than 1/10 sec with positive reflections in the anterior chest leads. Additionally, there is right axis deviation, suggesting left posterior hemiblock. Although right axis deviation is present, the characteristic findings associated with a left bundle branch block (LBBB), including prolongation of the QRS complex and posterior rotation of the QRS vector, are not seen.

78. The answer is C. *(pp 361–362)* The chest roentgenogram that accompanies the question represents the end-stage manifestations of chronic mitral regurgitation. There is a double density along the right cardiac border representing the right and left atrium. Along the left cardiac border, there is the classic four-bump heart consisting of the following cardiac structures: aortic arch, pulmonary artery, left atrial appendage, and left ventricle. Multiple Kerley's B lines are present and are especially noticeable in the right lower lung field. These correlate with a mean pulmonary artery wedge pressure greater than 20 mmHg. The findings of pulmonary hemosiderosis or ossification are indicative of long-standing pulmonary hypertension, which may be seen in mitral stenosis.

79. The answer is D. *(p 369)* Calcific constrictive pericarditis is represented by the chest roentgenogram that accompanies the question. The lateral view shows heavy calcification of the pericardium and left atrial enlargement with posterior displacement of the barium-filled esophagus. A calcified aortic or mitral valve annulus is not seen. Restrictive cardiomyopathy is not typically characterized by the development of myocardial or pericardial calcification.

80. The answer is E. *(pp 370–371)* The patient described in the question presents with classic risk factors for epicardial coronary artery disease. The lateral chest roentgenogram represents coronary artery calcification of all three major epicardial coronary arteries (*a* = left anterior descending artery, *c* = circumflex artery, *r* = right coronary artery, and *p* = posterior descending branch of the right coronary artery). A history suggestive of myocardial ischemia in combination with coronary calcification predicts a 90 percent chance of obstruction of the major epicardial coronary arteries.

81. The answer is B.   *(pp 371–373)*   The radiograph that accompanies the question identifies two leaflets of a St. Jude metallic prosthesis. When open, the valve leaflets form parallel lines. A Bjork-Shiley valve is characterized by a single metallic leaflet and a radiographically opaque sewing ring. The ball cage valve (Starr-Edwards) is readily identified both on plain films and under fluoroscopy. Tissue valves, including the bovine paricardial valve, are characterized by a metallic sewing ring; however, the valve leaflet structures themselves are radiolucent.

82. The answer is A.   *(pp 365–367)*   The posteroanterior and lateral chest roentgenograms that accompany the question provide an example of an anterior displacement of the esophagus. This is due to a retro-esophageal aberrant subclavian artery arising from an aortic diverticulum. In this "common" type of right-sided aortic arch, the left subclavian passes behind the esophagus, and there is a minimal increase in associated congenital cardiac defects. However, in individuals with the "common" type of right-sided aortic arch who also have congenital cardiac defects, tetralogy of Fallot and atrial or ventricular septal defects are most commonly detected.

In contradistinction, the "avian" right-sided aortic arch is identified by anterior placement of the arch in front of the trachea and esophagus. With this configuration, there is a 90 percent incidence of heart defects, most commonly tetralogy of Fallot. This abnormality derives its name by being the most common anatomical configuration in birds. Left atrial enlargement is identified by a double density along the right cardiac border, a bulging left atrial appendage, and an elevated left main stem bronchus. Radiographic characteristics of tetralogy of Fallot include a small boot-shaped heart (*coeur en sabot*) with decreased pulmonary blood flow. In Holt-Oram syndrome, a secundum atrial septal defect is common. Hypoplastic, fingerlike or absent thumbs are frequently seen.

83. The answer is A.   *(pp 375–376, 414)*   The echocardiogram is a valuable diagnostic tool providing early and accurate diagnosis for a variety of cardiac problems. It is biologically safe without any cumulative effects. Both anatomic (from two-dimensional imaging) as well as physiological (from Doppler) information about cardiac structure, function, and great vessel anatomy can be obtained. However, delineation of complete cardiac anatomic information is possible in only 80 to 90 percent of studies. The equipment is mobile and, therefore, can be moved to the patient's bedside, an advantage in the critical care setting. Serial examinations can be performed and changes can be monitored over an extended period of time. The test can be performed quickly (usually over 15 to 45 min) and is relatively inexpensive.

84. The answer is B.   *(p 402)*   Echocardiography is a sensitive method for diagnosing hypertrophic obstructive cardiomyopathy. The classic finding is asymmetric septal hypertrophy in which the ratio of the septal to posterior wall thickness is 1.3 to 1.0 or greater. Symmetric hypertrophy as well as other patterns may be seen. There is systolic anterior motion of the mitral valve. The left ventricular cavity is usually decreased in size, and there often is a dilated left atrium. Midsystolic notching or closure of the aortic valve is also a reliable sign.

85. The answer is C.   *(pp 402–403)*   The usual echocardiographic features of restrictive cardiomyopathies, including amyloidosis, are ventricular wall hypertrophy with normal cavity size, dilated atria, normal or reduced systolic function, and abnormal diastolic function. Amyloidosis is also associated with an abnormal glittering appearance of the ventricular walls. The cardiac valves and interatrial septum are usually thickened in amyloidosis.

86. The answer is C.   *(pp 361–363)*   The radiograph that accompanies the question identifies a patient with chronic right-sided heart failure from Ebstein's anomaly. The feature of right-sided heart failure includes a decrease in pulmonary vasculature, radiolucent lung fields, and right ventricular enlargement. A normal size of the cardiac silhouette and pulmonary edema in a "butterfly pattern" are the hallmarks of acute left-sided heart failure. Acute right-sided heart failure is suggested by lateralization of pulmonary blood flow and centralization of the pulmonary vasculature dilatation. Chronic left-sided heart failure is characterized by cephalization of the pulmonary vasculature and development of Kerley's B lines.

87. The answer is D. *(pp 404–405)* Both valve motion and morphology should be used to provide a better diagnostic definition of mitral valve prolapse. Some valves are voluminous, thick, redundant, and prolapsed in every view, whereas others are only prolapsed in the parasternal long axis view and are small, thin, and relatively normal in appearance. A normal mitral valve and saddle-shaped mitral annulus may produce an apparent bowing of the leaflets toward the atrial side of the annulus in the apical four-chamber view. Mitral valve prolapse is, therefore, best defined as leaflet displacement above the plane of the mitral annulus in the parasternal long axis view. The morphology of the mitral valve has prognostic importance, and patients with thickened and redundant leaflets have a higher incidence of endocarditis, severe regurgitation, and death.

88. The answer is B. *(p 405)* The aortic valve in valvular aortic stenosis usually shows reduced mobility of the leaflets. The leaflets are often thickened and calcified. There is usually concentric left ventricular hypertrophy and a dilated aortic root. Two-dimensional echocardiography is inaccurate in quantitating the aortic valve area because of difficulty in accurately planimetering the valve due to increased echogenicity of the valve cusps and irregular valve orifice. Severe aortic stenosis is usually excluded when the cusps are separated by more than 12 mm. Cusp separation of less than 7 mm is only suggestive of severe aortic stenosis. The Doppler accurately determines peak and mean pressure gradients across the aortic valve and calculation of the aortic valve area.

89. The answer is B. *(pp 431–438)* Exercise testing is best used in a population with an intermediate probability of having coronary disease. A young woman is much more likely to have a false-positive result than a true positive, because the prevalence of coronary disease in young women is very low. In general, exercise testing has a 60 to 70 percent sensitivity for diagnosing angiographically significant coronary disease. Therefore, 30 to 40 percent of people with coronary disease will have a normal treadmill response. The ability to exercise for 12 min on a Bruce protocol without ST-segment depression is evidence for an overall good prognosis, irrespective of the severity of coronary disease. Angiotensin-converting enzyme (ACE) inhibitors can decrease blood pressure at rest and during exercise and can increase exercise capacity in patients with chronic heart failure; however, they should not have much of an effect on exercise duration in patients with coronary disease and good left ventricular function. Digitalis is a common cause of a false-positive electrocardiographic (ECG) response to exercise testing. Beta blockers and calcium blockers can delay the time to ischemia and improve exercise capacity. A 60-year-old man with exertional chest pain and a history of hypertension is likely to have coronary disease, and a normal treadmill ECG response probably represents a false-negative result.

90. The answer is A. *(p 451)* The hemodynamic tracing that accompanies the question indicates a large v wave usually associated with acute or subacute mitral regurgitation. It should be recognized that the enlarged left atrium seen with chronic mitral regurgitation decreases the magnitude of the v wave. Large v waves, whose height exceeds the mean by 10 mmHg, have been described in ventricular septal defect, chronic coronary artery disease, and aortic valvular disease. However, the large v wave is not classically seen in patients with either aortic insufficiency or stenosis.

91. The answer is A. *(pp 407–408)* Echocardiography is a useful technique to visualize infective vegetation. Vegetations are usually mobile, irregular, and echo-dense structures attached to the valve leaflets. The presence and size of the vegetations are not in themselves indications for surgery, though there is an increased risk of embolic events when the vegetations are large. The absence of a vegetation on echocardiography does not exclude endocarditis. Complications of endocarditis, including leaflet rupture, shunt lesions, and valve ring abscesses, can also be detected by echocardiography.

92. **The answer is C.** *(p 443)*   In congestive heart failure (CHF), the total lung capacity is decreased, the functional residual capacity is normal, and the residual volume is normal or increased. Parenchymal lung disease leads to uniformly decreased volumes. Neuromuscular disease is characterized by a decreased inspiratory capacity with a preserved residual volume. Obesity is characterized by a decreased expiratory reserve volume.

93. **The answer is C (2, 4).** *(pp 207–209)*   The pain of pericarditis is usually sharp and located in the anterior chest and neck; it is aggravated by the supine position and relieved by sitting upright. A pulmonary embolus is usually associated with dyspnea rather than pain. If pain does develop, it is usually pleuritic and located in the lateral chest. The pain associated with a dissecting aortic aneurysm is usually "tearing" and located in the posterior thorax. It may radiate as the dissection progresses. Severe tricuspid regurgitation may cause the sensation of a shirt collar being "too tight."

94. **The answer is A (1, 2, 3).** *(p 208)*   Patients with pulmonary hypertension secondary to mitral stenosis, pulmonary infarction, conditions resulting in Eisenmenger's physiology, or aortic aneurysm may experience hemoptysis. The anterior chest discomfort associated with pulmonary hypertension is frequently aggravated by exertion and has been historically attributed to dilatation of the pulmonary artery but may actually represent right ventricular ischemia. The temporal relationship between the development of edema and dyspnea is important. The dyspnea associated with left ventricular dysfunction, mitral stenosis, or cor pulmonale (each of which may be associated with significant pulmonary hypertension) usually precedes the development of peripheral edema. Patients with Cheyne-Stokes respirations exhibit periods of hyperpnea alternating with periods of apnea. This respiratory pattern is seen in patients with cerebrovascular disease or left ventricular dysfunction and may occasionally be observed as a "normal variant" in newborns.

95. **The answer is C (2, 4).** *(p 213)*   Hemochromatosis results in a bronze tint to the skin. A bluish coloration of the skin appears in patients with a right-to-left intracardiac shunt. Sudden flushing of the skin, occasionally precipitated by the use of alcohol, is seen in patients with carcinoid heart disease. Jaundice is seen in patients with hemolysis and severe aortic stenosis. Hepatic congestion from congestive heart failure seldom results in jaundice. In and of itself, congestive heart failure (CHF) with resulting hepatic congestion produces jaundice. An occasional side effect of amiodarone is the production of a slatelike color of the skin of the hands and nose.

96. **The answer is B (1, 3).** *(pp 217–222)*   A ventricular septal defect is a common manifestation of congenital heart disease. It is seen in combination with other defects in the cardiofacial and Cornelia de Lange syndromes. Other manifestations of the cardiofacial syndrome include unilateral, partial, lower facial weakness, which is most apparent when the patient is crying. A seventh nerve palsy has also been described. Other cardiovascular manifestations of the Cornelia de Lange syndrome include patent ductus arteriosus, pulmonary stenosis, anomalous pulmonary venous return, and atrial septal defect. The other two syndromes described, Ellis–van Creveld and rubella, are associated with an atrial septal defect. Other findings seen in the Ellis–van Creveld syndrome include polydactyly, dysplastic teeth and nails, and multiple frenulae that bind the upper lip to the alveolar ridge. An atrioventricular canal may also be seen. A patient whose mother had a rubella infection during pregnancy may have cataracts, nystagmus, and deafness.

97. **The answer is A (1, 2, 3).** *(pp 222–223)*   Peripheral manifestations of bacterial endocarditis include Osler's nodes, Janeway's lesions, clubbing of the fingers, and splinter hemorrhages of the nails and petechiae. Osler's nodes are nonhemorrhagic, tender lesions located on the distal pad of the finger or toe. Janeway's lesions are hemorrhagic but nontender and appear on the plams or soles. Splinter hemorrhages are black, linear hemorrhages located in the distal third of the fingernail. Jaccoud's arthritis is usually due to repeated attacks of rheumatic fever and resembles the peripheral manifestations of rheumatic heart disease with ulnar deviation of the fourth and fifth fingers and flexion of the metacarpal phalangeal joint. A discriminating feature from rheumatoid arthritis is that the fingers can be moved freely back into correct alignment.

98. The answer is E (all). *(pp 217–229)* Kawasaki's disease is characterized predominantly by a widespread erythematous rash. However, an early manifestation of the disease is a sterile inflammation of the conjunctiva. Myocarditis is a cardiac manifestation. Blue sclerae are seen in osteogenesis imperfecta and Marfan's syndrome. The cardiovascular manifestations include aortic and mitral valve regurgitation. In Wilson's disease, an abnormality of copper metabolism results in the development of golden-brown corneal rings known as Kayser-Fleischer rings. The cardiovascular abnormalities include interstitial fibrosis and perivascular myocarditis. Patients with Down's syndrome (trisomy 21) have Brushfield's spots of the iris. Additional characteristics include a small head, shallow orbit, epicanthal folds, low-set ears, widely spaced eyes, transverse palmar creases, and a ventricular septal or atrioventricular canal defect.

99. The answer is E (all). *(p 227)* Congenital complete heart block is occasionally seen in children born to mothers with systemic lupus erythematosus. Jervell and Lange-Nielsen independently described congenitally deaf children with a long QT syndrome, which predisposes them to ventricular dysrhythmias and sudden cardiac death. Deafness is also a feature of congenital rubella and Klippel-Feil syndromes. The congenital long QT syndrome not associated with auditory manifestations is known as Romano-Ward syndrome. Sarcoidosis may cause an infiltrative myocardial disease resulting in conduction disturbances. The Emery-Dreifuss syndrome is characterized by sinus node dysfunction, atrial paralysis, elbow contractures, and humeroperoneal weakness.

100. The answer is D (4). *(p 232)* Pulsus paradoxus (≥ 12 mmHg fall in systolic blood pressure with inspiration) is seen in patients with cardiac tamponade, constrictive pericarditis, restrictive cardiomyopathy, and severe obstructive lung disease. Pulsus alternans is seen in patients with severe left ventricular dysfunction. Aortic stenosis results in a decrease in the pulse pressure, and aortic insufficiency results in an increase in pulse pressure. An unequal pulse pressure between the arms is seen in infants with supravalvular aortic stenosis and adults with subclavian steal syndrome.

101. The answer is A (1, 2, 3). *(pp 255–264)* An atrial septal defect is characterized by a constellation of abnormal heart sounds. The tricuspid component of the first heart sound (S_1) is usually increased due to high flow across the tricuspid valve, which holds the valve open. The fixed splitting of the second heart sound (S_2) is a hallmark auscultatory finding of an atrial septal defect. With inspiration, there is normal delay of the pulmonary component of S_2. This delay is maintained with expiration due to decreased left ventricular ejection time. A pulmonary vascular ejection click is present due to dilatation of the pulmonary artery. An aortic vascular ejection click is not seen with an isolated atrial septal defect.

102. The answer is E (all). *(pp 285–305)* A loud murmur or cardiac noise may occasionally be heard by a patient or family member. Although these sounds are usually heard in a quiet room, they may at times be heard at a considerable distance. Hamman's sign, also known as a mediastinal crunch, is due to air in the mediastinum. It has been described variously as crackles, squeaks, or crunching sounds heard with each heartbeat. It can be mistaken for either pleural or pericardial friction rubs. The "cooing dove" sound is frequently heard as a regurgitant murmur due to a ruptured or retroverted aortic cusp. The systolic "honk" may be heard in patients with mitral valve prolapse. When a ventricular septal defect is associated with a large left-to-right shunt, a loud murmur may be auscultated without the use of a stethoscope.

103. The answer is B (1, 3). *(pp 267–274)* The second heart sound (S_2) consists of two components: the aortic and pulmonic valve closure sounds. Normal physiological splitting is due to a prolongation of right ventricular and a decrease in left ventricular ejection periods. This results in an early aortic closure sound (A_2) and delayed pulmonic closure sound (P_2). The pulmonary component of S_2 is inscribed with the incisura of the pulmonary artery pressure tracing. A_2 is generally much louder than P_2, and its intensity exceeds that of P_2 even in the pulmonic area. Transmission of P_2 to the apex is usually abnormal in adults but is occasionally normal in children.

104. The answer is A (1, 2, 3). *(pp 269–273)* Reversed or paradoxical splitting of the second heart sound (S_2) results in a narrow splitting with inspiration and separation of the components with expiration. This abnormality can be due to early excitation of right ventricular ejection or a delay in left ventricular ejection. A hemodynamic cause of paradoxical splitting is severe aortic stenosis or hypertrophic obstructive cardiomyopathy. An electrical etiology of paradoxical splitting is right ventricular premature depolarization or a delay due to a left bundle branch block (LBBB). Pulmonary stenosis results in a wide physiological splitting of S_2.

105. The answer is A (1, 2, 3). *(pp 259–305)* In acute severe aortic regurgitation, the first heart sound (S_1) may be soft or absent because of premature closure of the mitral valve. The Austin Flint murmur, due to rapid streaming of blood across the anterior leaflet of the mitral valve is typically seen. The third heart sound (S_3) is inscribed due to overwhelming diastolic regurgitant flow across the incompetent aortic valve. A fourth heart sound (S_4), which is typically due to either decreased ventricular compliance or excessive rapid late diastolic filling due to atrial systole, is not typically seen.

106. The answer is C (2, 4). *(pp 285–305)* Isometric handgrip increases systemic vascular resistance, thereby increasing the intensity of murmurs associated with aortic or mitral regurgitation. Due to ventricular dilatation, it decreases the obstruction in hypertrophic obstructive cardiomyopathy and increases leaflet "coadaptation" in patients with mitral valve prolapse. Phase II of the Valsalva maneuver increases intrathoracic pressure, thereby decreasing venous return and left ventricular volume, which increases the murmurs of hypertrophic obstructive cardiomyopathy and mitral valve prolapse. Amyl nitrite results in vasodilatation and a reflex increase in heart rate and venous return, thereby increasing ejection murmurs associated with left ventricular outflow tract obstruction but decreasing the murmurs of mitral or aortic regurgitation or ventricular septal defect. Squatting simultaneously increases venous return and systemic vascular resistance, thereby decreasing the right-to-left shunt across the ventricular septal defect in tetralogy of Fallot and increasing the volume of blood ejected across the right ventricular outflow tract obstruction.

107. The answer is A (1, 2, 3). *(p 316)* Hypoxia and hypercapnia function as local retinal vasodilators, resulting in retinal and disk edema. The dark blood column is secondary to hypoxia. Arterial venous nicking is not a common manifestation of an acute exacerbation of cor pulmonale.

108. The answer is A (1, 2, 3). *(pp 268–274)* The splitting of the second heart sound (S_2) depends on consideration of three separate intervals: the electromechanical coupling interval, the duration of ventricular mechanical systole, and the impedance, or hangout, interval. In patients with pulmonary hypertension, the hangout interval is decreased. The prolongation of right ventricular ejection with normal ventricular performance results in a narrow physiological split S_2 during expiration. As right ventricular dysfunction develops, the splitting of S_2 increases in duration.

109. The answer is C (2, 4). *(pp 276–279)* The pathological third heart sound (S_3) has had three proposed explanations: the valvular, ventricular, and impact theories; however, the valvular theory, which proposed diastolic tensing of the atrial ventricular valves, is no longer accepted. The ventricular theory proposes that S_3 is due to the interaction of the force of blood entering the left ventricle and the ability of the left ventricle to receive it; that is, the left ventricle can suddenly reach the limits of its distensibility, thereby decelerating the flow of blood. The impact theory proposes that S_3 is due to the dynamic impact of the heart with the chest wall. The root theory has not been used to explain the genesis of S_3.

110. The answer is E (all). *(p 326)* In classic electrocardiographic teaching, the development of a Q wave signifies transmural myocardial infarction. Further investigation has shown that Q waves may develop in unstable angina pectoris, Prinzmetal's angina, exercise-induced ischemia, and hypertrophic cardiomyopathy. The development of Q waves associated with acute myocardial infarction may "disappear" due to shrinking of the zone of infarction, successful reperfusion of an acute myocardial infarction, development of an intraventricular conduction delay, "contracoup" left ventricular infarction, or hypertrophy of adjacent myocardial fibers. Q waves are seen in one-half to three-fourths of patients with myocardial infarction.

111. The answer is A (1, 2, 3). *(pp 361–363)* A decrease in the size of the cardiac silhouette is frequently encountered in the conditions of chronic obstructive pulmonary disease (COPD), Addison's disease, and anorexia nervosa. The cardiothoracic ratio in these conditions is less than the normal mean value in adults of 44 percent. In COPD, the increase in size of the thoracic cavity decreases the relative size of the cardiac silhouette. In Addison's disease and anorexia nervosa, weight loss and decreased intravascular volume may lead to the diminished cardiac silhouette. The definition of a small cardiac silhouette is best made retrospectively when comparison to chest roentgenograms taken after therapy can be made. Biventricular hypertrophy is present in hemochromatosis.

112. The answer is E (all). *(p 329)* Diffuse PR-segment changes, especially in the presence of a new atrial arrhythmia in a patient with an acute large ventricular myocardial infarction, suggest coexisting atrial infarction. PR-segment changes have been noted to include elevation in lead I or the left chest leads with reciprocal depression in the right chest leads or lead III.

113. The answer is B (1, 3). *(p 443)* Exercise testing in patients with significant cardiac disease is characterized by a measurable maximum oxygen uptake ($\dot{V}_{O_2}$ max) below normal, preserved oxygen saturation, attainment of the anaerobic threshold, and a highest minute ventilation below 50 percent of the maximum voluntary ventilation (MVV). In pulmonary disease, the $\dot{V}_{O_2}$ and anaerobic threshold are usually not attained while systemic oxygen saturation falls. The MVV is nearly achieved at maximum effort. In obesity, $\dot{V}_{O_2}$ max is normal and is attained at a low work load.

114. The answer is E (all). *(p 451)* Serious and life-threatening complications associated with pulmonary artery catheterization occur in less than 5 percent of patients. The most common complication is conduction disturbances, including ventricular arrhythmias during flotation of the balloon catheter to the right ventricle and complete heart block when a catheter is inserted in a patient with a complete left bundle branch block (LBBB). Other complications include: pneumothorax, pulmonary infarction, pulmonary artery rupture, and septicemia.

115. The answer is A (1, 2, 3). *(pp 452–453)* Hemodynamic monitoring is not routinely performed unless there are clear indications. The assessment of therapeutic intervention in patients with altered hemodynamics, including the discontinuation of inotropic and vasopressor agents, is frequently facilitated by pulmonary artery catheterization. It is recommended to keep patients relatively hypovolemic with the clinical diagnosis of noncardiogenic pulmonary edema. Patients who remain hypotensive despite adequate fluid resuscitation also may require hemodynamic monitoring. Routine insertion for patients with acute myocardial infarction is not necessary.

116. The answer is D (4). *(p 330)* The electrocardiogram that accompanies the question represents diffuse epimyocarditis or pericarditis. Representative abnormalities include diffuse epicardial injury (ST-segment elevation and PR-segment depression in V_2–V_6). Electrocardiographic abnormalities have arbitrarily been divided into four stages: 1, ST-segment elevation; 2, ST-segment resolution to baseline; 3, T-wave inversion, and 4, T-wave resolution to baseline. Inferior and lateral myocardial infarction are associated with reciprocal ST-segment changes that are not seen in this electrocardiogram. The electrocardiographic changes seen with pulmonary embolism include: sinus tachycardia, $S_1Q_3T_3$, an incomplete right bundle branch block (RBBB), and signs of right ventricular ischemia.

117. The answer is B (1, 3). *(pp 335–337)* In the figure that accompanies the question, a left bundle branch block (LBBB) has classically concealed the electrocardiographic signs of myocardial infarction. However, the presence of an anteroseptal myocardial infarction can be diagnosed by the presence of small Q waves in leads I, V_5, and V_6. Cabrera's sign refers to the notch in the ascending limb of the predominant negative deflection in leads V_3 and V_4. This finding is a less sensitive finding of complete LBBB with myocardial infarction. A right bundle branch block (RBBB) may be concealed when there are additional conduction disturbances in the left bundle branch, the anterior-superior division of the left bundle branch, or the free wall of the left ventricle.

118. The answer is A (1, 2, 3). *(pp 357, 365)* There are three structures in the intercostal space: the intercostal arteries, intercostal veins, and intercostal nerves. Any of these three may enlarge, resulting in rib notching. With coarctation of the aorta, the intercostal arteries enlarge. With superior vena cava syndrome, the intercostal veins may enlarge. With neurofibromatosis, rib notching may be produced by numerous intercostal neurofibromas. Osteodysplasia is defined as the abnormal development of bone. This is not associated with rib notching.

119. The answer is B (1, 3). *(pp 337–341)* The electrocardiogram that accompanies the question is from a patient with Wolff-Parkinson-White syndrome, the classic characteristics of which include a short PR interval, a delta wave, and wide QRS complex. Excitation through an accessory pathway of the Kent bundle type accounts for these abnormalities due to bypassing the usual delay in the atrioventricular (AV) node. Patients who have preexcitation due to conduction through Mahaim (nodal-ventricular) fibers have a normal PR interval without a distinct delta wave when in sinus rhythm.

120. The answers are: A-Y, B-N, C-Y, D-Y, E-N. *(pp 209–211)* "Two-pillow" orthopnea may be seen with both severe heart failure and chronic disease. The patient needs to sleep propped up on two pillows to avoid the perception of shortness of breath. While the symptom of paroxysmal nocturnal dyspnea may indicate severe left ventricular dysfunction, it may also occur in patients with hyperventilation syndrome, chronic lung disease, anxiety, or pulmonary emboli. Patients who have received a chronic high dose of nitroglycerin may develop methemoglobinemia. Methemoglobin cannot effectively carry oxygen and, therefore, the patients appear cyanotic with normal arterial blood oxygenation. The symptoms of methemoglobinemia include dyspnea, fatigue, and headache. This condition is usually benign and self-limited once the diagnosis is made and the medication discontinued. Cheyne-Stokes respirations are characterized by a pattern of hyperpnea alternating with periods of apnea. They are usually seen in patients with left ventricular dysfunction and cerebral vascular disease but may occasionally be seen as a normal variant in newborns. Thyrotoxicosis is associated with dyspnea due to a high metabolic rate.

121. The answers are: A-N, B-Y, C-N, D-Y, E-Y. *(pp 240–247)* Kussmaul's sign is an inspiratory increase in jugular venous pressure and is seen in conditions with resistance to right ventricular filling such as right ventricular infarction, restrictive cardiomyopathy, and constrictive pericarditis. Tietze's syndrome is characterized as tenderness over the sternum in the costochondral, chondrosternal, and xiphisternal joints. Palpation of these areas may reproduce the patient's chest discomfort. Mondor's disease is swelling of the superficial veins on the anterior chest wall. It too may be a cause of chest discomfort. Tricuspid regurgitation is characterized as a fusion of the C and V waves that produces a "CV" wave. Pulsations in the epigastrium may be associated with an abdominal aortic aneurysm or right ventricular hypertrophy due to chronic lung disease.

122. The answers are: A-N, B-N, C-N, D-N, E-N. *(pp 287–304, 504)* Graham Steell murmur is an early diastolic murmur heard at the left lower sternal border associated with an accentuated pulmonary closure sound, clinical or echocardiographic evidence of right ventricular hypertrophy, and large pulmonary arteries on chest roentgenogram. This is associated with pulmonary regurgitation due to pulmonary hypertension. The Austin Flint murmur or rumble is seen with moderate-to-severe aortic regurgitation and is due to the regurgitant steam "hitting" the anterior leaflet of the mitral valve. Duroziez's murmur describes the systolic and diastolic murmurs heard over peripheral arteries in patients with aortic regurgitation. The Carey Coombs murmur is described in acute rheumatic carditis. It is heard in middiastole, following the third heart sound (S_3), is low pitched, and ends prior to the first heart sound (S_1). It is due to the rapid flow across the mitral valve and, therefore, can be heard in any high-output condition. Still's murmur is an innocent systolic ejection murmur of vibratory quality and is frequently auscultated in children.

123. The answers are: A-N, B-Y, C-N, D-N, E-Y. *(pp 363, 368)* Acute right-sided heart failure can be associated with the following radiographic characteristics: lateralization of pulmonary flow (Westermark's sign) and, in its chronic form, pulmonary opacifications due to pulmonary infarction. The "butterfly pattern" is seen in acute left-sided heart failure. With acute right-sided heart failure commonly due to pulmonary embolism, the right-sided heart chambers are enlarged. Pulmonary parenchymal calcifications are seen in the various manifestations of chronic left-sided heart failure.

124. **The answers are: A-Y, B-Y, C-Y, D-N, E-N.** *(p 381)* M-mode echocardiography begins with a search for the mitral valve. To understand the pattern produced by the anterior mitral valve leaflet, it is important to remember that all motion is relative to a fixed point on the anterior chest wall. The point of maximum excursion of the anterior leaflet is designated the E point. The nadir of the initial diastolic closing of the valve is designated the F point. The middiastolic closing motion, referred to as the EF slope, represents the velocity of blood moving from the left atrium in to the left ventricle. The peak of the leaflet opening during atrial systole is the A point. Complete closure of the leaflet during ventricular systole marks the C point.

125. **The answers are: A-N, B-Y, C-Y, D-Y, E-Y.** *(pp 274–276)* An opening snap is the hallmark of mitral stenosis. It has, however, been recorded in patients with tricuspid stenosis as well as in patients who have high flow across atrioventricular valves. The latter condition has been seen in patients with large atrial or ventricular septal defects, tricuspid atresia with large atrial septal defects, and thyrotoxicosis. The immobile leaflets associated with severe calcific mitral stenosis may diminish or eliminate the opening snap.

126. **The answers are: A-N, B-Y, C-N, D-Y, E-Y.** *(p 413)* The area of opening of the aortic valve and the pattern of leaflet motion provide qualitative information about left ventricular stroke volume. The aortic leaflets open abruptly in low-cardiac output states and severe mitral regurgitation. Premature opening of the aortic valve suggests elevated left ventricular end-diastolic pressure, as in severe aortic regurgitation. Very early systolic partial closure is evidence of outflow obstruction due to a discrete membranous subvalvular aortic stenosis. Early to midsystolic partial or complete closure is evidence for hypertrophic obstructive cardiomyopathy.

127. **The answers are: A-N, B-Y, C-N, D-Y, E-N.** *(pp 400–401)* Although the diagnosis of cardiac tamponade should be made primarily by clinical and hemodynamic criteria obtained at the bedside, two-dimensional echocardiography can be used to provide additional diagnostic information. Collapse of the right atrial and right ventricular walls during diastole is commonly seen in tamponade. Diastolic collapse of the right ventricle, however, is only a marker for equalization of the right ventricular diastolic and pericardial pressures, and its absence does not exclude tamponade. The right ventricle is usually small, indicating poor filling of that chamber. The size of the effusion is not an indicator for tamponade. A small effusion can be associated with tamponade when it accumulates rapidly, and conversely, a large effusion that accumulates over a long period of time may not cause hemodynamic compromise. Plethora of the inferior vena cava with blunted respiratory variation is a marker of a hemodynamically significant pericardial effusion.

128. **The answers are: A-N, B-Y, C-Y, D-Y, E-N.** *(p 435)* Exercise testing can be used to determine prognosis following myocardial infarction. The presence of several parameters can be used to predict an increased severity of coronary disease and a poor prognosis if not treated. The inability to complete stage II of a Bruce protocol predicts an overall poor response to medical therapy and, in general, coronary bypass surgery is usually recommended in patients with multivessel disease who cannot achieve greater than 6.5 METs of work load. Symptoms that develop at a low heart rate or work load suggest severe coronary disease. Significant ST-segment depression greater than 2 mm, postexercise duration of ST-segment depression for greater than 6 min in recovery, or the presence of ST depression in multiple leads are all associated with an increased severity of coronary disease. Exercise-induced U-wave inversion has been reported as a potentially important marker of left main stenosis. Exercise-induced hypotension has a predictive value of about 50 percent for left-main or triple-vessel disease. It can also occur in patients with significant valvular heart disease or cardiomyopathy.

129–131. The answers are: 129-D, 130-D, 131-C. *(p 365)*   Acute right- or left-sided heart failure is not associated with the development of a pleural effusion. Chronic left-sided heart failure is most commonly associated with a right pleural effusion. Bilateral pleural effusions are seen with chronic left- and right-sided heart failure or noncardiac etiologies.

132–135. The answers are: 132-B, 133-C, 134-D, 135-A. *(pp 217–222)*   Patients with fetal alcohol syndrome have maxillary hypoplasia, which results in the appearance of an underdeveloped central face. Additional characteristics include a small and upturned nose, micrognathia, and a thin upper lip and vermilion. Although many cardiac defects have been described, atrial and ventricular septal defects are particularly common.

Diagnostic features of Noonan's syndrome include ptosis, low-set ears, downward slanting eyes, a webbed neck, hypertelorism (widely spaced eyes), low posterior hairline, short stature, mental retardation, and a normal chromosomal configuration.

Marfan's syndrome was originally described by a Parisian pediatrician. This entity is characterized by an arm span greater than body height, disproportionately long legs with a resulting ratio of upper segment to lower segment of no more than 0.85, kyphoscoliosis, and pectus excavatum or carinatum. Aortic dilatation and mitral and tricuspid regurgitation are commonly associated cardiac defects. Blue sclerae have been described. The chromosomal configuration is normal.

Patient's with Turner's syndrome may have a webbed neck, short stature, low posterior hairline, pigmented moles, widely spaced nipples, normal intelligence, and a single sex chromosome. A murmur consistent with pulmonary stenosis may be heard and coarctation of the aorta is frequently seen.

136–140. The answers are: 136-D, 137-C, 138-A, 139-E, 140-B. *(p 360)*   The five chest roentgenograms that accompany the question represent five different pulmonary blood flow patterns. Figure A shows cephalization of the pulmonary vasculature, showing dilatation of the upper vessels with constriction of the lower vessels. Figure B shows a patient with marked pulmonary trunk and central segments of the pulmonary arteries with rapid pruning of the peripheral branches. Figure C shows a massive pulmonary embolus on the left pulmonary artery resulting in enhanced blood flow to the right lung with decreased blood flow to the left (Westermark's sign). Figure D shows a large pulmonary arteriovenous fistula localized in the right lower lobe. Figure E illustrates collateralization, which is decreased pulmonary blood flow that results in the formation of bronchial arterial collaterals with numerous small tortuous vessels in the upper and middle lung fields.

141–145. The answers are: 141-B, 142-D, 143-E, 144-C, 145-A. *(pp 357–364)*   Patients with acute myocardial infarction may occasionally have radiographic signs of acute pulmonary edema due to left ventricular decompression. The radiographic signs of this abnormality include bilateral increase in pulmonary vascular markings with a normal size cardiac silhouette (butterfly pattern).

Lateralization of pulmonary blood flow is seen in a patient with a massive pulmonary embolus, resulting in obstruction of the left main pulmonary artery but dilatation of the right pulmonary artery and an increased flow (Westermark's sign).

The radiographic signs of tetralogy of Fallot include the characteristic boot-shaped heart (*coeur en sabot*).

Coarctation of the aorta has several distinct radiographic findings, including a figure-three sign of the dilated descending aorta and an E sign of the barium-filled esophagus. In addition, the left ventricle is enlarged.

A left ventricular aneurysm is identified by a "bulge" along the left cardiac border.

III. The Major Cardiovascular Symptoms

DIRECTIONS: Each question below contains five suggested responses. Select the **one best** response to each question.

146. Ischemic chest pain in the absence of atherosclerosis may be due to all the following EXCEPT

    (A) hypertrophic cardiomyopathy
    (B) mitral valve prolapse
    (C) systemic arterial hypertension
    (D) acute aortic regurgitation
    (E) severe chronic aortic stenosis

147. In patients with symptomatic extrasystolic beats, the actual sensation of a palpitation is due to the patient's perception of the

    (A) preextrasystolic beat
    (B) extrasystolic beat
    (C) postextrasystolic beat
    (D) premature atrial contraction
    (E) premature ventricular contraction

148. A reversible ischemic neurologic disability (RIND) refers to

    (A) a migraine headache with facial paresthesias that last less than 3 hours
    (B) brief, transient paresthesias of the lower extremities after sitting for a prolonged period with the legs crossed
    (C) an abrupt onset of motor or sensory deficit that lasts longer than a few minutes but less than 24 hours before complete recovery
    (D) a distinctive episode of motor or sensory deficit that persists more than 24 hours but completely resolves within 3 weeks
    (E) a repetitive motion injury such as disability due to computer keyboard use that resolves within 3 weeks of rest

DIRECTIONS: Each question below contains four suggested responses of which **one or more** is correct. Select

A	if	**1, 2, and 3**	are correct
B	if	**1 and 3**	are correct
C	if	**2 and 4**	are correct
D	if	**4**	is correct
E	if	**1, 2, 3, and 4**	are correct

149. Features associated with chest discomfort from myocardial ischemia include the acute development of

(1)   a new heart murmur
(2)   new pulmonary rales
(3)   hypotension
(4)   new pulsus alternans

150. In patients who have recurrent symptoms of apparent loss of consciousness, cardiac syncope should be suspected over a seizure disorder when

(1)   an apneic phase is followed by labored breathing
(2)   a consistent pattern of motor or autonomic activity is evident
(3)   there is a precedent aura
(4)   the episode has a variable course each time

151. Headaches that occur in patients with systemic arterial hypertension

(1)   usually localize to the temporal region
(2)   have a poor correlation between severity and level of blood pressure in moderate cases
(3)   are often accompanied by tinnitus
(4)   are the most frequent presenting symptom in malignant hypertension

152. Significant pedal edema may be caused by

(1)   kwashiorkor
(2)   cirrhosis of the liver
(3)   therapy with minoxidil
(4)   congestive heart failure (CHF)

DIRECTIONS: Each question below contains five suggested responses. For **each** of the **five** responses listed with every question, you are to respond either YES (Y) or NO (N). In a given item **all, some, or none of the alternatives may be correct.**

153. Correct statements regarding coronary artery disease include which of the following?

   (A) Men with exertional chest discomfort relieved with rest have less than a 50 percent chance of having significant epicardial coronary artery disease
   (B) Angina due to myocardial ischemia usually lasts less than 1 min
   (C) The resting electrocardiogram (ECG) is normal in 25 to 50 percent of patients with stable angina pectoris
   (D) Spontaneous pneumothorax is most often seen in older debilitated women
   (E) Asymptomatic myocardial infarction may occur in as many as 30 percent of patients

154. Correct explanations for the dyspnea seen in patients with congestive heart failure (CHF) include which of the following?

   (A) There is a direct correlation between dyspnea and the pulmonary capillary wedge pressure
   (B) Stimulation of chemoreceptors in patients with CHF relate to dyspnea
   (C) Direct stimulation of the respiratory receptors in patients with CHF contributes to dyspnea
   (D) The low cardiac output in patients with CHF contributes to dyspnea
   (E) The dyspnea of patients with anemia is related to increased oxygen-carrying capacity

155. Correct statements regarding the fatigue associated with heart disease include which of the following?

   (A) Exercise-induced fatigue in patients with congestive heart failure (CHF) is always related to decreased skeletal muscle blood flow
   (B) Exercise-induced fatigue is due to the anaerobic metabolism of skeletal muscles
   (C) Exercise-induced fatigue in patients with CHF can be reversed with cardiac rehabilitation
   (D) Exertional fatigue in patients with known coronary artery disease is a risk factor for the development of myocardial infarction
   (E) Malaise may be a prodromal symptom of acute myocardial infarction

DIRECTIONS: Each group of questions below consists of four lettered headings followed by a set of numbered items. For each numbered item select

A	if the item is associated with	(A) **only**
B	if the item is associated with	(B) **only**
C	if the item is associated with	**both** (A) and (B)
D	if the item is associated with	**neither** (A) nor (B)

Each lettered heading may be used **once, more than once, or not at all.**

Questions 156–159

(A) Mechanoreceptor
(B) Chemoreceptor
(C) Both
(D) Neither

156. Congestive heart failure (CHF)

157. Length-tension inappropriateness

158. Acidoses

159. Lung disease

Questions 160–163

(A) Orthopnea
(B) Paroxysmal nocturnal dyspnea
(C) Both
(D) Neither

160. Stimulation of chemoreceptors

161. Stimulation of mechanoreceptors

162. Stimulation of respiratory receptors

163. Stimulation of cerebral receptors

DIRECTIONS: The group of questions below consists of lettered headings followed by a set of numbered items. For each numbered item select the **one** lettered heading with which it is **most** closely associated. Each lettered heading may be used **once, more than once, or not at all.**

Questions 164–168

For each type of pain listed below, select the medical entity most likely to be responsible for it.

(A) Aortic dissection
(B) Reflux esophagitis
(C) Pneumonia
(D) Anxiety
(E) Herpes zoster

164. Brief, lightninglike pain

165. Heartburn

166. Sudden onset of tearing pain

167. Pleuritic pain

168. Bandlike pain

III. The Major Cardiovascular Symptoms

Answers

146. **The answer is B.** *(pp 463–464)*   There are multiple etiologies for myocardial ischemia in the absence of atherosclerosis, including hypertrophic cardiomyopathy, pulmonary hypertension, aortic regurgitation, and chronic aortic stenosis. All of these conditions are characterized by a relative imbalance between myocardial oxygen supply and demand. Patients with pulmonary hypertension have chest discomfort from right ventricular ischemia due to pressure overload on the right ventricle. The pain of aortic regurgitation results from increased ventricular dimensions from volume overload resulting in increased myocardial oxygen demand and an inadequate coronary blood flow. Acute aortic stenosis results in myocardial ischemia from acute left ventricular volume overload. The chest discomfort due to mitral valve prolapse is usually not secondary to myocardial ischemia.

147. **The answer is C.** *(p 475)*   A palpitation is a symptom defined by patients as an unpleasant awareness of the heart beat. It may be caused by a variety of abnormalities of the cardiac rhythm. When extrasystolic beats are present, the patients are more commonly aware of the postextrasystolic beat (i.e., the beat following the extrasystolic beat) than of the premature beat itself. This is due to the increased stroke volume resulting from the compensatory pause in the postextrasystolic beat.

148. **The answer is D.** *(p 481)*   A cerebrovascular attack or episode refers to changes in motor or sensory function caused by an alteration in cerebral blood flow to a portion of the brain. The commonly used term, transient ischemic attack (TIA), refers to an abrupt onset of an episode of motor or sensory deficit that lasts longer than a few minutes but less than 24 hours before complete recovery. A recent term, reversible ischemic neurologic disability (RIND), is used to describe a motor or sensory deficit that persists for more than 24 hours but that resolves within 3 weeks. Paresthesias of the lower extremities after sitting with the legs crossed and repetitive motion injuries are not true neurologic disabilities related to ischemia but are variations of compression injuries. The constellation of symptoms that occur with a migraine headache are related to dynamic vascular changes.

149. **The answer is E (all).** *(pp 459–462)*   Chest discomfort from myocardial ischemia may result in severe left ventricular systolic dysfunction. This may result in the development of new pulmonary rales, hypotension, and pulsus alternans. The development of a new heart murmur due to papillary muscle dysfunction is also a feature of myocardial ischemia.

150. **The answer is D (4).** *(pp 476–477)*   A clear distinction between syncope, a brief loss of consciousness, and a seizure disorder may occasionally be difficult, but careful analysis of symptoms and clinical events surrounding the episode is important to differentiate the two possibilities. Seizures are usually preceded by

a characteristic aura, but they may also occur abruptly and without warning and usually follow a consistent pattern of motor or autonomic activity. With recurrent episodes, the course is usually identical each time. With cardiac syncope, the motor and autonomic activity and course are variable. Following a seizure, an apneic phase is followed by labored breathing. In cardiac syncope, breathing is usually fast and shallow with no apparent apneic phase.

151. **The answer is C (2, 4).** *(p 482)*   Headaches may be a relatively common symptom occurring in patients with systemic arterial hypertension. However, in patients with moderate hypertension, there is a poor correlation between the level of blood pressure and the perception of a headache. However, headache is the most frequent symptom of patients presenting with severe or malignant hypertension. Classically, the headache in patients with systemic arterial hypertension is occipital or frontal in location but commonly may be generalized. It does not usually localize in the temporal region.

152. **The answer is E (all).** *(pp 482–483, Table 22-1)*   Although pedal edema is one of the primary signs of congestive heart failure (CHF), the presence of pedal edema does not always indicate CHF. A large variety of disease entities may cause edema, including cirrhosis of the liver, renal disease, nutritional deficiencies such as kwashiorkor, hormonal abnormalities, and mechanical problems such as venous or lymphatic obstruction. In addition, increased capillary permeability due to a variety of mechanisms may cause significant edema. Nifedipine and minoxidil are vasodilators that are known to have the side effect of pedal edema.

153. **The answers are: A-N, B-N, C-Y, D-N, E-Y.** *(pp 461–465)*   The presence of exertional chest discomfort relieved by rest is highly predictive of myocardial ischemia due to significant obstruction of the epicardial coronary arteries as identified by angiographic studies in more than 90 percent of patients. This symptom has a greater predictive value in men than in women. Angina pectoris usually lasts between 1 and 15 min. The relief of angina with nitroglycerin is typically seen in less than 5 min. The resting electrocardiogram (ECG) is normal in 50 percent of patients with stable angina pectoris. Spontaneous pneumothorax is seen in young men (between 30 and 50 years of age) who are otherwise healthy. The presence of asymptomatic Q-wave myocardial infarctions are identified in up to 30 percent of patients, especially in older patients and patients with diabetes mellitus.

154. **The answers are: A-N, B-Y, C-N, D-Y, E-N.** *(pp 471–473)*   Dyspnea in patients with congestive heart failure (CHF) is multifactorial. This may be due in part to stimulation of mechanoreceptors as a result of elevation of pressures in the right atrium or ventricle, pulmonary artery, or left atrium; however, there is poor correlation between the pulmonary capillary wedge pressure and the feeling of dyspnea. An imbalance between myocardial oxygen supply and demand in the respiratory muscles due to impaired cardiac output stimulation of the chemoreceptors may also play a role. Acidosis due to low cardiac output may stimulate chemoreceptors, which alter the respiratory rate. The dyspnea associated with anemia is thought to be secondary to decreased oxygen-carrying capacity.

155. **The answers are: A-N, B-Y, C-N, D-Y, E-Y.** *(p 469)*   Fatigue has been observed in approximately 25 percent of patients with congestive heart failure (CHF) despite adequate skeletal muscle blood flow. Fatigue in this circumstance is due to the anaerobic metabolism of skeletal muscle. Cardiac rehabilitation, which holds promise, has not yet been shown to be a definite benefit in patients with CHF. Fatigue in a patient with known coronary artery disease may be considered a risk factor for the development of acute myocardial infarction or sudden cardiac death. Generalized malaise may antecede myocardial infarct. It has been postulated that this symptom reflects the inflammatory nature of atherosclerosis in its acute stages.

156–159. The answers are: 156-A, 157-A, 158-B, 159-D. *(p 470)*   Various stimulants to respiratory drive include mechanoreceptors, chemoreceptors, and pulmonary receptors. Mechanoreceptors are sensitive to increased volume in the right atrium and ventricle, pulmonary artery, and left atrium. Patients with congestive heart failure (CHF) have an increased respiratory rate due to the stimulation of mechanoreceptors. Length-tension inappropriateness involves stimulation of the mechanoreceptors in the respiratory muscles and diaphragm through proprioceptive signals to increase the respiratory rate. Acidosis, hypoxia, and hypercapnia are chemoreceptor stimulants to increase the respiratory rate. Lung disease stimulates pulmonary receptors in the parenchyma to increase the respiratory drive.

160–163. The answers are: 160-D, 161-C, 162-D, 163-D. *(pp 472–473)*   Supine breathlessness (orthopnea) and breathlessness that occurs at night and is relieved by the upright position (paroxysmal nocturnal dyspnea) are due to stimulation of mechanoreceptors. This results from a shift of blood volume from the periphery to the pulmonary vasculature.

164–168. The answers are: 164-A, 165-B, 166-C, 167-D, 168-E. *(pp 461–465)*   Chest discomfort secondary to anxiety is short (i.e., less than 1 min) and of lightninglike quality. It occurs at rest or in the evening after work. The pain of reflux esophagitis is epigastric or retrosternal and is described as a burning pain (i.e., "heartburn"), especially after eating or with postural changes. The chest discomfort associated with aortic dissection is sudden, tearing, and widely radiated. The pain of pneumonia is pleuritic and results from pleural irritation; it is sharp and frequently accompanied by reduced inspiratory effort. Herpes zoster is characterized as a bandlike pain across the chest.

IV. Heart Failure

DIRECTIONS: Each question below contains five suggested responses. Select the **one best** response to each question.

169. A 43-year-old man complains of dyspnea on exertion and exertional chest pain. Echocardiographic studies suggest an aortic valve orifice area of less than 0.70 cm², making it most appropriate to schedule the patient for

   (A) aortic valve replacement
   (B) coronary angiography to search for significant coronary artery disease prior to valve surgery
   (C) follow-up evaluation with echocardiography in 6 months
   (D) follow-up evaluation with echocardiography in 1 year
   (E) an exercise test to rule out concomitant coronary disease

170. Supportive evidence that left-sided failure is present includes all the following EXCEPT

   (A) abnormally elevated filling pressures as detected by right heart catheterization
   (B) a cardiac index of 3.5 liters/min/m²
   (C) a reduction in maximum oxygen consumption determined noninvasively by exercise
   (D) the presence of pulmonary rales on physical examination
   (E) low left ventricular ejection fraction at rest on echocardiography

171. All the following statements regarding resting state measures of myocardial function are true EXCEPT

   (A) the ejection fraction is the percentage of end-systolic volume that is ejected
   (B) the fractional shortening is the percentage shortening of the ventricular end-diastolic diameter
   (C) the mean circumferential fiber shortening is normally greater than 1.2 circumferences per second
   (D) the ejection fraction determined by echocardiography is sensitive to changes in afterload
   (E) there is good correlation between ejection fractions obtained by echocardiography when compared with measurements made by angiography

172. The response to exercise is determined primarily by

   (A) adaptation of the skeletal muscle
   (B) cardiovascular reflexes
   (C) cardiac output
   (D) motivation
   (E) adaptation of the peripheral vascular bed

173. All the following statements regarding exercise capacity and heart failure are true EXCEPT

(A) exercise testing is highly useful in evaluating symptoms in patients with chronic cardiomyopathy

(B) exercise testing is helpful when determining if a patient requires cardiac transplantation

(C) exercise testing is contraindicated in patients with dilated cardiomyopathy

(D) the maximum oxygen consumption equals the product of the cardiac output and the arteriovenous oxygen difference

(E) the best index of maximal exercise capacity is maximum oxygen consumption

174. Physical findings typical of the hyperdynamic states (high cardiac output states) include all the following EXCEPT

(A) an increased resting heart rate of 125 to 130 beats per minute

(B) a cervical venous hum

(C) wide pulse pressure

(D) a midsystolic murmur in the second or third left intercostal space

(E) a third heart sound (S_3)

175. Correct statements regarding high cardiac output states include all the following EXCEPT

(A) it is important to recognize high cardiac output states as a cause for congestive heart failure (CHF) because many of these conditions are curable

(B) some high cardiac output states may be aggravated by conventional therapy such as vasodilator drugs

(C) the increased cardiac output of the hyperdynamic states results from increased cardiac output alone

(D) reduced left ventricular afterload is present in many of the high cardiac output states

(E) hyperthyroidism, anemia, and systemic arteriovenous fistula may all be associated with high cardiac output states

176. Circulatory congestion refers specifically to

(A) inadequacy of the cardiovascular system due to inadequate blood volume

(B) inadequacy of the cardiovascular system due to decreased venous return

(C) congestion due to either heart failure or noncardiac circulatory overload

(D) congestion due to inadequate oxyhemoglobin

(E) edema of any cause

177. All the following statements regarding left- and right-sided failure are true EXCEPT

(A) one does not observe left heart failure without biochemical consequences in the right ventricle

(B) increases in diastolic pressure in one ventricle may influence pressure in the other

(C) the most common cause of right heart failure is chronic obstructive pulmonary disease (COPD)

(D) right heart failure is clinically characterized by an increase in systemic venous pressure

(E) enclosure by the pericardium contributes to ventricular interdependence

178. All the following statements regarding the pathophysiology of heart failure are true EXCEPT

(A) hypertension is the most common primary cause of heart failure

(B) the left ventricle in heart failure is preload-independent and afterload-dependent

(C) diastolic dysfunction appears to have a better prognosis than systolic dysfunction

(D) in the early stages of left ventricular dysfunction, the Frank-Starling curve shifts downward and to the right

(E) when the left ventricle is enlarged, less shortening of the fiber is required to eject a normal stroke volume

179. All the following disorders can be diagnosed from an endomyocardial biopsy EXCEPT

(A) cardiac amyloidosis

(B) carcinoid heart disease

(C) cardiac hemochromatosis

(D) dilated cardiomyopathy

(E) cardiac sarcoidosis

180. All the following statements regarding the pharmacological effects of digoxin are true EXCEPT

(A) high digoxin requirements may be the result of extensive metabolism to dihydro metabolites in the intestine

(B) patients with short-bowel syndrome do not have a significant decrease in the absorption of digoxin tablets

(C) the inotropic effect of digoxin is related to its binding to the sodium (Na^+), potassium (K^+)–activated membrane adenosine triphosphatase (ATPase) of the heart, which increases intracellular calcium (Ca^{2+})

(D) digoxin enhances both the effects of the parasympathetic and sympathetic nervous system of cardiac tissue

(E) digoxin may lead to increases in systemic, pulmonary, and coronary vascular resistance

181. Common complications seen in patients using potassium-sparing diuretics include all the following EXCEPT

(A) a potential complication of spironolactone is life-threatening hyperkalemia

(B) caution should be used in patients with diabetes and renal insufficiency when prescribing a potassium-sparing diuretic

(C) physicians should avoid using potassium-sparing diuretics, potassium supplements, and angiotensin-converting enzyme (ACE) inhibitors concurrently

(D) metabolic acidosis is commonly seen with the administration of spironolactone

(E) gynecomastia can be seen as a side effect of spironolactone

182. Complications of thiazide diuretics include all the following EXCEPT

(A) hypokalemia
(B) hypoglycemia
(C) hyperuricemia
(D) hyperlipidemia
(E) hypercalcemia

183. All the following statements regarding thiazide diuretics are true EXCEPT

(A) thiazide diuretics in high doses are useful as first-line antihypertensive agents

(B) an advantage of thiazide diuretics is low cost

(C) thiazide diuretics are less potent than loop diuretics in inducing salt and water excretion

(D) thiazide diuretics cause frequent metabolic side effects

(E) thiazides are relatively ineffective in patients with renal failure

184. Intra-aortic balloon pump insertion is indicated in all the following clinical situations EXCEPT

(A) ventricular septal defect that accompanies acute myocardial infarction

(B) acute mitral regurgitation that accompanies myocardial infarction

(C) acute aortic regurgitation with congestive heart failure (CHF) secondary to bacterial endocarditis

(D) unstable angina pectoris unresponsive to medical therapy

(E) with cardiomyopathy in a patient who is unresponsive to medical therapy and is awaiting transplantation

185. Complications of immunosuppressive therapy include all the following EXCEPT

(A) opportunistic infections
(B) lymphoproliferative malignancy
(C) graft muscle rejection
(D) toxic bone marrow suppression due to azathioprine
(E) nephrotoxicity due to cyclosporine

186. Contraindications to cardiac transplantation include all the following EXCEPT

(A) age above 60 years or neonates
(B) active malignancy
(C) human immunodeficiency virus (HIV)
(D) diet-controlled diabetes mellitus
(E) severe peripheral vascular disease

DIRECTIONS: Each question below contains four suggested responses of which **one or more** is correct. Select

A	if	**1, 2, and 3**	are correct
B	if	**1 and 3**	are correct
C	if	**2 and 4**	are correct
D	if	**4**	is correct
E	if	**1, 2, 3, and 4**	are correct

187. The high cardiac output state caused by hyperthyroidism is likely to be accompanied by

(1)   increased total body oxygen consumption
(2)   increased arteriovenous oxygen difference
(3)   increased systolic blood pressure
(4)   increased peripheral vascular resistance

188. Pathophysiologic consequences of a myocardial infarction include

(1)   increased systolic load due to the akinetic segment
(2)   decreased ejection fraction that approximates the amount of muscle loss
(3)   hypertrophy of the noninfarcted myocardium
(4)   decreased end-diastolic volume

189. Conditions with normal systolic function and decreased diastolic function include

(1)   systemic arterial hypertension
(2)   myocarditis
(3)   hypertrophic cardiomyopathy
(4)   congestive cardiomyopathy

190. True statements regarding ischemic heart disease include

(1)   diastolic dysfunction is a late manifestation of myocardial ischemia
(2)   a *hibernating myocardium* refers to persistent loss of contractile activity for hours or days despite return of blood flow and the absence of necrosis
(3)   ventricular remodeling commonly involves a reduction in chamber volume
(4)   hypertrophy is an almost invariable accompaniment of the remodeling process

191. In the setting of left ventricular dysfunction, which of the following neurohormonal factors would be activated?

(1)   Norepinephrine
(2)   Endothelin
(3)   Arginine vasopressin
(4)   Endothelial-derived relaxing factor

192. Regarding the assessment of heart failure,

(1)   changes in end-diastolic volume with time are not a good correlate of the course of heart failure
(2)   determination of maximum oxygen consumption (V_{O_2} max) is not helpful in patients with left ventricular dysfunction who are apparently asymptomatic
(3)   in advanced stages of heart failure, V_{O_2} max correlates very well with the ejection fraction
(4)   ventricular arrhythmias are an independent risk factor

193. Correct statements regarding the uses of digoxin include which of the following?

(1)   Digoxin can be administered to most patients with sinus bradycardia or asymptomatic sinus pauses without further decreasing sinus rate or accentuating the post-tachycardia pauses
(2)   Digoxin is efficacious in the therapy of supraventricular arrhythmias primarily because of the prolongation of conduction in atrial muscle
(3)   Myocardial ischemia enhances the arrhythmogenic effects of digoxin
(4)   Digoxin is as effective as dobutamine in improving cardiac output and reducing preload after myocardial infarction

194. True statements regarding dobutamine include

(1) there are specific dobutamine receptors in the renal vascular beds responsible for increased urine output with high-dose infusions of dobutamine

(2) dobutamine is not the inotropic agent of choice in the setting of significant hypotension

(3) unlike dopamine, dobutamine is not associated with ventricular arrhythmias

(4) the prolonged clinical benefits of short-term infusion of dobutamine are most probably related to long-lasting effects on the peripheral circulation rather than on the myocardium

195. True statements regarding the phosphodiesterase type III–inhibiting inotropic agents include

(1) there is a synergistic effect with the use of amrinone with dobutamine

(2) the cardiac inotropic effect of amrinone is identical to that of theophylline, another phosphodiesterase inhibitor

(3) the infusion rate of amrinone should be decreased in the setting of renal failure

(4) amrinone prolongs conduction in the AV node

196. In the family of drugs used to control vascular resistance and capacitance, agents that directly relax vascular smooth muscle include

(1) sodium nitroprusside

(2) clonidine

(3) hydralazine

(4) labetalol

197. Absolute contraindications to placement of a ventricular assist device (VAD) include patients with

(1) severe peripheral vascular disease of both carotid and femoral vessels

(2) age greater than 70 years and a recent history of a thoracotomy

(3) left ventricular dysfunction secondary to coronary disease and chronic obstructive lung disease (COPD) and a recent history of cardiotomy

(4) end-stage cardiomyopathy and the recent onset of oliguria and a creatinine of 2.1 mg/dL

DIRECTIONS: Each question below contains five suggested responses. For **each** of the **five** responses listed with every question you are to respond either YES (Y) or NO (N). In a given item, **all, some, or none of the alternatives may be correct.**

198. The ejection fraction may be unreliable as a measure of evaluating myocardial contractility in which of the following conditions?

    (A) Acute aortic regurgitation
    (B) Acute mitral regurgitation
    (C) Acute hypertension
    (D) Chronic hypertension
    (E) Chronic mitral regurgitation

199. True statements regarding the high cardiac output state associated with anemia include which of the following?

    (A) Many patients with heart failure due to anemia have underlying heart disease
    (B) In anemia, cardiac output is usually increased when the hemoglobin is 9 g/dL of blood
    (C) Heart failure from anemia alone is unlikely unless the hemoglobin is below 5 g/dL of blood
    (D) Beta blockade prevents the increase of cardiac output with anemia
    (E) Rapid correction of anemia should be instituted for congestive heart failure (CHF) secondary to anemia

200. True statements regarding the treatment of heart failure include which of the following?

    (A) Patients with heart failure should be urged to continue to exercise up to their symptomatic limit
    (B) The SOLVD trial showed a statistically significant reduction in mortality in the group treated with enalapril
    (C) In the SAVE trial, the group treated with captopril exhibited a statistically significant reduced mortality during follow-up
    (D) Aneurysmectomy significantly improves left ventricular performance in the majority of patients
    (E) Patients with a dilated cardiomyopathy and heart failure should be anticoagulated in the absence of a specific contraindication

201. Correct statements regarding drug interactions with digoxin include which of the following?

    (A) Both cholestyramine and metoclopromide decrease the bioavailability of digoxin administered orally and lower serum digoxin levels
    (B) Both erythromycin and tetracycline cause elevation of serum digoxin levels when digoxin is administered orally
    (C) Amiodarone decreases the serum concentration of digoxin
    (D) Digoxin-specific sheep Fab antibody fragments promptly cause a marked decrease in serum digoxin levels
    (E) In patients with renal failure, the digoxin-Fab antibody complex may dissociate, causing renewed intoxication

202. True statements regarding cardiac inotropic agents include

    (A) all the catecholamine derivatives exert a positive inotropic effect by altering myosin ATPase activity
    (B) all the catecholamine derivatives except dobutamine have some alpha$_1$-adrenergic receptor stimulation
    (C) unlike isoproterenol and dopamine, dobutamine has very little positive chronotropic effect on the heart
    (D) although amrinone acts primarily as a phosphodiesterase inhibitor, it also possesses direct arteriolar vasodilating properties that improve cardiac output
    (E) amrinone generally causes tachycardia and significant lowering of blood pressure

203. Which of the following statements characterize angiotensin-converting enzyme (ACE) inhibitors?

(A) The primary mode of action to inhibit vasoconstriction is by inhibiting the production of the vasoactive decapeptide angiotensin I

(B) ACE inhibitors have a vasodilator effect that lowers systemic vascular resistance

(C) ACE inhibitors have a natriuretic effect that inhibits aldosterone secretion

(D) A secondary effect of ACE inhibitors is to stimulate bradykinin production directly for an additional vasodilator effect

(E) The currently available ACE inhibitors enalapril and lisinopril have an active sulfhydryl group as part of their structure

IV. Heart Failure

Answers

169. The answer is B. *(p 495)*   An adult with symptoms of significant aortic stenosis (i.e., dyspnea, angina pectoris, or syncope) in whom echocardiographic features suggest critical aortic stenosis should have cardiac catheterization performed promptly. Cardiac catheterization not only confirms that critical aortic valve narrowing is present but can also assess further left ventricular function. In men over 35 years of age, coronary angiography is indicated to search for concomitant coronary atherosclerosis. Generally, if critical aortic stenosis is present in a symptomatic patient, aortic valve replacement should be performed after a thorough preoperative evaluation. Exercise testing in a patient with severe aortic stenosis could be quite hazardous. Abnormal exercise-induced ST changes could be due to either concomitant coronary disease or left ventricular hypertrophy due to the aortic stenosis, making depression of the ST segment with exercise nondiagnostic.

170. The answer is B. *(p 487)*   Left-sided heart failure is evidenced by the presence of abnormally elevated left-sided filling pressures sufficient to cause pulmonary venous congestion on chest roentgenogram and rales on auscultation of the chest. In addition, a low cardiac index (less than 2.4 liters/min/m^2) is supportive evidence of heart failure. In heart failure, the heart is unable to produce a normal increase in cardiac output with exercise. This is reflected by an abnormally low maximum oxygen consumption determined noninvasively during exercise. Poor left ventricular function at rest determined by echocardiography is usually present. Abnormal ventricular function at rest does not necessarily indicate that overall heart failure is present, nor does the absence of overall cardiac failure necessarily mean that ventricular function is normal.

171. The answer is A. *(p 493)*   Resting stage measurements of left ventricular function include the ejection fraction, fractional shortening, and the mean circumferential shortening. The ejection fraction, the percentage of the end-diastolic volume that is ejected, is normally greater than 55 percent. The percentage shortening of the ventricular end-diastolic diameter, or fractional shortening, should be greater than 28 percent normally. The mean velocity of internal diameter or circumferential fiber shortening should be greater than 1.2 circumferences per second. These "ejection phase" measures are sensitive to changes in afterload. These measurements can be determined noninvasively and are comparable to those made with angiography.

172. The answer is C. *(p 492)*   The response to exercise is determined primarily by the exercise cardiac output. However, other factors, including adaptation of the skeletal muscles, adaptation of the peripheral vascular beds, cardiovascular reflexes, motivation, and drug therapy, can also affect exercise tolerance.

173. The answer is C. *(p 438)*   Exercise capacity can be determined from the maximum work load achieved by the patient and is highly useful for evaluating the significance of symptoms in chronic cardiomyopathy objectively. Respiratory gas exchange during exercise provides a useful approach for characterizing cardiac function class based on maximum oxygen consumption. The maximum oxygen consumption equals the product of the cardiac output and the arteriovenous oxygen difference. Exercise testing with measurement of respiratory gas exchange is useful when making decisions concerning cardiac transplantation and also for following responses to vasodilator therapy in chronic heart failure.

174. **The answer is A.** *(p 504)* The heart rate at rest is usually slightly increased in the range of 85 to 110 beats per minute. A cervical venous hum over the internal jugular vein is commonly heard. The pulse pressure is typically wide. Pistol-shot sounds and Duroziez's murmur may be heard over the femoral arteries, and carotid artery bruits are often present. A midsystolic murmur may be present over the second or third intercostal space. A third (S_3) and fourth (S_4) heart sound can be heard.

175. **The answer is C.** *(p 503)* Hyperthyroidism, systemic arteriovenous fistula, anemia, and beriberi are among the causes of high cardiac output states, many of which are curable. However, these conditions may cause congestive heart failure (CHF) that is refractory to conventional therapy. In patients with reduced afterload, vasodilator therapy for CHF may aggravate the condition. The increased cardiac output in these states is primarily a result of increased cardiac output and reduced left ventricular afterload.

176. **The answer is C.** *(p 515)* Circulatory failure is inadequacy of the cardiovascular system in providing nutrition to the cells of the body and inadequate retrieval of breakdown by-products of metabolism. The causes may be either cardiac (pump failure) or noncardiac. Noncardiac causes include inadequate oxyhemoglobin, inadequate blood volume, increased capacity of the vascular system, and peripheral vascular abnormalities.

   Circulatory congestion is excess blood volume from either cardiac or noncardiac causes. Noncardiac causes include conditions in which there is an increase in blood volume (salt-retaining steroids, excess fluid administration, and renal insufficiency) and then conditions in which there is increased venous return or decreased peripheral resistance (AV fistulae, beriberi, severe anemia, and end-stage cirrhosis).

177. **The answer is C.** *(p 519)* *Left heart failure* and *right heart failure* are clinical terms used for conditions in which the primary impairment is of the left side or of the right side of the heart, respectively. These are very useful conceptual terms, but we must recognize that the heart is a circuit and it is apparent that one side cannot pump significantly more than the other side for any length of time in the absence of shunts or other abnormal communications. Experimentally produced pure failure of one ventricle may produce hemodynamic and biochemical abnormalities of the other ventricle even without the usual hemodynamic manifestations of ventricular failure. The pericardium restrains both right and left ventricles and contributes to ventricular interdependence. This is most purely seen in cases of cardiac tamponade. With an intact pericardium, increases in diastolic pressure in one ventricle may influence the diastolic pressure in the other—a reverse Bernheim phenomenon. The most common cause of right heart failure is left heart failure. In patients with progressive right heart failure, the most striking clinical finding is that of elevated central venous pressure with increased jugular venous pressure, as well as ascites and edema.

178. **The answer is A.** *(pp 559–560)* In the past, hypertension has been one of the most common cofactors in the development of heart failure. Effective therapy of hypertension has greatly reduced the incidence of hypertension as a primary cause of heart failure in many populations. In the early stages of left ventricular dysfunction, a shift downward and to the right of the Frank-Starling curve occurs (i.e., there is a lower stroke volume for any given filling pressure). The performance of the ventricle becomes progressively more impaired as afterload is increased. Therefore, a shift occurs from a preload-dependent and afterload-independent ventricle in the normal heart to a preload-independent and afterload-dependent ventricle in the setting of heart failure. Patients with diastolic dysfunction appear to have a better prognosis than patients with systolic dysfunction. Patients with left ventricular dilatation can generate a greater stroke volume and thus maintain cardiac output than would be possible if the amount of fiber shortening were constant and the volume of the ventricle smaller.

179. The answer is D. *(pp 637–642)* Although problems can arise in diagnosis due to small sample size and variable pathological interpretations, endomyocardial biopsy can obtain myocardial samples reliably and safely for diagnosis. Specific pathological findings and staining techniques permit identification of certain disorders, including carcinoid heart disease, allograft rejection, amyloidosis, hemochromatosis, sarcoidosis, cardiac tumors, and endocardial fibroelastosis. Although myocyte hypertrophy and occasionally some fibrosis can be seen in idiopathic dilated cardiomyopathy, there are no pathognomonic histological or biochemical features using current methods.

180. The answer is D. *(pp 573–576)* Digoxin is unstable in highly acidic solutions and may be inactivated by hydrolysis if delayed gastric emptying is present with an intragastric pH of less than 2. About 10 percent of patients demonstrate extensive intestinal metabolism of digoxin to inactive dihydro derivatives, causing high digoxin requirements. This may be partially corrected by use of an encapsulated, highly bioavailable preparation of liquid digoxin. Patients with malabsorption due to short-bowel syndrome or jejunoileal bypass do not have poor absorption of digoxin tablets. The mechanism of the inotropic effect of digoxin is unclear. Digoxin binds to the sodium (Na^+), potassium (K^+)–activated membrane adenosine triphosphatase (ATPase) of the heart, which may lead directly to increased calcium (Ca^{2+}) influx. It is also possible that ATPase-binding causes a decrease in Na^+-pump activity, leading to an increased intracellular Ca^{2+}. The next result is an increased intracellular concentration of Na^+, which favors an exchange for extracellular Ca^{2+}, causing an inotropic effect. Digoxin enhances parasympathetic activity by a number of mechanisms. It increases arterial baroreceptor reflex such that afferent signals are augmented, resulting in increased vagal tone and decreased sympathetic tone. Digoxin also increases the sensitivity of the cardiac fibers to acetylcholine. These parasympathomimetic effects account for the efficacy of digoxin in supraventricular arrhythmias. Digoxin also causes contraction of isolated human arteries and veins. This is blocked by Ca^{2+} antagonists but not by α-adrenergic blockade. The net result is increased coronary systemic and pulmonary vascular resistance, which may worsen heart failure, especially if digoxin is given as a bolus.

181. The answer is D. *(p 601)* Hyperkalemia is a side effect of potassium-sparing diuretics. Patients with diabetes and renal insufficiency are more prone to life-threatening hyperkalemia. Physicians should avoid the concurrent administration of angiotensin-converting enzyme (ACE) inhibitors, potassium-sparing diuretics, and potassium supplements. Even though these diuretics also inhibit hydrogen ion (H) excretion, metabolic acidosis is rare. Gynecomastia is a common complication of spironolactone administration.

182. The answer is B. *(pp 599–600)* Thiazide diuretics are associated with hypokalemia. They can increase serum cholesterol by 10 percent and reduce the urinary excretion of calcium (Ca^{2+}) by 40 to 50 percent. Hyperuricemia occurs in thiazide-treated patients due to circulatory volume contraction. Hyperglycemia is also associated with thiazide diuretics.

183. The answer is A. *(p 600)* Thiazide diuretics are relatively inexpensive and orally active. Disadvantages of thiazide diuretics include frequent metabolic side effects and a lower potency than loop diuretics in inducing salt and water exertion. Low doses of thiazide diuretics can be useful as adjunctive agents in hypertension, thus avoiding some of the metabolic side effects of the drug. Thiazides become less effective in renal insufficiency at a serum creatinine above 3 mg/dL.

184. The answer is C. *(p 625)* Inflation of a balloon pump during diastole displaces a volume of blood equal to balloon volume, thus raising aortic diastolic pressure and augmenting coronary perfusion. Thus, patients with unstable angina unresponsive to medical therapy will benefit. Deflation during systole allows the heart to pump against a reduced arterial impedance, thus benefiting patients with cardiomyopathy and patients with mitral regurgitation. Patients with a ventricular septal defect improve by increased ventricular function and by decreasing the left-to-right shunt. Intra-aortic pump insertion is contraindicated in patients with acute aortic regurgitation because of the bacterial endocarditis and because diastolic inflation increases the aortic regurgitation.

185. The answer is C. *(pp 633–635)* Without immunosuppressive agents, such as azathioprine, cyclosporine and prednisone, localized graft rejection due to lymphoid infiltration of the cardiac muscle occurs. Recognized side effects of all immunosuppressive agents administered chronically include an increased incidence of lymphoproliferative malignancies and opportunistic infections. Accelerated graft coronary disease occurs in long-term cardiac allograft graft survivors and is an independent process from cardiac muscle rejection. Compared to naturally occurring atherosclerosis, the process tends to be more diffuse and involves even small penetrating intramyocardial vessels. Long-term cyclosporine use is associated with hypertension and nephrotoxicity. Prednisone use is associated with glucose intolerance, osteoporosis, cataracts, and bone fractures. Azathioprine is usually associated with dose-related bone marrow suppression.

186. The answer is D. *(pp 630–631)* Excellent pediatric cardiac transplant programs are now able to offer transplantation to younger patients, even neonates with irreparable heart disease. The excellent results of cardiac transplants in older age-groups have expanded the upper age limits from 50 to 55 years of age to above age 60 in patients who have no other problems and are physiologically younger than their chronological age. Insulin-dependent diabetes is considered a major contraindication by most programs due to the accelerated cerebrovascular and renal disease in these patients. However, diet-controlled diabetic patients without end-organ damage are not excluded from consideration merely on that basis. Concomitant illnesses that decrease the likelihood of survival after transplantation or predispose to complications, such as infection or acceleration of the underlying disease process, are felt to be contraindications. These include human immunodeficiency virus (HIV), chronic lung disease, severe peripheral vascular disease, and advanced hepatic or renal dysfunction.

187. The answer is B (1, 3). *(pp 504–505)* Hyperthyroidism usually increases cardiac output. The total body oxygen consumption is increased by 25 to 75 percent, and the arteriovenous oxygen difference is decreased. Systemic vascular resistance is reduced, tachycardia is present, and stroke volume may be increased, each tending to increase cardiac output. Systolic blood pressure is increased with a moderate reduction in diastolic blood pressure.

188. The answer is A (1, 2, 3). *(pp 517–518)* Many changes in chamber mechanics occur after myocardial infarction. These changes include an increase in systolic load on the normal myocardium due to the akinetic myocardium. There is a decrease in ejection fraction that approximates the amount of myocardium loss, and there is a compensatory hypertrophy of the nonischemic myocardium in patients that have myocardial infarctions to compensate for the loss of muscle mass. With increasing systolic load, there is an increase in the diastolic volume, which causes wall tension to be increased with any given pressure and the nonischemic myocardium to hypertrophy.

189. The answer is B (1, 3). *(p 518)* There are two forms of failure of the left ventricle, one due to systolic dysfunction and another due to diastolic dysfunction. Patients with increased chamber stiffness due to hypertrophy or infiltrative states tend to manifest forms of diastolic dysfunction. Diastolic dysfunction in the absence of systolic dysfunction occurs in systemic arterial hypertension and hypertrophic myopathy. Myocarditis and congestive cardiomyopathy usually are manifested by combined systolic and diastolic dysfunction. Patients with hypertension and hypertrophic myopathy can develop systemic dysfunction at end-stage.

190. The answer is D (4). *(p 558)* Both systolic and diastolic dysfunction are early manifestations of myocardial ischemia since even modest reduction of blood flow may deprive the myocardium of adequate nutrition for generation of muscle contraction and muscle relaxation. In humans the induction of ischemia through obstruction of a coronary artery results in a loss of contraction in the region involved. If blood flow is restored to the region before necrosis occurs, contractile activity does not return for hours or days. This persistent loss of contractile activity despite return of blood flow and the absence of necrosis is termed *stunning*. *Hibernating myocardium* refers to myocardium with a contractile dysfunction resulting from a chronic inadequacy of blood flow without histologic evidence of myocardial infarction. Ventricular remodeling is an adaptive process in which the ventricle is reshaped by structural changes; it results in an increased chamber volume and increased myocardial mass.

191. The answer is A (1, 2, 3). *(pp 560–561)* In the setting of left ventricular dysfunction, neurohormonal systems are activated regardless of the etiology. Activation of the sympathetic nervous system occurs and is manifested by elevated plasma norepinephrine levels. The renin-angiotensin system also becomes activated in heart failure. Arginine vasopressin, or antidiuretic hormone, also is increased in many patients with heart failure. Atrial natriuretic peptide, a hormone released from the atrium, circulates in higher than normal levels in patients with heart failure. There is also evidence for an increased level of endothelin, which is a potent vasoconstrictor released by the endothelium. Release of other tissue hormones is impaired, such as endothelial-derived relaxing factor (EDRF) and nitric oxide, which is a potent vasorelaxing factor.

192. The answer is D (4). *(pp 561–562)* In patients with heart failure, estimation of end-diastolic volume, especially as it changes with time, is an important marker of the course of heart failure. In general the separation of disability due to heart disease from that due to physical deconditioning in a patient with heart failure is a problem that can be resolved to some degree by performing gas-exchange measurements during an exercise test. A maximum oxygen consumption (V_{O_2} max) can be determined. In apparently asymptomatic patients with considerable ventricular dysfunction, a modest reduction in V_{O_2} max may be demonstrated. In the later stages of heart failure, V_{O_2} max is poorly related to ejection fraction since a major component of the limitation of exercise then results from peripheral mechanisms contributing to abnormal skeletal muscle flow and metabolism. Asymptomatic ventricular premature beats and runs of nonsustained ventricular tachycardia are common in patients with left ventricular dysfunction. It is important to keep in mind, however, that the ventricular arrhythmias contribute independently to the risk of dying from heart failure.

193. The answer is B (1, 3). *(pp 577–580)* Administration of digoxin to patients with ventricular failure often results in slowing of the sinus rate because of improvement of ventricular performance with a decrease in sympathetic tone. Digoxin can be administered to most patients with sinus bradycardia or asymptomatic sinus pauses without further decreasing sinus rate. Digoxin has little chronotropic effect on the sinoatrial (SA) node. However, in the presence of sick sinus syndrome, digoxin may lengthen the sinus node recovery and SA conduction time and may cause an exacerbation of symptoms. Digitalis modifies the critical relation between the conduction time and the refractory period of the slow and fast pathways in the atrioventricular (AV) node and can terminate paroxysmal supraventricular tachycardia (PSVT). However, because of its short half-life and high efficacy, intravenous adenosine is probably the current drug of choice for terminating PSVT. The arrhythmogenic effects of digoxin are complex; possible mechanisms include delayed afterpotentials and intracellular calcium (Ca^{2+}) overload. The magnitude of delayed afterpotentials and susceptibility to triggered activity may be enhanced in the presence of ischemia at digoxin concentrations that are not toxic in the absence of ischemia. One study of myocardial infarction and cardiac failure demonstrated that dobutamine markedly increased cardiac output, decreased filling pressure, and relieved pulmonary congestion, whereas digoxin did not affect either preload or afterload. Thus, an inotropic drug in combination with a diuretic is preferred therapy for patients with an acute infarct and congestive heart failure (CHF).

194. The answer is C (2, 4). *(pp 591–592)* There are no specific dobutamine receptors. There are, however, specific dopaminergic receptors in both the mesenteric and renal vascular beds that are responsible for arterial vasodilatation when dopamine is used in low doses. Infusion of dopamine at 3 µg/kg/min or less may lead to dopaminergic renal arterial vasodilation and increased renal blood flow and thus promote sodium excretion. In the setting of acute myocardial infarction complicated by significant hypotension, dobutamine is not the inotropic agent of choice. Stimulation of beta$_2$ receptors that occurs with dobutamine may be detrimental. Dopamine or norepinephrine may be required in this setting to maintain adequate blood pressure through alpha$_1$ vasoconstriction. Beta$_2$ receptors result in arteriolar vasodilation. Dobutamine does not overtly worsen myocardial ischemia. It reduces left ventricular filling pressure and decreases heart size.

This offsets the increased myocardial contractility occurring with dobutamine such that increased myocardial oxygen requirements resulting from increased contractility are balanced by decreased oxygen requirements resulting from decreased filling pressure. Infusion of dobutamine for short periods of time may result in long-term improvement of cardiac function in patients with congestive heart failure. Down regulation of beta receptors in the failing myocardium affects primarily beta$_1$ receptors, while the sensitivity and number of beta$_2$ receptors are only minimally affected. Thus activation of the beta$_2$ receptor may be responsible for a substantial portion of the inotropic actions of dobutamine. The fate of beta$_2$ receptors after long-term administration of dobutamine is unknown. The mechanisms of prolonged clinical benefits of dobutamine after termination of infusion are probably related to long-lasting effects on the peripheral circulation rather than on the myocardium.

195. The answer is B (1, 3). *(pp 592–593)* The activity of the phosphodiesterase type III inhibitors appears to be more selective within the cardiac cell than that of theophylline, which may contribute to the relatively greater inotropic action of amrinone compared with theophylline. The positive inotropic action of the phosphodiesterase type III agents may result from increased sensitivity of contractile proteins for Ca^{2+}. Of therapeutic interest, the positive inotropic actions of these phosphodiesterase type III agents may vary with the level of cyclic AMP present in the cardiac cell and may therefore be more apparent after beta$_1$-adrenergic stimulation. The concomitant use of amrinone with dobutamine may therefore have a synergistic inotropic cardiac effect and improve cardiac output more than dobutamine alone. Amrinone is metabolized via conjugative pathways. Up to 40 percent of amrinone is excreted unchanged in the urine. Therapy with amrinone should be initiated with an intravenous bolus of from 0.75 to 3 mg/kg and followed by a continuous infusion at a rate of from 4 to 10 μg/kg/min. In patients with severe renal insufficiency, the rate of infusion should be decreased to prevent toxic plasma levels and adverse reactions such as hypotension and ventricular arrhythmias. Amrinone shortens the functional refractory period and the conduction time of the canine AV node.

196. The answer is B (1, 3). *(pp 613–617, Tables 30-2 and 30-3)* Drugs that directly relax vascular smooth muscle include nitrates, sodium nitroprusside, hydralazine, minoxidil, and diazoxide. Clonidine has a central inhibitory effect by stimulating central alpha$_2$ receptors, resulting in decreased sympathetic outflow and reduced sympathetic vasoconstrictor activity. Guanabenz and guanfacine also have a similar action. Labetalol is a beta-adrenoceptor blocker, which also exerts alpha-adrenoceptor blocking activity.

197. The answer is B (1, 3). *(pp 624–625)* Ventricular assist devices (VADs) are approved for recovery support after open heart surgery, myocardial infarction, or transplantation, and as bridging support in patients with refractory heart failure who are candidates for cardiac transplantation. Primary cerebrovascular disease, malignancy, chronic obstructive lung disease (COPD), liver failure, blood dyscrasia, and concomitant infection are exclusion criteria for placement of a VAD. In transplant patients, infection, renal insufficiency, and respiratory failure all predict a negative outcome but are not absolute contraindications with some devices. Likewise, age above 70 and renal insufficiency predict a poor outcome in postcardiotomy patients after VAD implantation.

198. The answers are: A-Y, B-Y, C-Y, D-Y, E-Y. *(p 493)* In acute mitral regurgitation or aortic regurgitation, in acute hypertension and in long-standing hypertension, the ejection fraction may become unreliable for evaluating myocardial contractility since a reduced ejection fraction may be secondary to afterload mismatch. The systolic unloading of the left ventricle in chronic mitral regurgitation may yield a normal ejection fraction when myocardial contractility is actually depressed.

199. The answers are: A-Y, B-N, C-Y, D-N, E-N. *(pp 507–508)* Patients who have an underlying hyperdynamic state and congestive heart failure (CHF) often have underlying heart disease. Cardiac output may be increased in anemia but usually not until the hemoglobin is below 7 g/dL of blood. Patients rarely develop heart failure from anemia alone unless the hemoglobin is below 5g/dL of blood. The increased cardiac output is primarily due to reduced peripheral vascular resistance, though contractility is increased somewhat. Beta blockade does not prevent the increased cardiac output associated with anemia. CHF caused by anemia should be treated with diuretics and sodium (Na+) restriction. The anemia should be corrected gradually as transfusing packed red blood cells too rapidly may cause pulmonary edema.

200. The answers are: A-Y, B-N, C-Y, D-N, E-N. *(pp 568–570)* Patients with heart failure should be encouraged to exercise. Whereas in the past patients with heart failure were told to lead a sedentary existence, it is now common practice to advise patients to exercise up to their symptomatic limits. Studies have explored the use of ACE inhibitors in patients with left ventricular dysfunction. In the Studies of Left Ventricular Dysfunction (SOLVD) trial, over 4,000 patients within an ejection fraction of less than 35 percent in the absence of heart failure symptoms were randomly assigned to placebo or enalapril therapy. The trend toward reduction in total mortality in the group treated with enalapril did not reach statistical significance, but there was a striking delay in the onset of overt congestive heart failure in that group. In the Survival and Ventricular Enlargement Trial (SAVE) over 2,000 patients from 3 to 16 days after an acute myocardial infarction and with an ejection fraction of less than 40 percent were randomly assigned to receive placebo or captopril therapy. The group treated with captopril exhibited a statistically significant reduced mortality during follow-up. In patients with a left ventricular aneurysm, aneurysmectomy often combined with coronary artery bypass surgery may significantly improve left ventricular performance, but only in selected patients. In patients with heart failure (in the absence of atrial fibrillation and especially when patients are fairly active), there appears to be no strong indication for anticoagulation unless a previous thrombotic event has occurred. The decision to anticoagulate should be individualized.

201. The answers are: A-Y, B-Y, C-N, D-N, E-Y. *(pp 580–581)* Many drugs interact with digoxin, causing marked changes in serum levels and bioavailability. Cholestyramine binds digoxin when orally administered and may lower effective digoxin levels. By administering cholestyramine 8 hours after digoxin, this effect can be avoided. Metoclopromide increases intestinal motility and decreases the bioavailability of digoxin. Both erythromycin and tetracycline inactivate gut flora and increase the bioavailability of digoxin, leading to elevated levels. Amiodarone decreases renal and total body clearance of digoxin and may lead to markedly elevated digoxin levels; in general, the digoxin dose should be decreased by one-half when these drugs are administered together. Presently, the treatment of choice for massive digoxin overdose is administration of digoxin-specific Fab fragment antibodies that bind and neutralize both digoxin and digitoxin. These Fab fragments bind to digoxin and rapidly accelerate the removal of digoxin from cellular membranes. A dramatic rise in serum digoxin levels ensues, but this digoxin is bound and, therefore, pharmacologically inactive. Fab fragments have a low molecular weight, and rapid renal excretion of digoxin bound to these fragments ensues, resulting in a half-life of digoxin of less than 5 hours. The safety and efficacy of these fragments are documented. Immunogenicity may be a problem if the patient requires a second dose at a later date. In patients with renal failure, the half-life of the Fab fragments may be as high as 330 hours. After administration of Fab fragments to patients with renal failure, plasmapheresis can remove the antigen-antibody complexes, thus minimizing the later return of toxicity.

202. The answers are: A-N, B-N, C-Y, D-Y, E-N. *(pp 589–593)* It is unlikely that inotropic agents exert their effect by altering myosin ATPase activity because of their rapid onset of action. It is generally believed that positive inotropic action is mediated by increased delivery of calcium at the contractile apparatus or increased affinity of the contractile apparatus for calcium. For example, norepinephrine attaches to cell-surface inotropic receptors and activates adenylcyclase. This catalyzes the conversion of ATPase to $3'5'$-cyclic AMP. This leads to an increased number of calcium channels resulting in increased calcium flux into the cell. The synthetic catecholamine dobutamine appears to be the ideal agent to use as an inotrope in the setting of acute myocardial infarction. It exerts strong beta$_1$-receptor stimulation with mild beta$_2$-agonist activity. It also possesses alpha$_1$-agonist activity but this is less than that of dopamine or norepinephrine. The only catecholamine derivative that possesses alpha$_1$ activity is isoproterenol (Isuprel). Unlike dopamine or norepinephrine, dobutamine has very little chronotropic effect and the mechanism of this is not well understood. Amrinone is a phosphodiesterase inhibitor and leads to increased intracellular cyclic AMP and consequent positive inotropic action. This agent also possesses arteriolar dilating properties that are enhanced by other vasodilators. Thus, even in patients experiencing minimal improvement in cardiac contractility, arteriolar vasodilation induced by amrinone substantially improves left ventricular performance. Myocardial oxygen requirements are diminished by these beneficial hemodynamic effects. Amrinone improves cardiac output and diminishes left ventricular filling pressure in patients with heart failure without causing tachycardia or changes in blood pressure.

203. The answers are: A-N, B-Y, C-Y, D-N, E-N. *(p 618)* Angiotensin-converting enzyme (ACE) inhibitors act by inhibiting the production of the strong vasoactive octapeptide angiotensin II from the decapeptide angiotensin I. Suppression of angiotensin II, a potent constrictor of arteriolar resistance vessels, results in a significant vasodilatory effect, which lowers systemic vascular resistance. In addition, ACE inhibitors have a natriuretic effect by inhibiting aldosterone secretion. A secondary vasodilatory effect is provided by the inhibition of bradykinin degradation (not the direct stimulation), which results in increasing levels of circulating bradykinin. The currently available ACE inhibitors are somewhat different in their individual structures and pharmacokinetic actions. Captopril is the only one that has a sulfhydryl group as part of its structure.

V. Disorders of Rhythm or Conduction

DIRECTIONS: Each question below contains five suggested responses. Select the **one best** response to each question.

204. Identify the cardiac abnormality illustrated in the electrocardiogram (ECG) below, and choose the correct first line of treatment.

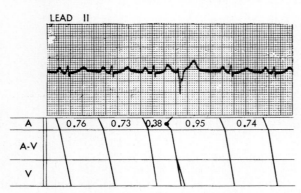

(A) Premature atrial depolarization (beta blocker)
(B) Premature atrial depolarization (amiodarone)
(C) Premature atrial depolarization (reassurance)
(D) Premature ventricular depolarization (sotalol)
(E) Premature ventricular depolarization (procainamide)

205. The rhythm strip below illustrates

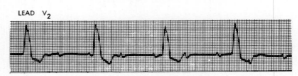

(A) first-degree AV block
(B) type I second-degree AV block
(C) type II second-degree AV block
(D) complete third-degree atrioventricular (AV) block
(E) accelerated junctional rhythm

206. The phase of the cardiac Purkinje fiber action potential that represents slow repolarization is

(A) phase 0
(B) phase 1
(C) phase 2
(D) phase 3
(E) phase 4

207. All the following statements concerning the rhythm strip below are true EXCEPT

MONITOR LEAD

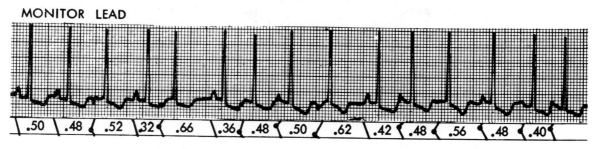

(A) it may be seen in a patient with chronic obstructive pulmonary disease (COPD)
(B) it may be seen in a patient whose aminophylline level is 25 μm/dL (normal 10–20 μm/dL)
(C) it illustrates an automatic mechanism
(D) it illustrates a reentrant mechanism
(E) it exhibits varying degrees of atrioventricular (AV) block

208. The rhythm strip shown below has which of the following characteristics?

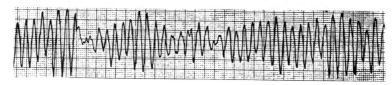

(A) Its mechanism is due to triggered activity
(B) It is seen as a complication of patients with Romano-Ward syndrome
(C) It is seen as a complication in patients with Lown-Ganong-Levine syndrome
(D) It is seen as a complication of patients who have an intracranial lesion
(E) It is seen as a complication of phenothiazine therapy

---

209. The dominant pacemaker rate of the heart is the

(A) atrial pacemaker rate of 20 to 40 beats per minute
(B) ventricular pacemaker rate of 60 beats per minute
(C) sinus node rate of 60 to 100 beats per minute
(D) atrioventricular (AV) nodal rate of 20 beats per minute
(E) His-Purkinje rate of 20 beats per minute

210. Select the arrhythmogenic mechanism below that is correctly matched with the electrical stimulation that identifies it.

(A) Automaticity and termination by overdrive pacing
(B) Reentry and initiation by electrical stimulation
(C) Delayed afterdepolarization–triggered activity and entrainment during overdrive pacing
(D) Early afterdepolarization–triggered activity and entrainment during overdrive pacing
(E) Automaticity and initiation by overdrive pacing

211. The electrocardiographic (ECG) tracing below is most compatible with

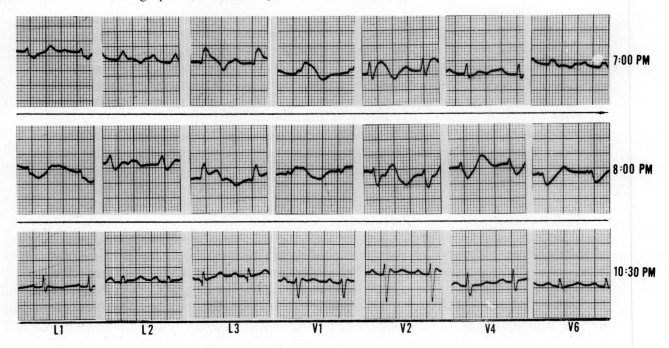

(A)   acute myocardial infarction
(B)   dilated cardiomyopathy
(C)   pericarditis
(D)   hyperkalemia
(E)   supraventricular arrhythmia

212. The electrocardiogram (ECG) tracing below is most compatible with the diagnosis of

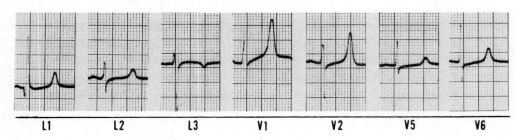

(A)   hypocalcemia
(B)   hypercalcemia
(C)   hyperkalemia
(D)   hyperkalemia and hypocalcemia
(E)   hyperkalemia and hypercalcemia

213. A 65-year-old man with a history of hypertension and known left bundle branch block (LBBB) presents with symptoms suggestive of an acute myocardial infarction. Electrocardiogram (ECG) shows more pronounced ST elevation in the anterior anterolateral leads than at baseline. The patient is treated with thrombolytics, aspirin, heparin, and nitroglycerine. His blood pressure is 140/70, and his heart rate is 80 and regular. All the following actions are indicated EXCEPT

(A) intravenous metoprolol followed by oral metoprolol
(B) temporary intravenous bipolar pacing wire
(C) initiation of an angiotensin-converting enzyme (ACE) inhibitor to minimize left ventricular remodeling
(D) admission to an intensive care unit (ICU)
(E) immediate catheterization and revascularization if pain does not respond to thrombolytics

214. A 42-year-old man develops Lyme disease. He presents to the emergency room with complete heart block, hypotension, and lightheadedness. The cardiologist places a transvenous pacemaker without difficulty. The next morning, the nurse notes a change in the paced QRS axis, but the leads were not changed nor was the monitor switched on. Which of the following causes should be suspected?

(A) New development of a left bundle branch block (LBBB)
(B) Ventricular tachycardia
(C) Migration of the pacing lead and impending dislodgement
(D) Inadvertent decrease in the pacemaker output
(E) Oversensing of a native QRS complex

215. Inappropriate ventricular pacing can lead to ventricular fibrillation when the ventricular spike occurs during the vulnerable period of the T wave. All the following conditions are associated with low fibrillation thresholds EXCEPT

(A) digitalis toxicity
(B) acutely after valve replacement surgery
(C) sick sinus syndrome
(D) acute myocardial infarction
(E) acutely after coronary bypass grafting

216. In a patient with a unipolar temporary pacing lead, which of the following tools can be used to indicate perforation of the pacing tip?

(A) Making the pacemaker less sensitive and seeing if it continues to pace
(B) Recordings made from the lead with an alligator clip connected between the lead and V_1 lead of the electrocardiogram (ECG) showing ST inversion on the tip electrode
(C) Switching the left arm lead with the pacing lead and seeing if the ST vector points towards the septum
(D) Sudden decrease in the pacing threshold
(E) Lack of motion of the ring artifact on the portable chest roentgenogram

217. All the following are indications for temporary cardiac pacing EXCEPT

(A) new-onset right bundle with left axis deviation in association with an acute anteroseptal infarct
(B) new-onset complete atrioventricular (AV) block with stable blood pressure in the setting of an acute inferior infarct
(C) symptomatic bradycardia associated with infranodal block
(D) torsades de pointes associated with drug-induced QT prolongation
(E) atrial pacing following cardiac surgery

218. Correct preprocedural interventions prior to cardioversion include all the following EXCEPT

(A) hypokalemia should be corrected to prevent arrhythmic complications
(B) elective cardioversion should be deferred for 72 hours prior to the procedure if the patient takes digitalis regularly
(C) elective cardioversion should be deferred if digitalis excess is suspected until the problem is corrected
(D) elective cardioversion should be done in the morning after an overnight fast
(E) the patient should be observed for 24 hours on a monitor to avoid complications, especially when drug toxicity is suspected

219. Correct statements concerning anticoagulation following cardioversion include all the following EXCEPT

(A) anticoagulation with warfarin for 3 weeks in a patient with atrial fibrillation is indicated prior to cardioversion in the setting of chronic atrial fibrillation
(B) prior to cardioversion, a prothrombin time of 1.3 to 1.5 times the control level or an international normalized ratio (INR) of 2.0 to 3.0 should be maintained prior to cardioversion
(C) treatment with warfarin may be discontinued following cardioversion and the prothrombin time allowed to return slowly to baseline
(D) continued anticoagulation should be prescribed for patients with prosthetic valves or cardiomyopathy
(E) anticoagulation for 3 weeks is not considered necessary if the onset of atrial fibrillation has been present for less than 2 to 3 days

220. In cases of intractable atrial fibrillation, restoration of normal sinus rhythm, atrial transport, and reduction of thromboembolic risk may be achieved by a surgical technique such as

(A) the corridor procedure
(B) the left atrial isolation procedure
(C) the maze procedure
(D) endocardial catheter fulguration
(E) His bundle ablation

221. Correct statements regarding iatrogenic complications of electrophysiological studies include all the following EXCEPT

(A) complete heart block in patients with pre-existing left bundle branch block (LBBB) can occur during right ventricular catheterization
(B) in a patient with Wolff-Parkinson-White syndrome and paroxysmal supraventricular tachycardia (PSVT), atrial fibrillation should be initiated early to assess ventricular response over the accessory pathway
(C) patients with a prior history of atrial fibrillation are more prone to developing sustained atrial fibrillation in the laboratory
(D) the overall complication rate is very low with an almost negligible mortality when right-sided heart catheterization is done for electrophysiological studies
(E) deep venous thrombosis, pulmonary embolism, infection, pneumothorax, and perforation of cardiac chambers have been reported during electrophysiological studies

DIRECTIONS: Each question below contains four suggested responses of which **one or more** is correct. Select

A	if	**1, 2, and 3**	are correct
B	if	**1 and 3**	are correct
C	if	**2 and 4**	are correct
D	if	**4**	is correct
E	if	**1, 2, 3, and 4**	are correct

222. The cardiac action potential is characterized by which of the following statements?

   (1) Most cardiac cells have fast action potentials
   (2) Fast action potentials in the heart are generated by an inward rush of sodium (Na^+)
   (3) The Na^+ channel is blocked by tetrodotoxin
   (4) Purkinje fibers are the prime example of a slow action potential

223. The initiation and propagation of the cardiac impulse are characterized by which of the following statements?

   (1) Normally, spontaneous impulse generation is much faster in the sinus node than in the His-Purkinje system
   (2) Activation of ventricular muscle spreads from epicardium to endocardium
   (3) His bundle fibers conduct faster than atrial muscle
   (4) Atrial specialized fibers are usually capable of repetitive spontaneous self-excitation

224. Statements that accurately describe triggered action include which of the following?

   (1) It is a form of automaticity
   (2) It is one of the mechanisms responsible for cardiac arrhythmias
   (3) It can be initiated by early but not delayed afterdepolarization
   (4) It is single or repetitive firing of a cell or group of cells initiated by an afterdepolarization

225. Conditions under which early afterdepolarizations can occur include

   (1) hypokalemia
   (2) quinidine therapy
   (3) slow heart rate
   (4) amitriptyline therapy

226. Sinus bradycardia may be due to

   (1) appropriate vagal tone
   (2) increased automaticity
   (3) decreased automaticity
   (4) activation and delayed afterdepolarization

227. Reentry, an abnormality of impulse conduction, explains which of the following cardiac arrhythmias?

   (1) Ventricular tachycardia
   (2) Torsades de pointes
   (3) Atrial flutter
   (4) Preexcitation

228. The clinical situations represented by the lead II rhythm strip below could include

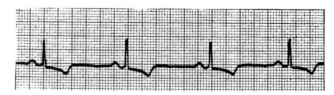

   (1) a well-trained athlete
   (2) a patient with inferior wall myocardial infarction
   (3) a patient with increased intracranial pressure
   (4) a patient taking antihistamines containing ephedrine

229. Anticoagulation in patients with atrial fibrillation is recommended

   (1)   to eliminate the possibility of embolization

   (2)   for patients with concomitant valve disease but not for patients with ischemic heart disease *and* atrial fibrillation

   (3)   for patients with no structural heart disease but with short paroxysms of atrial fibrillation

   (4)   for the persistent "lone" atrial fibrillation

230. Which of the following clinical circumstances can potentiate the cardiotoxic effect of hyperkalemia?

   (1)   Hyponatremia

   (2)   Acidosis

   (3)   Hypocalcemia

   (4)   Hypercalcemia

231. Correct statements regarding the electrophysiological effects of potassium include which of the following?

   (1)   Hyperkalemia can produce right axis deviation on the electrocardiogram (ECG)

   (2)   Hypokalemia increases the rate of repolarization of the cardiac cell

   (3)   At potassium plasma levels of 6.0 to 6.5 mEq/L, atrioventricular (AV) conduction is accelerated, but at levels of 7.5 mEq/L or higher, conduction is depressed

   (4)   With advanced hypokalemia, the T-wave amplitude decreases and may become inverted, and the ST segment becomes elevated while the U-wave amplitude increases

232. Correct statements concerning intracellular magnesium (Mg^{2+}) and the heart include which of the following?

   (1)   Intracellular Mg^{2+} deficiency may be associated with an increase in intracellular sodium (Na^+) and calcium (Ca^{2+}) and a loss of potassium (K^+)

   (2)   In patients with a prolonged QT interval and torsades de pointes, administration of intravenous magnesium sulfate may abolish the arrhythmias even if the initial Mg^{2+} level is normal

   (3)   Isolated Mg^{2+} derangements are rare

   (4)   Hypermagnesemia may predispose to digitalis toxicity

233. The use of emergency cardiac pacemaking in the presence of acute myocardial infarction is indicated in which of the following situations?

   (1)   Development of new right bundle branch block (RBBB)

   (2)   Development of a new left bundle branch block (LBBB)

   (3)   Development of a new type I second-degree atrioventricular (AV) block

   (4)   Development of a new RBBB with superior QRS axis with AV block

234. A patient has ventricular arrhythmia that is not associated with acute myocardial infarction, not due to a remediable cause, not controlled by medical therapy, and not amenable to ablation. Under which of the following conditions would an implantable cardioverter-defibrillator (ICD) be indicated?

   (1)   One or more episodes of spontaneously occurring and *inducible* ventricular fibrillation

   (2)   Spontaneously occurring but *noninducible* documented syncopal or hypotensive ventricular tachycardia

   (3)   One or more episodes of spontaneously occurring and *inducible* syncopal or hypotensive ventricular tachycardia

   (4)   Symptomatic ventricular tachycardia or ventricular fibrillation occurring within 2 days of an acute myocardial infarction

235. The rhythm strip below exhibits which of the following characteristics?

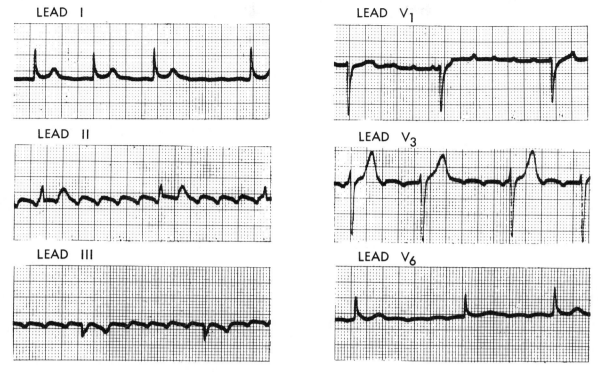

LEAD I

LEAD V₁

LEAD II

LEAD V₃

LEAD III

LEAD V₆

(1) It is commonly seen in patients with no structural heart disease
(2) It is an example of a reentry rhythm
(3) It is not influenced by rapid atrial pacing
(4) It may be converted with rapid atrial pacing

236. Use of esophageal leads in electrocardiography (ECG) may be applied to

(1) detect or confirm reentrant atrioventricular (AV) nodal tachycardia
(2) provide temporary ventricular pacing
(3) record the timing of retrograde P waves obscured by the QRS complex in the Wolff-Parkinson-White syndrome
(4) provide temporary atrial pacing

DIRECTIONS: Each question below contains five suggested responses. For **each** of the **five** responses listed with every question you are to respond either YES (Y) or NO (N). In a given item, **all, some, or none of the alternatives may be correct.**

237. The treatment of a symptomatic patient with the rhythm strips below (at baseline and during tachycardia) may involve the use of which of the following agents?

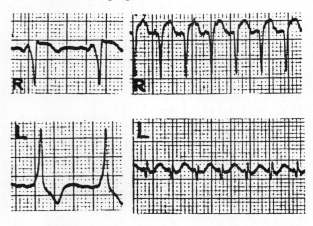

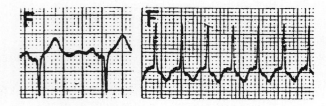

(A) Edrophonium chloride
(B) Digoxin
(C) Verapamil
(D) Propranolol
(E) Lidocaine

238. Pacemakers must be used in which of the following settings of atrioventricular (AV) block?

(A) First-degree AV heart block
(B) Type I second-degree AV block
(C) Type II second-degree AV block
(D) Acquired asymptomatic type III AV block
(E) Asymptomatic patients with a bifascicular block

239. The abnormality illustrated in the rhythm strip below

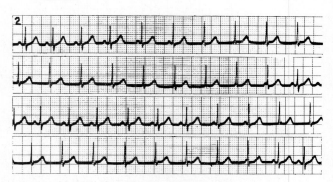

(From Marriott HJL: Workshop in electrocardiography. Tampa Tracings, 1972.)

(A) represents accelerated idioventricular rhythm
(B) is frequently seen in acute myocardial infarction
(C) is frequently seen in digitalis toxicity
(D) may be effectively treated with atropine
(E) is usually symptomatic

240. Correct statements regarding esophageal pacing include which of the following?

(A) Esophageal pacers can be used to diagnose atrial arrhythmias
(B) The patient must be intubated to use an esophageal pacing wire
(C) The esophageal pacing systems can sense but are not sufficiently capable of overdrive pacing of atrial flutter
(D) The standard esophageal pacing lead is a unipolar electrode
(E) Esophageal pacing is better suited for atrial pacing than ventricular pacing because of the geographic closeness of the left atrium to the esophagus

241. Temporary transvenous pacing wires are often inserted to treat hemodynamically significant bradyarrhythmias. Correct statements regarding the insertion of temporary pacing wires include which of the following?

(A) Standard pacing wires are typically inserted through the femoral artery into the left ventricle

(B) If a permanent pacer is to be placed using the subclavian approach, the groin should be used for placement of the transvenous pacer

(C) The insertion site should be well shaved and prepared with a sterile solution

(D) The pacing wire can be left in for 7 to 10 days before being changed

(E) Temporary atrial pacing catheters placed from the groin run a higher risk of dislodgement and loss of capture than ventricular leads

242. Correct statements regarding electrophysiological testing for conduction system disease include which of the following?

(A) Asymptomatic patients with sinus node dysfunction should be evaluated by electrophysiological studies

(B) The sinus node recovery time is the most frequently performed test to evaluate sinus node function

(C) Patients with sinus node dysfunction frequently have coexisting atrioventricular (AV) conduction problems

(D) Patients with infra-Hisian block tend to have an unpredictable course and permanent pacing is usually desirable

(E) Symptomatic patients with third-degree heart block should undergo electrophysiological testing to localize the site of the block

243. Correct statements regarding the pacemaker syndrome include which of the following?

(A) It is a physiological disturbance caused by ventricular inhibited (VVI) pacing

(B) Primary symptoms include chest pain and depression

(C) It can be caused by undesirable stimulation of the skeletal muscles

(D) The problem can be rectified by pacing the atrium prior to the ventricle

(E) The problem can be exacerbated with ventricular rate-responsive (VVIR) pacing

244. True statements regarding the evaluations of ST segments and T waves by ambulatory electrocardiography (ECG) include which of the following?

(A) Ambulatory ECG is less reliable in evaluating myocardial ischemia than cardiac arrhythmias

(B) ST-segment and T-wave changes caused by hyperventilation do not affect the interpretation of myocardial ischemia by ambulatory ECG

(C) A one-lead system is equally as effective as a two-lead system when evaluating myocardial ischemia

(D) Anxiety does not affect the interpretation of the ST segment and T wave

(E) Ambulatory ECG monitoring is superior to exercise testing in detecting Prinzmetal's variant angina

245. Correct statements regarding the technique of intracardiac electrophysiological studies include which of the following?

(A) Routine electrophysiological studies require left-sided heart catheterization

(B) Continuous heparinization is used for left-sided catheterization to avoid thromboembolic complications

(C) For the induction of ventricular tachycardia the sensitivity of different pacing protocols seems to be related directly to the number of extra stimuli used

(D) The induction of polymorphic ventricular tachycardia is a highly specific event and predicts an overall poor prognosis

(E) Incremental pacing can be used to induce a tachycardia or produce an atrioventricular (AV) block

246. Correct statements regarding the prognostic value of signal-averaged electrocardiograms (SAECGs) include

(A) patients who have an abnormal SAECG after myocardial infarction have an increased likelihood of spontaneous ventricular tachycardia or sudden cardiac death

(B) restoration of artery patency with thrombolytic therapy seems to be associated with a lower incidence of late potentials

(C) regional or global left ventricular function is independent of the presence of an abnormal SAECG

(D) most patients with abnormal SAECGs do not develop serious ventricular arrhythmias

(E) in the absence of demonstrable structural heart disease, patients with ventricular tachycardia rarely have late potentials

DIRECTIONS: Each group of questions below consists of four lettered headings followed by a set of numbered items. For each numbered item select

A	if the item is associated with	(A) **only**
B	if the item is associated with	(B) **only**
C	if the item is associated with	**both** (A) and (B)
D	if the item is associated with	**neither** (A) nor (B)

Each lettered heading may be used **once, more than once, or not at all.**

Questions 247–250

   (A)   Early afterdepolarizations
   (B)   Delayed afterdepolarizations
   (C)   Both
   (D)   Neither

247. Torsades de pointes

248. Effective termination with verapamil

249. Toxicity with type III antiarrhythmic agents

250. Digitalis toxicity

Questions 251–254

   (A)   Reentry mechanism
   (B)   Automatic mechanism
   (C)   Both
   (D)   Neither

251. Sinus tachycardia

252. Atrial tachycardia

253. Right ventricular outflow tachycardia

254. Ventricular tachycardia

Questions 255–258

   (A)   Ordered reentry
   (B)   Random reentry
   (C)   Both
   (D)   Neither

255. Atrial flutter

256. Atrial fibrillation

257. Ventricular tachycardia

258. Accelerated idioventricular rhythm

Disorders of Rhythm or Conduction

Answers

204. The answer is C. *(pp 713–714)* The rhythm strip that accompanies the question identifies a premature atrial depolarization with aberrant intraventricular conduction. Even if this is symptomatic, the best treatment is reassurance. If intervention is needed, a beta blocker may be used. Membrane-active agents such as class IA or III antiarrhythmic agents should be avoided. Correct identification of the premature beat as that originating within the atria is essential. The P wave is "buried" in the preceding T wave, and the compensatory pause is less than complete.

205. The answer is D. *(pp 748–751)* In first-degree atrioventricular (AV) block, AV conduction is prolonged (i.e., the PR interval is greater than 0.20 sec), but all impulses are conducted to the ventricle. Type I second-degree AV block is characterized by progressive AV block until a P wave fails to elicit a QRS complex. The cycle then recurs. In type II second-degree AV block, conduction usually proceeds from the sinus node to the ventricles; however, occasionally, P waves are not followed by a QRS complex. The block is infranodal (i.e., a manifestation of bilateral bundle branch block), permanent, and usually progresses to complete AV block. In complete third-degree AV block, the ventricular complexes are independent of P-wave influence and occur at a slow rate—that is, less than 45 beats per minute. The rhythm strip that accompanies the question represents a ventricle with AV disassociation. The inherent rate of the junction is 30 beats per minute; it represents a complete (third-degree) heart block. Treatment for symptomatic patients includes the use of atropine, isoproterenol (except in the setting of acute MI), and a temporary or permanent pacemaker.

206. The answer is C. *(pp 647–648)* The cardiac Purkinje fiber action potential has five phases: phase 0, rapid depolarization; phase 1, immediate rapid repolarization; phase 2, slow repolarization or plateau; phase 3, rapid repolarization; and phase 4, the diastolic interval.

207. The answer is D. *(pp 720–722)* The rhythm strip that accompanies the question is recorded from a patient with chronic obstructive pulmonary disease (COPD) and is a multiform (chaotic) atrial tachycardia. The patient also has evidence of varying atrioventricular (AV) block. The mechanism of this rhythm is automatic. It is recorded in patients with chronic lung disease, in patients with aminophylline or digoxin toxicity, and in patients with metabolic or electrolyte abnormalities. Treatment with beta or calcium channel blockers has been tried but is frequently unrewarding. The most effective treatment is correction of the underlying abnormality.

208. The answer is C. *(p 744)* The rhythm strip that accompanies the question identifies a particular form of polymorphic ventricular tachycardia called torsades de pointes (twisting of the points). The electrocardiographic (ECG) features include varying polarity of the QRS axis back and forth around the baseline. Additionally, the QT interval is prolonged. Although still debated, the current mechanism is thought to be triggered activity. Any pharmacological intervention or condition associated with prolongation of the QT interval may result in this abnormality. These include congenital prolongation of the QT interval seen in Romano-Ward or Jervell and Lange-Nielson syndromes or as a complication of increased intracranial pressure. Lown-Ganong-Levine syndrome is a form of accelerated atrioventricular conduction with a normal QRS configuration.

209. The answer is C. *(p 659)* The dominant pacemaker of the heart is in the sinus node, which fires at a rate of 60 to 100 beats per minute. The normal rate of atrial tissue, the atrioventricular (AV) node and the His-Purkinje system, is 40 to 60 beats per minute. Distal myocardial cells are capable of an intrinsic rhythm of approximately 20 to 40 beats per minute.

210. The answer is B. *(p 697)* Electrical stimulation of arrhythmias can be used frequently to identify the underlying physiological mechanism. Stimulation of an arrhythmia by electrial pacing indicates that the arrhythmia is caused by either reentry or delayed afterdepolarization–triggered activity. Termination of an arrhythmia by overdrive pacing is indicative of reentry or delayed afterdepolarization–triggered activity. Entrainment is seen with reentry mechanisms and is not expected in other mechanisms. An automatic rhythm is neither terminated nor induced by overdrive pacing.

211. The answer is D. *(pp 763–764)* The electrocardiogram (ECG) that accompanies the question illustrates the current of injury that can be seen occasionally in hyperkalemia. In this patient, the plasma potassium level was 9.1 mEq/L. The P wave is of low amplitude, and the PR is prolonged. There is a diffuse intraventricular conduction delay. The current of injury simulates acute myocardial infarction. The intraventricular conduction delay in the presence of hyperkalemia can be differentiated from the classic QRS widening of the bundle branch blocks by the fact that hyperkalemia induces uniform depression of conduction, thereby resulting in aberration of both the initial and terminal portions of the QRS complex.

212. The answer is D. *(p 769)* The electrocardiographic (ECG) tracing that accompanies the question shows a prolonged QT interval due to hypocalcemia and the tented T wave of hyperkalemia. This is characteristic of the hypocalcemia and hyperkalemia seen in chronic renal failure.

213. The answer is B. *(pp 807–808)* In the setting of an acute myocardial infarction with a known left bundle branch block (LBBB), the electrocardiogram (ECG) is often difficult to interpret. Occasionally, an immediate catheterization is necessary to confirm the diagnosis of myocardial infarction. In patients with known LBBB and an acute infarct, temporary pacing is not necessary. The risk of progression to high-grade complete atrioventricular (AV) block is low. However, the risk increases if an alternating LBBB and right bundle branch block (RBBB) are present or if a prolonged PR interval is also present. Beta blockers, angiotensin-converting enzyme (ACE) inhibitors, and admission to an intensive care unit (ICU) have all been shown to be beneficial in patients with acute myocardial infarctions.

214. The answer is C. *(p 809)* A change in the pacing axis on an ECG suggests migration of the pacing tip or impending dislodgement. On occasion, the axis can change from a left bundle to a right bundle; this suggests interventricular septal perforation of the pacing wire. One should check the insertion site for infection, check the pacing and sensing thresholds daily, and insure that all connections are tight.

215. The answer is C. *(p 809)* Temporary ventricular pacing should be set up so that the pacer is inhibited appropriately when a native QRS complex occurs. Adequate sensing in a temporary transvenous lead is just as important as in a permanent pacing system. Sensing failure of a temporary pacer can lead to pacing spikes that occur randomly throughout the cardiac cycle. When these occur on top of the T wave, ventricular fibrillation can occur. Conditions that lead to a low fibrillation threshold and make the patient more susceptible to ventricular fibrillation include digitalis toxicity, acute myocardial infarction, and acutely after cardiac surgery. The sick sinus syndrome is not associated with changes in fibrillatory thresholds.

216. The answer is B. *(pp 809–810)* Several things can suggest sudden perforation of the pacing electrode. These include loss of capture, inadequate sensing, inadequate pacing secondary to a sudden increase in the pacing threshold, a change in the paced QRS morphology. Chest roentgenogram and echocardiography are merely adjunctive tests that may or may not show lead misplacement. Unipolar recordings made from the lead with an alligator clip connected between the lead and the V_1 lead of the electrocardiogram (ECG) can be used. Normally this will show a more pronounced ST elevation on the tip than on the proximal electrode. ST inversion on the tip electrode is associated with perforation. See the figure below.

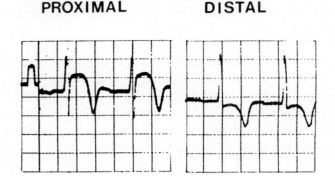

PROXIMAL   **DISTAL**

217. The answer is B. *(p 807)* Indications for temporary cardiac pacing in association with acute infarct have changed over the last decade. Multifascicular block, such as infranodal right bundle with left axis deviation associated with an anterior infarct and higher degrees of atrioventricular (AV) block associated with infarct, is an indication for temporary cardiac pacing. This type of acute-onset conduction system disease often precedes infranodal complete heart block, and an abrupt transition from 1:1 conduction to high-grade block or asystole can occur. Heart block associated with inferior myocardial infarction is often secondary to ischemia of the AV node. Usually there is a good ventricular escape, but on occasion, hemodynamically significant bradycardia can occur. If atropine does not restore the sinus mechanism and adequate blood pressure, temporary pacing may be necessary. Temporary pacemakers serve as a bridge to permanent pacing in patients with symptomatic bradycardia and can also help control ventricular tachyarrhythmias, such as torsades de pointes, in patients who have long QT syndromes or drug-induced torsades. Temporary pacing is also used after cardiac surgery to maintain an adequate cardiac output. Occasionally the atrial wires can be used to overdrive atrial flutter into normal sinus rhythm.

218. The answer is B. *(p 843)* Elective cardioversion should be performed in the morning following an overnight fast, but urgent cardioversion should be delayed as long as possible following a prior meal. Electrolytes, blood urea nitrogen (BUN), creatinine, and digoxin levels (where applicable) should be checked prior to cardioversion. Hypokalemia should be corrected, if present, to prevent complications from arrhythmias. If the patient is taking digoxin but there is no evidence of digitalis excess, the dose should be withheld only on the day of cardioversion. If digitalis excess is present, the process must be reversed prior to proceeding with elective cardioversion. Blood pressure and rhythm should be monitored for 24 hours following the procedure to avoid late arrhythmic complications, especially in the setting of digitalis, quinidine, or other antiarrhythmic drug excess.

219. The answer is C. *(pp 843–844)* Anticoagulation prior to cardioversion is recommended for atrial fibrillation but not for atrial flutter or supraventricular tachycardia (SVT) since atrial fibrillation is the arrhythmia most likely to be associated with embolism during cardioversion. Anticoagulation should be used when there are no contraindications since the incidence of emboli decreases by following this practice. Anticoagulation with warfarin should be started 3 weeks prior to elective cardioversion in a patient with chronic atrial fibrillation. The prothrombin time should be maintained at 1.3 to 1.5 times the control levels or at an international normalized ratio (INR) of 2.0 to 3.0. Following cardioversion, warfarin should be maintained for at least 4 weeks since the atria may not contract normally for several weeks despite the return of normal sinus rhythm. Anticoagulation may be continued for a greater time in patients at continued risk for emboli or recurrence of atrial fibrillation—that is, patients with prosthetic valves, cardiomyopathy, atrial or ventricular clot, or a prior history of emboli. If the atrial fibrillation is of new onset (i.e., less than 3 days), heparinization is adequate to prevent thrombus formation prior to cardioversion. Warfarin should be started if the situation is likely to recur.

220. The answer is C.   *(pp 867–868; Guiraudon, Circulation 72 (Suppl. 3): 220, 1985; Cox, J Thorac Cardiovasc Surg 101: 584–592, 1991)*   The left atrial isolation procedure is capable of confining atrial fibrillation to the left atrium, but it has not been applied routinely to control the detrimental clinical effects of atrial fibrillation. The corridor procedure introduced by Guiraudon in 1985 involves using a strip of atrial septum between the sinoatrial node and the atrioventricular (AV) node. Although helpful, this procedure only alleviates the rapid irregular ventricular response to atrial fibrillation. This procedure does not restore AV synchrony nor does it reduce the vulnerability of patients to thromboembolic phenomena. The maze procedure introduced by Cox in 1987 involves complex map-guided surgery to block atrial fibrillation foci. This procedure is able to restore AV synchrony and, thus, preserve atrial transport function. By this mechanism, it also may alleviate the possibility of thromboembolic phenomena.

221. The answer is B.   *(pp 890–891)*   Atrial fibrillation will obviously not permit study of other forms of supraventricular tachycardia (SVT); however, in patients with the Wolff-Parkinson-White syndrome and SVT, if atrial fibrillation must be initiated for diagnostic purposes, it should be performed at the end of the study. This allows complete diagnostic electrophysiological testing of the bypass tracts and supraventricular arrhythmias first. Frequently, atrial fibrillation develops during the initial placement of the catheters; therefore, excessive manipulation of catheters in the atria should be avoided. The mechanical irritation from the catheters can cause a variety of arrhythmias and conduction disturbances. In patients with underlying left bundle branch block (LBBB), complete atrioventricular (AV) block can occur as the catheter disturbs the right ventricular septum. In general, electrophysiological testing has a low complication rate; however, complications can occur even in the best laboratories. Development of electromechanical dissociation (EMD) in the laboratory should prompt a thorough search for pneumothorax or perforation of a cardiac chamber or coronary sinus.

222. The answer is A (1, 2, 3)   *(pp 647–650)*   Most cardiac cells have fast action potentials. These include the specialized atrial fibers, ventricular muscle cells, and the Purkinje fibers. The Purkinje fibers are the prime example of a fast fiber type. Fast action potentials in the heart are generated by an inward rush of sodium (Na^+) through an ionic channel that is selectively permeable to Na^+ ions when the cell activates. The Na^+ channel is blocked by tetrodotoxin, which is a channel-specific antagonist. Only one tetrodotoxin molecule binds to each Na^+ channel, and the binding has high affinity and specificity. The Na^+ channel is also blocked by many antiarrhythmic drugs with class I action.

223. The answer is B (1, 3)   *(pp 650–651)*   Normally the sinus node initiates the cardiac impulse, and the spontaneous impulse there is much faster (60 to 100 per minute) than in the His-Purkinje system (35 to 50 per minute). The specialized atrial tracts are capable of transmitting the cardiac impulse generated in the sinoatrial (SA) node to the atrioventricular (AV) node via internodal tracts. However, the specialized atrial tracts are not usually automatic; therefore, they are not capable of repetitive, spontaneous self-excitation under ordinary circumstances. Once the impulse leaves the AV node into the His bundle, conduction speeds dramatically through the bundle branches and the Purkinje network. In ventricular excitation, activation of ventricular muscle spreads from endocardium to epicardium.

224. The answer is C (2, 4).   *(p 652)*   Several mechanisms are thought to be responsible for cardiac arrhythmias. The three general categories are abnormalities of impulse generation, abnormalities of impulse conduction, and combined abnormalities of impulse generation and conduction. Triggered activity is an abnormality of impulse generation. It is not a form of automaticity; therefore, triggered activity is not self-excitatory but depends on a preceding action potential and afterdepolarization to initiate the process. Both early and delayed forms of afterdepolarization can initiate triggered activity.

225. The answer is E (all). *(p 653)* Early afterdepolarizations are depolarizations that occur before the cell fully repolarizes. They can occur in almost any type of heart cell and under conditions that cause significant delays in repolarization of the cells, such as hypokalemia, bradycardia, and drugs that are known to produce long QT intervals, such as quinidine and amitriptyline.

226. The answer is B (1, 3). *(pp 660–661)* Sinus bradycardia occurs when the sinus node pacemaker fires at a rate of less than 60 beats per minute. It may be normal due to the heightened vagal tone of a well-trained athlete or because of pharmacological suppression of automaticity (e.g., by a beta blocker or an antiarrhythmic agent). Heightened automaticity due to the use of epinephrine increases the sinus rate. Delayed afterdepolarizations do not cause sinus bradycardia.

227. The answer is B (1, 3). *(pp 659–663)* The model of reentry has three components: unidirectional block, a finite circuit, and an area of slow conduction. The limbs of the finite circuit have been arbitrarily labeled alpha and beta. The alpha limb conducts antegrade, and the beta limb, retrograde. Alpha pathways have faster conduction and longer refractory periods. This structure provides the necessary requirements for reentry to occur. This model has been used to explain the genesis of ventricular tachycardia and atrial flutter. Preexcitation of either the Wolff-Parkinson-White or Lown-Ganong-Levine types are due to accessory atrioventricular pathways. Torsades de pointes may be the result of triggered activity.

228. The answer is A (1, 2, 3). *(pp 746–747)* The rhythm strip that accompanies the question represents sinus bradycardia, which is defined as a sinus rate less than 60 beats per minute. The development of sinus bradycardia is not necessarily pathological. It was noted in 38 percent of 1000 healthy men in their twenties. Its frequency decreases with advancing age. Pathological sinus bradycardia is noted in several conditions: the convalescent period of typhoid fever or influenza, hypothermia, myxedema, obstructive jaundice, increased intracranial pressure, and depressed mental states. Pharmacological sinus tachycardia may result from the administration of ephedrine. Pathological sinus bradycardia can be seen in a patient with an inferior wall myocardial infarction. A physiological sinus bradycardia is seen in patients who are well-trained athletes.

229. The answer is D (4). *(pp 725–728)* Anticoagulation in patients with atrial fibrillation depends on the risk-benefit ratio. The risk of anticoagulation with warfarin is significant with an incidence of 4.3 percent major bleeding episodes per treatment year. This risk is accentuated when the prothrombin time is greater than 2.5 times the control. Full anticoagulation unfortunately does not totally eliminate the risk of embolization, which remains at approximately 1 percent per year. Anticoagulation is not indicated in patients with paroxysmal atrial fibrillation such as that seen after a motor vehicle accident or in patients with paroxysmal "lone" atrial fibrillation. Anticoagulation is recommended for patients with coronary heart disease with recurrent or chronic atrial fibrillation or those with chronic or persistent lone atrial fibrillation.

230. The answer is A (1, 2, 3). *(p 762)* In general, there is a fair correlation between the changes on the electrocardiogram (ECG) and plasma potassium level; however, this correlation depends on whether the hyperkalemia is induced experimentally or is the result of a clinical disorder such as renal failure. The ECG changes of hyperkalemia are amplified by the concomitant presence of acidosis and hyponatremia. A low calcium level in the presence of hyperkalemia increases the risk of atrioventricular (AV) block and ventricular fibrillation.

231. The answer is B (1, 3). *(pp 761–763)* Hyperkalemia produces both right axis and left axis deviations, as well as left bundle and right bundle branch blocks (LBBB and RBBB). Hyperkalemia can produce virtually any type of arrhythmia. These include bradyarrhythmias and complete heart block as well as tachyarrhythmias and ventricular fibrillation. Studies have shown that a dual effect of potassium on atrioventricular (AV) conduction can be achieved, depending on the level of potassium in the plasma. At plasma levels at 6 to 6.5 mEq/L, AV conduction is enhanced, but at levels greater than 7.5 mEq/L, conduction is generally depressed. Hyperkalemia affects the cardiac cell by decreasing the rate of repolarization, thus prolonging recovery time. Typically, the slope of phase II becomes steeper and that of phase III becomes less steep. All in all, the period of increased excitability is prolonged and the appearance of ectopic beats is enhanced. The ECG manifestation of hypokalemia includes an exaggerated U wave. With more severe hypokalemia, the amplitude of the T wave is reduced, the amplitude of the U wave is increased, and the ST segment is depressed. This gives the characteristic appearance of the ST-T-U wave complex.

232. The answer is A (1, 2, 3).   *(pp 770–771)*   Magnesium (Mg^{2+}) activates adenosine triphosphatase (ATPase), which is the energy source for the sodium (Na^+)-potassium (K^+) pump. Intercellular Mg^{2+} deficiency, which slows the pump, may result in an increase in intracellular Na^+ and calcium (Ca^{2+}) and loss of K^+. Hypomagnesemia appears to enhance digitalis-induced arrhythmias. Also torsades de pointes that occurs in patients with a prolonged QT interval can be suppressed by the administration of intravenous magnesium sulfate. This is thought to be due to Mg^{2+} inhibition of early afterdepolarizations. Isolated derangements of Mg^{2+} are rare because altered intracellular levels of Mg^{2+} affect Na^+, K^+, and Ca^{2+} concentrations.

233. The answer is D (4).   *(p 817)*   The presence of a new right bundle branch block (RBBB) in the setting of acute myocardial infarction has serious consequences. The RBBB receives its vascular supply in one of two ways. In 50 percent of patients, the right bundle has a dual blood supply from the atrioventricular (AV) nodal artery from the right coronary artery and the first septal perforator of the left anterior descending artery. In the remaining cases, it derives its blood supply solely from the first septal perforator. Therefore, the establishment of a new RBBB with or without a superior axis signifies that the vascular supply to the bundle is compromised from decreased perfusion of the first septal perforator. Prophylactic pacing is not recommended for an acquired left bundle branch block (LBBB) or a type I second-degree AV block because the typical location of these blocks is within the AV node, and progression to complete heart block is unusual. Third-degree AV block in the setting of inferior myocardial infarction may occur from AV nodal hypoperfusion or decreased perfusion of the proximal bundle branches in the septum. In either case, the extent of damage is not severe. In complete heart block complicating anterior myocardial infarction, extensive myocardial necrosis must have occurred to both bundle branches in the mid and distal branches of the conduction system. The use, however, of temporary pacemaking in this situation has not documented a change in long-term survival due to the extensive amount of myocardial necrosis.

234. The answer is A (1, 2, 3).   *(pp 849–850)*   Asymptomatic or symptomatic ventricular tachycardia or ventricular fibrillation associated with acute MI within 2 days is a circumstance in which an implantable cardioverter-defribillator (ICD) implantation is not indicated. ICD implantation is indicated for episodes of syncopal or hypotensive ventricular tachycardia regardless of whether they are inducible or noninducible as long as they are not associated with acute MI, not due to a remediable cause (i.e., drug toxicity, electrolyte derangement, or ischemia) and not controlled by acceptable drug therapy or definitive therapy such as surgical ablation. An ICD may be indicated, depending on patient characteristics, if there are one or more episodes of spontaneous and inducible ventricular fibrillation or syncopal or hypotensive ventricular tachycardia associated with an acute MI within 1 month but more than 2 days after the infarct, if there is no remediable cause or acceptable drug therapy and definitive ablation is unsuccessful.

235.   The answer is C (2, 4).   *(pp 722–724)*   The rhythm strip that accompanies the question illustrates atrial flutter with varying degrees of ventricular conduction. The rhythm is uncommon in the normal population; it was only found once among 67,000 Air Force personnel. When found, it is indicative of underlying structural heart disease. The mechanism is reentry. There are two types of atrial flutter. The classic form, type I, which has an atrial rate of 280 to 320 beats per minute, can be converted by rapid atrial pacing (entrainment). Type II flutter has a rate of 340 to 450 beats per minute and is unaffected by rapid atrial pacing.

236.   The answer is E (all).   *(pp 899–904, Table 48.3; Lubell, Am J Cardiol 27: 641–644, 1971; Burack, Am J Cardiol 23: 469–472, 1969)*   Use of esophageal leads in electrocardiography (ECG) may be applied to detect or confirm inapparent atrial activity and to evaluate the timing of retrograde P waves obscured by the QRS complex. The technique also has a therapeutic value. The atrium may be successfully paced 70 percent of the time at 20 to 30 mA to provide temporary support of atrial bradyarrhythmias or to revert atrial tachycardias. The esophageal route for ventricular pacing has been described and used by Lubell and by Burack and Furman. Although rarely necessary, it may be accomplished by using higher current levels of 50 mA in lower lead positions to record large ventricular deflections using the bipolar configuration.

237. **The answers are: A-Y, B-N, C-N, D-Y, E-N.** *(p 719)*   The rhythm strip that accompanies the question identifies the classic type of orthodromic tachycardia in Wolff-Parkinson-White syndrome. The reentrant pathway involves antegrade conduction in the atrioventricular (AV) conduction system and retrograde conduction via the accessory pathway. With this type of reentrant circuit movement, the QRS complexes during the tachycardia resemble the normal QRS configuration. Agents that slow antegrade conduction through the AV node would, therefore, be expected to result in slowing or termination of the circuit movement. Medications include those that act primarily as a result of increased vagal tone such as edrophonium chloride or phenylephrine hydrochloride. Other agents that slow the conduction of the AV node include propranolol, diltiazem, and class IA agents. Verapamil and lidocaine accelerate antegrade conduction through the AV node and, therefore, would be agents to avoid in this situation. Digoxin should be avoided because it may shorten the refractory period in the accessory pathway.

238. **The answers are: A-N, B-N, C-Y, D-Y, E-N.** *(pp 750–751)*   Pacemakers are rarely indicated for first-degree atrioventricular (AV) block. Occasionally HV prolongation could lead to first-degree block, and a pacemaker would be indicated. Type I second-degree AV block is seldom symptomatic; thus, insertion of a pacemaker in an asymptomatic patient with this conduction abnormality is not indicated. AV Wenckebach phenomenon is typically due to a block proximal to the bundle of His, usually within the AV node. These proximal conduction system defects are seldom associated with serious consequences, including progression to complete AV block. On the other hand, type II second-degree AV block typically occurs at or below the bundle of His. This block commonly progresses to third-degree heart block, and therefore, pacing is recommended whether the patient is symptomatic or not. It has been well-established that pacemakers are not indicated for patients who have asymptomatic bifascicular block. Studies have shown that progression to complete AV block is rare. A patient with acquired third-degree AV block, whether asymptomatic or not, represents a medical emergency. Pacing is mandatory and should be done immediately. If hemodynamic deterioration occurs prior to insertion of the pacemaker, the use of a sympathomimetic agent, such as isoproterenol, is advised. The value of pacing in congenital third-degree AV block is less well-established. Permanent pacing is indicated in all symptomatic patients. In asymptomatic patients, prognosis and the need for pacing may be established by ambulatory monitoring and electrophysiological studies.

239. **The answers are: A-Y, B-Y, C-Y, D-Y, E-N.** *(pp 728–730)*   The rhythm strip that accompanies the question identifies an accelerated idioventricular rhythm. This is most frequently seen in patients with acute myocardial infarction (especially those involving the inferior wall), digitalis toxicity, or metabolic or electrolyte abnormalities. The rhythm is seldom symptomatic and is usually of short duration. If symptomatic or persistent, then accelerating latent pacemakers with atropine is indicated. Suppression of the pacemaker with propranolol, digoxin, or procainamide would potentiate the secondary pacemaker.

240. **The answers are: A-Y, B-N, C-N, D-N, E-Y.** *(p 808)*   Esophageal pacing has been particularly helpful for diagnosing atrial tachyarrhythmias. In situations where it is impossible to tell if the rhythm is an atrial flutter, supraventricular tachyarrhythmia (SVT), or sinus tachycardia, the atrial electrode can be used to sense atrial electrical activity and provide a diagnosis. Furthermore, the esophageal pacing electrode can be used to overdrive pace regular atrial tachycardias such as atrial flutter. It is a standard bipolar electrode, but more recently, tip deflecting catheters have been used to improve capture. Although the esophageal pacing electrodes can be used for ventricular capture, they are best suited for atrial pacing because of the close proximity of the left atrium to the esophagus.

241. **The answers are: A-N, B-Y, C-Y, D-N, E-Y.** *(p 808)*   Standard transvenous pacing leads are often No. 4 or 5 French in size. They are inserted percutaneously through the femoral, internal jugular, or subclavian

veins. Temporary pacing wires can be inserted in the groin if the subclavian areas are to be used for permanent implantation. The groin is used to prevent contamination or thrombosis of the subclavian vein. As with all interventions, the insertion site should be shaved and prepared with a sterile solution. To prevent contamination, the site should be changed after no more than 3 to 4 days. Balloon-tipped, flow-directed catheters can be used without fluoroscopy but are often difficult to position in the right ventricular apex. A nonballoon catheter should be placed using a fluoroscope except in emergencies. Temporary pacing leads can also be placed in the atrium. The J-shaped lead, when placed from the subclavian or jugular vein, helps decrease the risk of dislodgement and loss of capture when placed in the right atrial appendage. Atrial leads placed through the femoral vein have a higher risk of dislodgement than do ventricular leads.

242. The answers are: A-N, B-Y, C-Y, D-Y, E-N.   *(pp 884–888)*   Electrophysiological studies can be used to detect sinus node dysfunction, especially in patients with presyncope, syncope, or those in whom the diagnosis cannot be made noninvasively. Asymptomatic patients with sinus node dysfunction or patients with obvious sinus node dysfunction on the surface electrocardiogram (ECG) do not generally need electrophysiological testing unless it is possible that another arrhythmia, such as ventricular tachycardia, could also be present. The most frequently performed test for sinus node function is the sinus node recovery time. The patient's atrium is paced for a period of approximately 30 sec at progressively shorter basic cycle lengths, and the pacing is suddenly interrupted. The escape interval that results is then measured. In most normal people, the corrected sinus node recovery time is less than 525 msec. Another way of measuring sinus node function is the sinoatrial (SA) conduction time. The specificity of these two tests combined is approximately 88 percent. It is also important to test the atrioventricular (AV) conduction in patients with sinus node dysfunction since AV conduction is also frequently abnormal in these patients. Asymptomatic patients with first-degree heart block do not need electrophysiological testing. However, in patients with second-degree AV block, it is important to localize the site of the block, as patients with infra-Hisian block tend to have an unpredictable course and often require permanent pacing. Asymptomatic patients with block localized to the AV node do not generally require permanent pacing. Patients with symptomatic third-degree heart block do not need electrophysiological testing because the diagnosis is already made, and permanent pacing is clearly indicated. If the patient's symptoms, however, cannot be explained by AV block, a search for another arrhythmia, such as ventricular tachycardia, may be necessary.

243. The answers are: A-Y, B-N, C-N, D-Y, E-Y.   *(pp 838–839)*   The pacemaker syndrome is a physiological disturbance caused by ventricular inhibited (VVI) pacing. Such pacing may result in a reduced cardiac output compared to a normal sinus rhythm. A particular form of pacemaker syndrome can occur in patients with intact ventriculoatrial conduction. In such situations, a P wave occurs after each ventricular pace beat, indicating the contraction of the atrium against the closed atrioventricular (AV) valves. This can result in further reduction in cardiac output and blood pressure. In some patients symptoms of lightheadedness and occasionally syncope may develop. The problem can be solved by pacing the atrium before the ventricle by using AV sequential (DVI) pacing or appropriately programmed fully automatic (DDD) pacing. The problem can be exacerbated by ventricular rate-responsive (VVIR) pacing.

244. The answers are: A-Y, B-N, C-N, D-N, E-Y.   *(pp 877–878)*   Long-term monitoring by electrocardiogram (ECG) does not provide the same degree of reliability in the interpretation of the pattern of the ST segment and T wave as in the detection of rhythm disturbances. The use of a two-lead system is more reliable in both the interpretation of ST-segment and T-wave changes and in the evaluation of rhythm disturbances than a one-lead system. Physiological limitations, including ST-segment and T-wave changes secondary to standing, hyperventilation, eating, anxiety, changes in the heart rate, and the effects of certain drugs make interpreting ST segments and T waves difficult. Long-term ECG recordings, however, are important in detecting angina at rest accompanied by ST-segment elevation (Prinzmetal's variant angina).

245. The answers are: A-N, B-Y, C-Y, D-N, E-Y. *(pp 881–884)*   Most electrophysiological studies are done through the right femoral vein. However, it is possible to perform such studies through peripheral veins and, at times, the subclavian and internal jugular. In general, most routine studies do not require left-sided heart catheterization; however, if searching for left-sided accessory pathways, then it is usually necessary to perform a left-sided heart catheterization. Continuous heparinization is used in these situations. The induction of ventricular tachycardia (VT) depends on the pacing protocol used. With multiple extrastimuli, polymorphic ventricular tachycardia and ventricular fibrillation can be induced at very short coupling intervals; however, it is at the expense of specificity of the test. The induction of sustained monomorphic ventricular tachycardia constitutes a specific response and is not generally seen in healthy patients. It is, however, possible to induce polymorphic ventricular tachycardia and fibrillation in an otherwise normal person if very short coupling intervals are used with multiple extrastimuli. Incremental pacing is used to induce a tachycardia or to precipitate atrioventricular (AV) block. This pacing protocol starts with a constant cycle length and gradually shortens the cycle length until the desirable event occurs. At very high pacing rates, a physiological AV node Wenckebach phenomenon occurs, but this is not pathological. Fixed cycle length pacing is also used to induce supraventricular tachycardias (SVTs), and to study ventriculoatrial conduction.

246. The answers are: A-Y, B-Y, C-Y, D-Y, E-Y. *(pp 895–896)*   Several prospective studies in patients post–myocardial infarction have demonstrated the prognostic significance of an abnormal signal-averaged electrocardiogram (SAECG). Abnormal SAECGs are found in 26 to 40 percent of patients soon after myocardial infarction. In patients with a history of myocardial infarction and an abnormal SAECG, 14 to 29 percent experience ventricular tachycardia during the first year compared to only 0.8 to 4.5 percent of those with a normal SAECG. Patients with a normal SAECG and an ejection fraction better than 40 percent are at a low risk for the development of ventricular tachycardia or sudden death. Although the negative predictive accuracy exceeds 95 percent, the positive predictive accuracy of the SAECG is not high; however, most patients with an abnormal recording do not develop serious ventricular arrhythmia. Successful thrombolytic therapy seems to correlate with a lower incidence of late potentials. An abnormal SAECG is independent of regional or global wall motion abnormalities.

247–250. The answers are: 247-A, 248-D, 249-A, 250-B. *(pp 661–662)*   Triggered rhythms are due to either early or delayed afterdepolarizations. Arrhythmias due to early afterdepolarizations, of which torsades de pointes is an example, may be due to a toxic response to type IA or type III antiarrhythmic agents. Digitalis toxicity rhythms are due to delayed afterdepolarizations. Neither rhythm is effectively blocked with the use of verapamil.

251–254. The answers are: 251-B, 252-C, 253-D, 254-C. *(p 660)*   Sinus tachycardia is due to a heightened automaticity. Both increased automaticity and reentry are mechanisms associated with atrial and ventricular tachycardia. The tachycardia associated with right ventricular outflow rhythm is thought to be due to triggered activity potentials of the delayed afterdepolarization mechanism.

255–258. The answers are: 255-A, 256-B, 257-A, 258-D. *(pp 662–663)*   The mechanism of reentry occurs when the conducted impulses from the sinus node pacemaker does not die out but continues to propagate and reactivate the heart, causing almost all clinically important tachyarrhythmias. Reentry may assume two forms: ordered or random. Ordered reentry is seen when the circulating wave front is continuously in a stable pathway. During random reentry, the wave front continually changes in size and location. Ordered reentry is seen in atrial flutter and ventricular tachycardia. Random reentry is the mechanism that explains the development of atrial fibrillation. Accelerated idioventricular rhythm is due to abnormal automaticity.

VI. Shock, Syncope, Sudden Death, and Cardiopulmonary Resuscitation

DIRECTIONS: Each question below contains five suggested responses. Select the **one best** response to each question.

259. The precipitating event in most sudden cardiac deaths is

    (A) ventricular tachycardia
    (B) asystole
    (C) electromechanical dissociation (EMD)
    (D) ventricular fibrillation
    (E) complete heart block

260. Which of the following statements regarding the mechanisms of blood flow during cardiopulmonary resuscitation (CPR) is true?

    (A) During chest compression (the systolic phase of CPR), the heart acts as a pump that directly increases blood flow to the brain
    (B) Intrathoracic pressure increases during chest compression as a direct result of the compression of lung tissue
    (C) Transesophageal echocardiography in humans during CPR shows that the mitral valve closes during chest compressions, thereby directing forward blood flow through the aortic valve
    (D) Greater sternal force during CPR augments myocardial and cerebral perfusion
    (E) The recommended rate for chest compression in adults is 60 beats per minute

261. All the following statements regarding cardiopulmonary resuscitation (CPR) are correct EXCEPT

    (A) with an excellent paramedical response team approximately 40 percent of all out-of-hospital cardiac arrest victims can be successfully resuscitated
    (B) the predominant cause of death in patients who are resuscitated in the field is cardiac rupture
    (C) predictors of successful CPR in the field include less than 4 min from collapse to initiation of CPR, less than 10 min to delivery of direct current cardioversion or defibrillation, and less than 7 min of total CPR
    (D) mortality rates for patients whose first rhythm is electromechanical dissociation (EMD) are higher than those for patients whose first rhythm is ventricular tachycardia
    (E) most patients who survive out-of-hospital cardiac arrest and who are eventually discharged from the hospital can return to gainful employment

DIRECTIONS: Each question below contains four suggested responses of which **one or more** is correct. Select

A	if	**1, 2, and 3**	are correct
B	if	**1 and 3**	are correct
C	if	**2 and 4**	are correct
D	if	**4**	is correct
E	if	**1, 2, 3, and 4**	are correct

262. Cardiovascular shock may occur as a result of

(1) tension pneumothorax
(2) myxoma
(3) septic shock
(4) right ventricular infarction

263. The compensatory physiological mechanisms that are activated in response to a shock syndrome may be destabilized by the

(1) absence of circulating leukotrienes
(2) release of prostaglandins
(3) impaired release of nitric oxide (NO)
(4) decreased red blood cell deformability

264. Effort-induced syncope associated with cardiac disease may be due to

(1) aortic stenosis
(2) primary pulmonary hypertension
(3) hypertrophic obstructive cardiomyopathy
(4) hypertensive cardiovascular disease

265. Therapeutic options in patients who have syncope as a result of the congenital long QT interval syndrome include

(1) permanent pacemaker implantation
(2) β-adrenergic blocking drugs
(3) left sympathetic stellectomy
(4) trial of phenytoin

266. Bystander-initiated cardiopulmonary resuscitation (CPR) significantly improves survival rates when

(1) the victim is less than 65 years old
(2) it is initiated within 5 min of collapse
(3) the initial rhythm is ventricular fibrillation
(4) it is maintained no longer than 12 min without advanced life support

267. In patients with coronary atherosclerotic heart disease or hypertension, factors that may increase the risk of sudden death include

(1) greater than 70 percent diameter obstruction in two or three coronary arteries
(2) unifocal premature ventricular contractions (PVCs) with early R-on-T phenomenon
(3) left ventricular ejection fraction of less than 40 percent
(4) nonspecific ST-segment and T-wave changes on resting electrocardiogram (ECG)

268. In patients with coronary atherosclerotic heart disease, measures to reduce the incidence of sudden death and improve survival may be achieved by treating

(1) asymptomatic significant left main obstruction with coronary artery bypass graft surgery
(2) symptomatic significant left main obstruction with coronary angioplasty
(3) asymptomatic ventricular ectopy with propranolol following Q-wave myocardial infarction
(4) symptomatic ventricular ectopy with mexiletine following Q-wave myocardial infarction

269. Direct current cardioversion and defibrillation are important means of correcting life-threatening arrhythmias during cardiopulmonary arrest. Correct statements regarding defibrillation and direct current cardioversion include which of the following?

(1) When defibrillating the patient with ventricular fibrillation, the paddles with 200 joules (J) should be discharged first, and if unsuccessful, they should be followed by a second defibrillation of 200 to 300 J and a third at 360 J

(2) Transthoracic impedance can be reduced by using firm pressure to hold the electrodes on the chest, by electrode gel or saline-soaked gauze pads between the electrodes and the skin, and proper electrode placement

(3) Although the transthoracic impedance can vary widely in adults, the average adults' impedance is somewhere between 70 and 80 ohms (Ω)

(4) Current flow through the chest is only dependent on the transthoracic impedance or resistance in the chest

270. Correct statements regarding electromechanical dissociation (EMD) include which of the following?

(1) Calcium chloride improves survival of patients with EMD

(2) Cardiorrhexis should be suspected if sudden EMD develops in a patient who has recently suffered an acute myocardial infarction

(3) Massive pulmonary embolism is unlikely to cause EMD

(4) Treatment of a patient with EMD involves an early search for treatable causes

DIRECTIONS: Each question below contains five suggested responses. For **each** of the **five** responses listed with every question you are to respond either YES (Y) or NO (N). In a given item, **all, some, or none of the alternatives may be correct.**

271. Correct statements regarding sudden cardiac death and its impact in the community include which of the following?

    (A)   The incidence is evenly divided between men and women

    (B)   There is an additional risk during exercise

    (C)   Over 75 percent of victims have coronary atherosclerotic heart disease

    (D)   Over 75 percent of victims are over age 65

    (E)   Less than 50 percent of victims have had prior manifestations of cardiovascular disease

272. Correct statements regarding the treatment of asystole or heart block during cardiopulmonary resuscitation (CPR) include which of the following?

    (A)   Patients with out-of-hospital cardiac arrest who present with asystole have a higher survival rate than patients who present with ventricular fibrillation

    (B)   Asystole that occurs during induction of general anesthesia is often due to vagal stimulation

    (C)   The use of temporary transvenous pacing is the best treatment for refractory asystole and continued bradycardia

    (D)   Occasionally, fine ventricular fibrillation may masquerade as asystole

    (E)   Atropine (10 to 20 mg intravenously) is the medical treatment of choice for patients with bradycardia and asystole

DIRECTIONS: Each group of questions below consists of lettered headings followed by a set of numbered items. For each numbered item select the **one** lettered heading with which it is **most** closely associated. Each lettered heading may be used **once, more than once, or not at all.**

Questions 273–276

For each clinical condition listed below, select the hemodynamic parameters that best identify the possible cardiogenic shock state (cardiac index = CI; pulmonary wedge pressure = PWP).

(A) CI = 5.0 L/min/m^2 and PWP = 8 mm
(B) CI < 2.2 L/min/m^2 and PWP < 15 mm
(C) CI < 2.2 L/min/m^2 and PWP > 18 mm
(D) CI > 2.2 L/min/m^2 and PWP > 18 mm
(E) CI > 2.2 L/min/m^2 and PWP < 15 mm

273. Acute renal failure

274. Acute mitral regurgitation following myocardial infarction

275. Massive pulmonary embolism

276. Critical aortic stenosis

Questions 277–280

For each clinical setting described below, select the type of syncope that is most likely to be associated with it.

(A) Vasodepressor syncope
(B) Vasovagal syncope
(C) Valsalva syncope
(D) Orthostatic syncope
(E) Carotid sinus syncope

277. A component of the Shy-Drager syndrome

278. Occurs after rapid ascent in an airplane

279. Occurs while shaving

280. A complication of bronchoscopy

VI. Shock, Syncope, Sudden Death, and Cardiopulmonary Resuscitation

Answers

259. The answer is D.   *(pp 947–948)*   Ventricular fibrillation is the precipitating event in most sudden cardiac deaths. Although recurrent, symptomatic ventricular tachycardia is a harbinger of sudden death, less than 5 percent of unexpected cardiac arrests are actually a result of ventricular tachycardia alone; nevertheless, ventricular tachycardia often may precede ventricular fibrillation. Asystole and complete heart block may occasionally precede ventricular fibrillation but are rarely the cause of sudden death. Electromechanical dissociation (EMD) is an end-stage mechanism whereby electrical activity is not accompanied by physiological maintenance of blood pressure.

260. The answer is D.   *(pp 959–963)*   The exact hemodynamic mechanisms that move blood out of the thorax to the vital organs during cardiopulmonary resuscitation (CPR) are not known with certainty. However, certain physiological facts are known. The relationship between aortic pressure, jugular venous pressure, and intrathoracic pressure are complex. In order for cerebral blood flow to occur during CPR, the carotid pressure must be greater than the venous pressure in the jugular veins. During the systolic phase of chest compression, the same pressure is transmitted to the carotid arteries and the greater veins. However, at the thoracic outlet, the veins collapse, preventing complete transmission of this pressure to the jugular veins and creating a pressure differential that promotes cerebral blood flow. Therefore, the heart itself simply acts as a passive conduit, not an active pump during CPR. Using a transesophageal probe during CPR has shown that the mitral valve both closes and stays open with chest compression. Thus, mitral valve closure, in itself, cannot be used to identify a primary mechanism of blood flow during CPR. Despite the uncertainties of the mechanism of blood flow during CPR, it is clear that more vigorous chest compression results in increased myocardial and cerebral perfusion. The current recommendations of the American Heart Association for CPR in adults is a compression rate of 80 to 100 beats per minute. These higher compression rates (i.e., 80 to 100 instead of 60 beats per minute) result in an overall chest compression duration of 50 percent of the cycle or more. The rise in thoracic pressure that occurs during chest compression is probably the result of small airway collapse with resultant air trapping. The air trapping in the small airways occupies volume in the lung that forces blood through the lungs during chest compression. This increase in thoracic pressure during chest compression is an important part of the CPR pump. Thus, pulmonary blood flow occurs via an indirect mechanism during chest compression. A similar mechanism operates during coughing. Indeed patients who can initiate repetitive coughs during an episode of ventricular tachycardia can maintain a blood pressure as long as they can sustain the coughing episode.

261. The answer is B.   *(pp 966–967)*   The likelihood of surviving cardiac arrest out of the hospital is most directly dependent on the number of bystanders who can initiate cardiopulmonary resuscitation (CPR), the response time of professional paramedical response teams, and the time until the first successful delivery of direct current cardioversion or defibrillation. Patients who have CPR begun in less than 4 min from time of collapse, who have less than 7 min of total CPR, and who have direct current cardioversion or defibrillation that is successful within 10 min of collapse have the best prognosis. In cities with a successful paramedical response system, up to 40 percent of patients with an out-of-hospital cardiopulmonary arrest can be resuscitated. The major cause of death for patients who are resuscitated in the field is anoxic encephalopathy. Most patients who survive out-of-hospital cardiac arrest and are discharged from the hospital are able to return to gainful employment.

262. **The answer is E (all).** *(p 908)* The etiologies of cardiovascular shock may be divided into four major categories: acute myocardial infarction, cardiac entities associated with inadequate ventricular function, cardiac obstruction or compression, and hypovolemia related to cardiovascular pathology (e.g., ruptured abdominal aortic aneurysm or hemorrhagic shock). Right ventricular infarction may complicate an acute myocardial infarction, particularly when the right coronary or circumflex systems are involved. Septic shock may cause myocardial dysfunction due to release of a variety of vasoactive substances such as histamine, various kinins, serotonin, prostaglandins, endorphins, proteases, free-oxygen radicals, activated complement components, and tumor necrosis factor. These compounds may cause direct depression of myocardial function. Tension pneumothorax and myxoma are pathophysiological problems that may create cardiac obstruction or compression. Other situations that cause cardiac obstruction or compression are pulmonary embolism, severe pulmonary hypertension, coarctation of the aorta, and severe hypertrophic cardiomyopathy.

263. **The answer is C (2, 4).** *(pp 908–909)* Activation of the sympathetic nervous system is the major homeostatic defense mechanism in shock. The volume-sensitive baroreceptors may be activated, vasopressin may be released, and transcapillary refill may be initiated as additional compensatory responses to shock. The particular benefits of sympathetic activation relate to peripheral events such as selective arteriolar vasoconstriction, increased heart rate, increased myocardial contractility, venoconstriction, increased release of adrenal hormones, and activation of the renin-angiotensin-aldosterone axis. Major decompensating factors relate to the loss of this adrenergic vasoconstriction due to the enhanced release of vasodilatin, prostaglandins, and nitric oxide (NO). In particular, NO, also known as endothelium-derived relaxing factor (EDRF), is produced by endothelial cells and macrophages, which may mediate the hypotensive effect of tumor necrosis factor. Microcirculatory phenomena that cause decompensation include increased capillary permeability, obstruction of the microvasculature by platelet and white-cell aggregates, decreased red blood cell deformability, and swelling of the endothelial cells. Lastly, myocardial depression may occur during shock due to a variety of factors, including a decrease in coronary perfusion secondary to systemic arterial hypotension and circulating coronary arterial vasoconstrictors such as leukotrienes.

264. **The answer is A (1, 2, 3).** *(p 936)* Effort-induced syncope may be a major symptom of aortic stenosis and hypertrophic obstructive cardiomyopathy. The latter disorder also has a nonexertional component that occurs in response to acute decreases in preload and afterload or in response to inotropic stimulation or transient arrhythmia. Effort-related syncope is an important presenting symptom of primary pulmonary hypertension, particularly in young patients without a cardiac murmur. It may also be present in patients with congenital heart disease and secondary pulmonary hypertension. Syncope in these situations occurs as a result of limits to right-sided cardiac output and a subsequent drop in left-sided output that is unable to respond to increased peripheral demand. Hypertensive cardiovascular disease without an obstructive component is not associated with effort-induced syncope.

265. The answer is A (1, 2, 3). *(pp 937–939)* The long QT interval syndrome may be congenital or acquired. Syncope with documented prolongation of the QT interval is almost always due to ventricular arrhythmia, which tends to be torsades de pointes ventricular tachycardia. The most frequent causes of acquired long QT interval syndrome are exposure to class I antiarrhythmic drugs or electrolyte disorders. The congenital long QT interval syndrome include the autosomal recessive Jervell and Lange-Nielson syndrome, and the autosomal dominant Romano-Ward syndrome. β-Adrenergic blocking agents usually control the symptoms. Left sympathetic stellectomy with or without beta-blocker therapy may be tried if syncope persists. Occasionally, permanent pacemaker implantation may be necessary. Class I antiarrhythmic agents such as phenytoin are contraindicated in the congenital long QT-interval syndrome because they can cause acquired long QT-interval syndrome.

266. The answer is C (2, 4). *(p 952)* There appears to have been a decline in the incidence of out-of-hospital cardiac arrest over the past decade. This may be a reflection of the substantial reduction in age-adjusted mortality attributed to coronary atherosclerotic heart disease. When sudden cardiac death occurs, the mortality and morbidity are insignificantly decreased by involvement of bystanders in the initiation of cardiopulmonary resuscitation (CPR) unless the CPR is initiated within 5 min after collapse and maintained for no longer than 12 min without advanced cardiac life support; in these cases, neurologic protection and eventual survival are significantly improved. The time of initiation of CPR is more important than the age of the victim or the initial cardiac rhythm.

267. The answer is E (all). *(pp 950–951)* There are four major characteristics associated with the enhanced risk of sudden cardiac death in patients with coronary atherosclerotic heart disease or hypertension. These characteristics are: ventricular electrical instability (particularly ventricular ectopy with early R-on-T depolarizations), extensive coronary arterial narrowing (particularly significant stenoses in two or three coronary vessels), abnormal left ventricular function, and electrocardiographic (ECG) conduction and repolarization abnormalities (e.g., advanced heart block, prolongation of the QT interval, and ST-segment and T-wave changes). Although these predictors can identify groups of patients at risk for sudden cardiac death, their sensitivity and specificity are sometimes suboptimal—a reflection of the erratic presentation of sudden cardiac death.

268. The answer is B (1, 3). *(pp 954–955; Cast Investigators: N Engl J Med 321: 406–412, 1984)* Studies comparing early randomized coronary artery surgery and medical trials have documented a poor, long-term outcome of significant left main coronary obstruction with medical therapy. Whether symptomatic or asymptomatic, patients with greater than 70 percent obstruction in the left main coronary artery have improved longevity with coronary artery bypass graft surgery. Coronary angioplasty is contraindicated in patients with significant unprotected left main obstruction in view of the impact of acute reclosure and late restenosis in this critical situation. Beta-blocker therapy, such as propranolol reduces mortality and morbidity following myocardial infarction due to a reduction of ventricular arrhythmia. The Cardiac Arrhythmia Suppression Trial (CAST) reported excessive mortality in patients treated with type I antiarrhythmic agents such as mexiletine, aprindine, flecainide, encainide, or moricizine; death resulted from proarrhythmia due to class I effects. Although this occurred in minimally symptomatic or asymptomatic patients, there are better antiarrhythmic agents than those listed to treat symptomatic ventricular ectopy following Q-wave myocardial infarction.

269. The answer is A (1, 2, 3). *(pp 964–965)* Defibrillation and direct current cardioversion are mainstays of therapy in ventricular tachycardia and ventricular fibrillation. One of the determinants for survival of out-of-hospital cardiac arrest is the time to first defibrillation. Successful defibrillation can be accomplished if adequate electrical current [amperes (amp)] is passed through the heart. The current flow through the heart is dependent on a number of factors including: the level of energy driving the current [joules (J)] and the transthoracic impedance [ohms (Ω)], which represents the resistance to current flow through the chest. Factors that affect this impedance include the level of energy selected, the electrode size, reducing the resistance at the skin-paddle interface with such materials as saline-soaked gauze or electrode gel pads, the time interval between previous shocks, the distance between the electrodes (i.e., the size of chest), the phase of ventilation, and the amount of pressure applied to the electrodes against the chest. Chest impedance in humans ranges from 15 to 150 Ω, but the average impedance is between 70 and 80 Ω. An understanding of the physics of defibrillation dictates that rapid successive defibrillation attempts at increasing energy levels are most effective if the other variables are kept constant. This is the reason the American Heart Association suggests rapid discharges at 200 to 300 J and then 360 J for a total of three successive shocks for ventricular fibrillation.

270. The answer is C (2, 4). *(pp 965, 1151)* Electromechanical dissociation (EMD), a poor prognostic sign in a patient with cardiopulmonary arrest, is defined as organized electrical activity on the surface electrocardiogram (ECG) at rates that support effective perfusion, yet no pulse or blood pressure can be documented. In treating patients with EMD, after initiating ventilation and cardiopulmonary resuscitation (CPR), treatable causes of this condition should be considered early, including hypovolemia due to hemorrhage, pericardial tamponade, massive pulmonary embolism, and tension pneumothorax. Cardiorrhexis, or cardiac rupture, is an uncommon complication of acute myocardial infarction. It usually occurs in the first 2 weeks following a myocardial infarction, and the peak incidence is probably between days 5 and 7; however, cardiac rupture may occur within the first 24 hours. Cardiorrhexis is more likely to occur in elderly women who are hypertensive but do not have signs of left ventricualr hypertrophy. EMD can be a sign of myocardial rupture. Despite aggressive therapy, including immediate pericardiocentesis and immediate surgical repair, survival from this catastrophic complication is rare. Studies do not support the use of calcium chloride in EMD.

271. The answers are: A-N, B-Y, C-Y, D-N, E-N. *(pp 947–948)* More than 75 percent of sudden cardiac deaths in the United States may be attributed to coronary atherosclerotic heart disease. Although most victims have had prior signs or symptoms of cardiovascular disease, 20 to 25 percent of cases present with cardiac arrest as the first manifestation. There is a predominance of men over women presenting with sudden cardiac death. Almost half of the victims of sudden cardiac death are under the age of 65. There appears to be an additional risk for sudden cardiac death during physical exertion, although sudden cardiac death may occur anytime during the routine activities of daily life. Thus, this should not deter cardiac patients from participating in carefully graded exercise programs.

272. The answers are: A-N, B-Y, C-Y, D-Y, E-N. *(p 965)* Patients who present with asystole or bradyarrhythmias in out-of-hospital cardiac arrest have a much worse prognosis than those who present with ventricular tachycardia or ventricular fibrillation. Therapy for this rhythm disturbance should begin promptly with basic life support followed by intravenous atropine. Atropine should be dosed in 0.5 mg boluses and repeated every 3 to 5 min until the maximum effective dose of 2 mg is reached. The optimal treatment for patients with asystole or symptomatic bradycardia is temporary transvenous pacing. In some patients, however, transcutaneous pacing may be an effective bridge until a temporary transvenous pacemaker can be positioned in the right ventricle. The reliability of transcutaneous pacing is variable and should not be considered a class I strategy of treatment. Occasionally, very fine ventricular fibrillation can appear to be asystole in the chest lead being monitored on the defibrillator oscilloscope. When the diagnosis of asystole is questionable, it is recommended that the leads being viewed on the screen be rotated by 90° by rotating the "quick look" paddles by 90° or by changing the lead selector knob on the defibrillator itself. If the diagnosis of fine ventricular fibrillation cannot be distinguished from asystole, the patient should be defibrillated since ventricular fibrillation is a more successfully treatable rhythm disturbance than asystole. The most common cause of asystole and bradyarrhythmias during the induction of general anesthesia is vagal stimulation. This is most easily treated with atropine followed by a pacemaker if necessary.

273–276. The answers are: 273-D, 274-C, 275-B, 276-C. *(pp 916–917; Forrester, N Engl J Med 295: 1404–1413, 1976)* Insertion of a flow-directed (Swan-Ganz) pulmonary artery catheter in critically ill patients with impending or overt cardiogenic shock allows the identification of hemodynamic subsets that may be used to direct diagnostic and therapeutic efforts. Forrester and his colleagues were the first to identify specific hemodynamic subsets based on the cardiac index (CI) and the pulmonary wedge pressure (PWP), and their seminal work still applies today.

Subset I: A CI < 2.2 L/min/m² and a PWP < 15 mm indicate a differential diagnosis of volume depletion, pericardial tamponade, tension pneumothorax, massive pulmonary embolism, right ventricular infarction, and early acute ventricular septal defect.

Subset II: A CI < 2.2 L/min/m² and a PWP > 18 mm are compatible with systolic pump failure, acute mechanical defect (e.g., mitral insufficiency, aortic insufficiency, or ventricular septal defect) and entities of critical aortic or mitral stenosis.

Subset III: A CI > 2.2 L/min/m² and a PWP > 18 mm indicate volume overload and diastolic pump failure. Such a scenario could follow an episode of acute renal failure where fluid input is not matched by output.

Subset IV: A CI > 2.2 L/min/m² and a PWP < 15 mm are compatible with non–cardiogenic shock such as sepsis or a drug overdose.

277–280. The answers are: 277-D, 278-A, 279-E, 280-B. *(pp 933–935; Bradbury and Eggleston, Am Heart J 1: 73–86, 1925; Shy and Drager, Ann Intern Med 82: 336–341, 1975)* All the pathophysiological states listed in the question are types of syncope that are not caused by cardiac disease. Orthostatic hypotension may be a result of absolute blood volume depletion due to hemorrhage or relative blood volume depletion due to venous pooling. In addition, postural hypotension may be a complication of various types of pharmacological agents or may be a result of an intrinsic neurogenic syndrome. Bradbury and Eggleston reported an idiopathic form of chronic autonomic failure in which postural hypotension is accompanied by a relatively fixed heart rate, heat intolerance, anhidrosis, nocturnal polyuria, urinary and anal sphincter dysfunction, and impotency. Recently this syndrome has been termed the idiopathic orthostatic hypotension (IOH) syndrome. Shy and Drager reported a syndrome of orthostatic hypotension accompanied by multiple central nervous system (CNS) manifestations. This syndrome is known as the Shy-Drager syndrome or multiple system atrophy (MSA).

The term vasodepressor syncope is a more accurate definition of the dramatic fall in peripheral vascular resistance mediated by inhibition of sympathetic neural responsiveness. The resultant postural shifts of blood volume to the lower extremities and a failure of cardiac output to compensate create the milieu for syncope. A bradycardia may occur that has vagal overtones, but this is not a primary cause of the syncope. This entity is the "common faint," which is seen in response to standing in a crowded poorly ventilated room, protracted military standing, emotional stress, venipuncture, or the sight of blood. Vasodepressor syncope may occur during jet flight, particularly when severe centrifugal force is applied causing pooling of blood in the lower extremities.

Carotid sinus syncope may be of a cardioinhibitory type, a vasodepressor type, or a mixed type. It is usually seen in elderly patients with a sensitive carotid sinus that may be inadvertently stimulated by a quick turn of the head during shaving or by wearing a tight collar.

Vasovagal syncope best describes the reflex type of syncope in which the vagal system primarily induces bradycardia. This may be seen as a response to vigorous instrumentation during bronchoscopy or esophagoscopy.

VII. Coronary Heart Disease

DIRECTIONS: Each question below contains five suggested responses. Select the **one best** response to each question.

281. All the following statements concerning hyper-triglyceridemia are true EXCEPT

    (A) triglyceride levels greater than 500 mg/dL are associated with pancreatitis
    (B) triglyceride levels greater than 500 mg/dL are seen in patients on calcium channel blocking agents
    (C) it is a component of familial combined hyperlipidemia
    (D) it is not present when a fasting triglyceride level of less than 200 mg/dL is present
    (E) it is a component of Frederickson's type V hyperlipidemia

282. All the following questions regarding the process of atherogenesis are true EXCEPT

    (A) fatty streaks consist almost exclusively of macrophages
    (B) the majority of atherosclerotic lesions progress through secretion of growth factors by the macrophages
    (C) platelet-derived growth factor increases the number of LDL receptors on smoooth muscle cells
    (D) both thromboxane A_2 and prostacycline are formed from arachidonic acid
    (E) diets high in eicosapentaenoic acid result in elevated production of thromboxane A_2

283. All the following statements regarding athero-genesis are true EXCEPT

    (A) endothelial cells are capable of producing particular types of collagen, prostacy-cline, factor VIII, and angiotensin converting enzyme
    (B) platelet-derived growth factor is the principal stimulant of smooth muscle in vitro
    (C) elevation of LDL serum levels results in an increasing number of LDL receptors on smooth muscle cells
    (D) elevated levels of LDL may promote proliferation of smooth muscle cells and components of connective tissue
    (E) prostacyclin produced by smooth muscle cells is an important thromboresistant factor to protect vascular surfaces from atherogenesis

284. All the following statements regarding coronary atherosclerotic plaques are true EXCEPT that they may be

    (A) concentric with relatively fixed narrowing
    (B) predominantly filled with lipid
    (C) eccentric with a fluctuating degree of narrowing
    (D) associated with a reactive hypertrophy of the underlying media
    (E) particularly prone to thrombosis if the plaque is soft

285. All the following statements concerning endothelial-dependent vasodilation are true EXCEPT

  (A) endothelial-derived relaxing factor (EDRF) is the key humoral factor promoting vasodilation in the normal endothelium
  (B) EDRF diffuses into underlying smooth muscle cells and increases cyclic guanosine monophosphate (cGMP), which results in dilatation
  (C) there is a similarity between EDRF and nitrous oxide (N_2O)
  (D) EDRF is easily degraded by oxygen-free radicals
  (E) acetylcholine causes dilatation with an intact endothelium and contraction when the endothelium is removed

286. Atherosclerosis creates a fundamental defect in endothelial-dependent vasodilation due to the proposed mechanism of

  (A) hyperactivity of endothelial-derived relaxing factor (EDRF)
  (B) suppression of EDRF by the amino acid arginine
  (C) inactivation of EDRF by superoxide dismutase
  (D) decreased production of nitrous oxide (N_2O) by the lipid-laden endothelium
  (E) increased degradation of nitric oxide (NO) by oxygen-free radical production

287. All the following statements regarding the clinical entity of angina with a normal coronary arteriography are true EXCEPT

  (A) it most commonly occurs in women
  (B) nitroglycerin frequently does not relieve the symptoms of chest pain rapidly
  (C) although excess lactate production with atrial pacing occurs, thallium perfusion defects are rarely seen
  (D) it can be associated with the development of cardiomyopathy
  (E) it is thought to be caused by an abnormality in coronary microvascular vasomotor control

288. All the following statements regarding the events produced by transient total coronary occlusion are true EXCEPT

  (A) decreased left ventricular compliance occurs within seconds
  (B) ischemic chest discomfort develops within 5 to 10 sec
  (C) contractile dysfunction leads to decreased ejection fraction
  (D) left ventricular filling pressure increases at 15 to 20 sec
  (E) ischemic changes on electrocardiogram (ECG) develop at about 20 sec

289. A 55-year-old man recently had his serum cholesterol checked at a health fair and was told it was 192 mg/dL. He further related that 2 months ago, he began to note he had a substernal pressurelike discomfort brought on by such activities as pushing a lawn mower or walking fast up an incline. The episodes are relieved with rest in a few minutes. Based on this history, the likelihood of this patient's symptoms representing angina pectoris is

  (A) 50 percent
  (B) 60 percent
  (C) 75 percent
  (D) 90 percent
  (E) 99 percent

290. A 42-year-old woman presents with a 3-month history of episodic substernal chest pain occurring at rest and variably with exertion. She has no known cardiovascular risk factors. An exercise tolerance test was performed, which demonstrated 3 mm horizontal ST depression in early stage III of the Bruce protocol. The predictive value of this finding in determining whether she has coronary artery disease is

  (A) 90 percent
  (B) 80 percent
  (C) 70 percent
  (D) 50 percent
  (E) 30 percent

291. All the following statements regarding the angiographic anatomy of coronary spasm are true EXCEPT

- (A) spasm occurs most commonly in the right coronary artery
- (B) spasm can involve saphenous veins or internal mammary bypass grafts
- (C) spasm is most often a diffuse rather than a focal process
- (D) spasm usually involves an atherosclerotic segment rather than one that appears smooth
- (E) spasm can be associated with either ST elevation or ST depression

292. The administration of ergonovine involves all the following factors EXCEPT

- (A) at least a 0.3-mg dose is required to induce coronary spasm
- (B) coronary spasm is induced in approximately 5 percent of patients with effort-related angina
- (C) it is relatively contraindicated in patients with a recent myocardial infarction
- (D) it is contraindicated in patients with severe hypertension
- (E) it is contraindicated in patients with significant left ventricular dysfunction

293. Characteristics of variant angina include all the following EXCEPT

- (A) the majority of patients with variant angina have a history of migraine headaches
- (B) it may at times be precipitated by exertion
- (C) it is commonly characterized by periods of spontaneous remission
- (D) it is frequently cyclic in nature, occurring at the same time of day
- (E) it is uncommonly associated with truly normal coronary arteries

294. Correct statements regarding ergonovine administration for the diagnosis of coronary spasm include all the following EXCEPT

- (A) it rarely produces refractory coronary spasm
- (B) it should only be given in a coronary care unit (CCU) to carefully selected patients with previously known low-risk coronary anatomy
- (C) it is contraindicated in patients with high-grade, fixed obstructions in a major coronary artery and unstable angina
- (D) a positive test may occur in 90 percent of patients with known variant angina
- (E) a positive test may occur in 25 percent of patients with atypical chest pain

295. The risk of acute myocardial infarction and death in patients presenting with unstable angina is a

- (A) 5 percent infarction rate and a 2 to 3 percent risk of death within 3 months
- (B) 7 to 8 percent infarction rate and a 5 percent risk of death within 3 months
- (C) 10 to 20 percent infarction rate and a 5 to 10 percent risk of death within 3 months
- (D) 20 to 40 percent infarction rate and a 30 percent risk of death within 3 months
- (E) 40 to 50 percent infarction rate and a 20 percent risk of death within 3 months

296. Clinical variables that are important in determining the early prognosis in patients with unstable angina pectoris include all the following EXCEPT

- (A) the presence of ischemic ST-segment and T-wave changes on the resting electrocardiogram (ECG)
- (B) poor exercise tolerance on exercise stress testing
- (C) the severity and frequency of the presenting anginal symptoms
- (D) the recurrence of angina after admission to the hospital
- (E) the presence of silent ischemia after hospital admission

297. Pharmacologic agents that have proved useful in the treatment of unstable angina include all the following EXCEPT

(A) aspirin
(B) intravenous heparin
(C) ticlopidine
(D) thrombolytic therapy
(E) intravenous nitroglycerin

298. Acute papillary muscle rupture with an acute myocardial infarction is best described by which of the following statements?

(A) The anterolateral papillary muscle is more susceptible to rupture than the posteromedial papillary muscle
(B) Half the patients with papillary muscle rupture have single-vessel disease
(C) Patients with large infarctions and diminished cardiac output are more prone to rupture
(D) The absence of a loud systolic murmur excludes papillary muscle rupture
(E) Papillary muscle rupture commonly occurs with anterior wall infarction

299. A 65-year-old man who presented with an acute anterior myocardial infarction after several days developed a pericardial friction rub and pleuritic chest pain that was difficult to control with narcotics or steroids. He then suddenly developed hypotension accompanied by marked jugular venous distention and electromechanical dissociation (EMD). No murmurs were audible. The most likely etiology of this patient's acute difficulty is

(A) acute mitral regurgitation due to rupture of the papillary muscle
(B) ventricular septal rupture
(C) external cardiac rupture
(D) extension of an acute myocardial infarction
(E) right ventricular infarction

300. All the following statements regarding the pathophysiology of myocardial ischemia (MI) are true EXCEPT

(A) transient occlusion of a coronary artery for less than 20 min is associated with no irreversible injury
(B) restoration of flow within 6 h of the onset of coronary occlusion is associated with significant salvage of myocardium
(C) transient coronary occlusion for 10 to 15 min may produce myocardial hibernation
(D) myocardial stunning may last 24 to 48 h
(E) reduction of coronary flow to about 5 percent of normal may be associated with regional myocardial wall dyskinesis

301. The most important prognostic determinant in patients with stable angina pectoris is the

(A) frequency of angina pectoris
(B) amount of exercise tolerance exhibited on a treadmill study
(C) amount of exercise-induced ventricular ectopy
(D) number of risk factors present
(E) amount of regular physical exercise in which the patient participates

302. All the following statements regarding the prognosis of patients with unstable angina pectoris are true EXCEPT

(A) patients who have had a prior history of stable angina have a worse prognosis than those who do not
(B) there is a significantly higher incidence of sudden death or myocardial infarction for 2 to 3 weeks after the onset of instability
(C) patients with transient ST-segment elevation during episodes of pain have a worse prognosis
(D) patients with Prinzmetal's angina have a high incidence of sudden death or infarction in the first 3 months after the onset of symptoms
(E) patients with isolated episodes of prolonged ischemic discomfort without evidence of infarction have the same mortality at 1 year as patients who have had a documented myocardial infarction

303. Important prognostic indicators in completed myocardial infarction include all the following EXCEPT

(A) the demonstration of normal exercise tolerance on exercise stress testing in the postinfarction period

(B) the demonstration of a left ventricular ejection fraction of greater than 50 percent

(C) the degree of ST-segment elevation occurring during the acute phase

(D) the development of overt heart failure during the acute period

(E) the development of recurrent angina early in the postinfarction period

304. All the following statements regarding atherogenesis are true EXCEPT

(A) diets high in saturated fat and cholesterol decrease hepatic low-density lipoprotein (LDL) receptors

(B) after smoking is discontinued, coronary risk decreases by 50 percent within 1 year

(C) radionuclide scans have determined that cigarette smoking induces regional disturbances of myocardial perfusion

(D) plasma fibrinogen levels are decreased by cigarette smoking

(E) cigarette smoking may limit the efficacy of antihypertensive therapy

305. Cigarette smoking has all the following effects on the vascular system EXCEPT

(A) thromboxane A_2 (TXA_2) release

(B) decreased prostacyclin (PGI_2) production

(C) increased α-adrenergic stimulation

(D) decreased vasopressin production

(E) increased platelet aggregation

306. Correct statements concerning systolic compression of a major coronary artery due to myocardial bridging include all the following EXCEPT

(A) it is a relatively rare angiographic finding

(B) it is presumably congenital in origin

(C) it may produce angina with exertion

(D) it may produce exercise-induced ventricular arrhythmias

(E) it usually requires surgical correction

307. The Multiple Risk Factor Intervention Trial (MRFIT) revealed a striking relationship between serum cholesterol levels and both coronary heart disease mortality and age-adjusted death rates in men. The increase in total mortality in people with very low serum cholesterols can best be explained by

(A) suicide

(B) trauma

(C) cancer

(D) side effect of cholesterol-lowering medication

(E) low levels of high-density lipoprotein (HDL) cholesterol

308. All the following congenital abnormalities of the coronary circulation may produce myocardial ischemia in the absence of atherosclerosis EXCEPT

(A) anomalous origin of the left main coronary artery from the right sinus of Valsalva

(B) anomalous origin of the left circumflex artery from the right sinus of Valsalva

(C) single coronary artery

(D) anomalous origin of a coronary artery from the pulmonary artery

(E) atresia of the coronary ostium

309. A drug that is contraindicated in patients with severe hypertriglyceridemia is

(A) probucol

(B) gemfibrozil

(C) lovastatin

(D) cholestyramine

(E) niacin

310. Coadministration of which of the following medications can lead to myopathy in a transplant patient taking cyclosporine?

(A) Probucol

(B) Gemfibrozil

(C) Lovastatin

(D) Cholestyramine

(E) Niacin

311. Treatment of an overdose with a beta blocker that is unresponsive to a beta agonist should include

    (A) norepinephrine
    (B) methoxamine hydrochloride
    (C) phentolamine mesylate
    (D) glucagon
    (E) propranolol

312. All the following statements regarding the action of lipid-lowering agents are true EXCEPT

    (A) bile acid sequestrants stimulate the synthesis of low-density lipoprotein (LDL) receptors
    (B) nicotinic acid inhibits the hepatic secretion of very low-density lipoprotein (VLDL)
    (C) fibric acids reduce the activity of lipoprotein lipase (LPL)
    (D) 3-hydroxy-3-methylglutaryl coenzyme A (HMG CoA) reductase inhibitors lead to an increased uptake of circulating VLDL remnants and LDL by the liver
    (E) probucol lowers the blood levels of LDL and HDL cholesterol

313. Which combination of beta blockers are highly lipid soluble, and, therefore, more prone to central nervous system (CNS) penetration?

    (A) Atenolol and esmolol
    (B) Labetalol and timolol
    (C) Propranolol and metoprolol
    (D) Sotalol and nadolol
    (E) Nadolol and timolol

314. The frequency of myocardial infarction in the perioperative period of coronary artery bypass grafting correlates best with

    (A) abnormality of left ventricular function
    (B) history of hypercholesterolemia
    (C) inability to achieve complete revascularization
    (D) poor distal artery reperfusion
    (E) a kink in the bypass graft with consequent slow flow

315. Correct statements concerning the clinical applications of calcium channel blockers include which of the following?

    (A) Only nifedipine and cardizem are effective in stable angina pectoris
    (B) The abrupt withdrawal of calcium antagonists is contraindicated in patients with stable effort-related angina
    (C) Diltiazem is more effective than verapamil in converting atrial fibrillation to normal sinus rhythm
    (D) Diltiazem and verapamil are effective in the treatment of the atrial fibrillation associated with the Wolff-Parkinson-White syndrome
    (E) Calcium antagonists have minimal use in the treatment of ventricular arrhythmia

316. The pharmacological properties of warfarin are best described by which of the following statements?

    (A) It crosses the placental barrier and is contraindicated in pregnancy
    (B) Because it appears in the milk of nursing mothers, patients on warfarin should not breast-feed
    (C) In fat malabsorption states, the anticoagulant effect of warfarin is reduced
    (D) Cholestyramine potentiates the anticoagulant effect of warfarin
    (E) When amiodarone is administered to patients receiving warfarin, the dose of warfarin should be increased

317. A 67-year-old man presents with unstable angina. On examination he is found to have a right carotid bruit. Subsequent evaluation reveals triple-vessel coronary disease along with an 85 percent right internal carotid stenosis. He has had no cerebrovascular symptoms. The best approach to this patient would be

    (A) continued medical therapy with heparin, aspirin, and nitrates
    (B) combined coronary artery bypass and carotid endarterectomy
    (C) carotid endarterectomy followed 2 weeks later by coronary artery bypass
    (D) coronary artery bypass followed by elective carotid endarterectomy
    (E) none of the above

318. Neurologic deficits secondary to air embolism during coronary bypass surgery have which of the following qualities?

(A) They are usually transient and resolve completely at a variable rate during the postoperative period

(B) They are usually devastating and resolution is unexpected

(C) They occur more frequently in younger patients as compared to the older population

(D) They have a better chance of resolution if high doses of steroids are used in the first 48 hours

(E) They should be treated with heparin

DIRECTIONS: Each question below contains four suggested responses of which **one or more** is correct. Select

A	if	**1, 2, and 3**	are correct
B	if	**1 and 3**	are correct
C	if	**2 and 4**	are correct
D	if	**4**	is correct
E	if	**1, 2, 3, and 4**	are correct

319. Low-density lipoprotein (LDL) receptors have which of the following characteristics?

(1) They increase with age

(2) The concentration of LDL in the blood is not dependent on the number of LDL receptors

(3) They are up-regulated by a diet high in saturated fat and cholesterol

(4) They are down-regulated by increased intrahepatic cellular cholesterol

320. Correct statements regarding apolipoproteins include which of the following?

(1) The presence of apolipoprotein B (apo B) is associated with severe coronary atherosclerosis

(2) Apolipoprotein A-1 (apo A-1) has a negative association with coronary atherosclerosis

(3) Lipoprotein[a] (Lp[a]) has a strong association with coronary atherosclerosis

(4) Lp[a] has a structure similar to fibrinogen

321. The pathophysiology of unstable angina pectoris is associated with

(1) platelet adhesion and activation at the coronary lesion site

(2) small areas of myocardial necrosis

(3) nonocclusive thrombi at the site of a fissured plaque

(4) varying vasomotor tone within the affected coronary vascular bed

322. The activation of lymphocytes and macrophages may compromise the structural integrity of the atherosclerotic plaque due to the release of substances such as

(1) oxygen-free radicals

(2) collagenase

(3) hydrogen peroxide (H_2O_2)

(4) haluronidase

323. Unstable angina and myocardial infarction are reflections of the molecular events at the atherosclerotic plaque level that initiate activated macrophages, which may produce

(1) anticoagulant factor that leads to plaque bleeding and fissure

(2) growth factors that stimulate vascular smooth muscle migration

(3) antiangiogenic factors that destabilize the vessel wall

(4) proteolytic agents that lead to tissue damage and disruption

324. Characteristics of a normal functioning arterial endothelium include

(1) an anti-inflammatory state due to control of the localization of circulating leukocytes

(2) endothelial-dependent vasoconstriction in response to stimuli

(3) a nonthrombogenic surface as a result of a balance of coagulation factors

(4) growth promotion of the medial layer to accommodate and stabilize the lumen

325. The threshold to evoke myocardial ischemia may be significantly lower in the early morning hours owing to

(1) the degree of fixed coronary stenosis

(2) variations in catecholamine secretion

(3) the physical conditioning of an individual

(4) variations in coronary vascular tone

326. Based on data accumulated from multiple randomized trials, coronary artery bypass surgery has been shown to have a clear-cut advantage over medical therapy in patients with class I or II angina who have

(1) three-vessel disease, moderately impaired left ventricular function, and no ischemia demonstrated on exercise stress testing

(2) two-vessel disease involving the right coronary artery and left circumflex artery, moderate left ventricular dysfunction, and mild ischemia on exercise stress testing

(3) three-vessel disease, normal left ventricular function, and moderate ischemia on exercise testing

(4) single-vessel disease, mild left ventricular dysfunction, and severe ischemia demonstrated on exercise stress testing

327. Measures that have proven useful in the treatment of angina pectoris due to vasospasm without significant obstructive coronary atherosclerosis include

(1) nitrates

(2) beta blockers

(3) calcium antagonists

(4) coronary artery bypass grafting

328. Potential candidates for thrombolytic therapy include which of the following?

(1) A 52-year-old man with left bundle branch block (LBBB) and symptoms of prolonged myocardial ischemia (MI) presenting within 3 h of the onset of symptoms

(2) An 80-year-old man presenting with prolonged ischemic chest pain and inferior ST-segment elevation within 4 h of the onset of symptoms

(3) A 42-year-old man with continuing ischemic chest pain and inferior ST-segment elevation presenting 8 h after the onset of symptoms

(4) A 48-year-old man with prolonged ischemic chest pain with ECG findings of inferolateral ST depression presenting within 2 h of the onset of symptoms

329. Criteria that are presently used as end points for stopping a predischarge exercise test following an acute myocardial infarction include

(1) achievement of a work load of 3.5 METs

(2) a heart rate of 120 to 140 beats per minute

(3) achievement of 60 percent of the age-predicted maximum heart rate

(4) presence of exercise-induced symptoms

330. Infectious diseases known to affect the coronary arteries include

(1) leprosy

(2) syphilis

(3) typhus

(4) Kawasaki's disease

331. Causes of coronary arterial aneurysms include

(1) congenital origin

(2) trauma

(3) atherosclerosis

(4) angioplasty

332. Beta blockers known to accumulate in patients with renal failure include

(1) atenolol

(2) esmolol

(3) nadolol

(4) metoprolol

333. Calcium antagonists are effective medications in the treatment of

(1) hypertensive emergencies

(2) silent myocardial ischemia

(3) hypertrophic cardiomyopathy

(4) acute myocardial infarction as prophylaxis in survivors

334. Characteristics of aspirin therapy include which of the following?

(1) Its major antithrombotic effect is its ability to inhibit platelet thromboxane A_2 (TXA_2) synthesis

(2) The oral administration of aspirin causes platelet inhibition in approximately 60 min

(3) Aspirin inhibits the secondary wave of aggregation induced by adenosine diphosphate (ADP) and epinephrine

(4) Aspirin reversibly inhibits cyclooxygenase

SUMMARY OF DIRECTIONS

A	B	C	D	E
1, 2, 3 only	1, 3 only	2, 4 only	4 only	All are correct

335. Characteristics of ticlopidine include which of the following?

   (1) Its main mechanism of action is the inhibition of prostaglandin

   (2) Neutropenia occurs in less than 1 percent of patients receiving ticlopidine and resolves upon discontinuation of the drug

   (3) Optimal efficacy in terms of inhibition of platelet function is usually reached within 24 hours

   (4) Ticlopidine is effective in reducing death and myocardial infarction in patients with unstable angina

336. The effects of urokinase administration include

   (1) it only activates fibrin-bound plasminogen

   (2) it activates plasminogen directly

   (3) it results in high levels of fibrinogen

   (4) it leads to extensive plasminogen activation and depletion of α_2-antiplasmin

337. The risks of coronary angioplasty include

   (1) mortality of 0.5 to 1 percent of patients

   (2) need for emergency bypass surgery in 2 to 3 percent of patients

   (3) restenosis rate of 30 to 50 percent

   (4) acute myocardial infarction (MI) in 2 to 4 percent of patients

338. Coronary artery bypass surgery is superior to medical therapy in treating patients with which of the following angiographic findings?

   (1) Left main stem disease greater than 50 percent

   (2) Proximal left anterior descending disease greater than 70 percent along with other significant coronary stenosis

   (3) Proximal three-vessel disease greater than 50 percent

   (4) Multivessel stenosis greater than 50 percent with moderate-to-severe left ventricular dysfunction

339. True statements regarding late coronary bypass patency include

   (1) approximately 50 percent of saphenous vein grafts are patent 10 years postoperatively

   (2) 10-year survival is the same in patients whether they receive an internal mammary graft or all saphenous vein grafts

   (3) approximately 90 percent of left internal mammary grafts to the left anterior descending artery are patent 10 years postoperatively

   (4) approximately 94 percent of saphenous vein grafts are patent 5 years postoperatively

DIRECTIONS: Each question below contains five suggested responses. For **each** of the **five** responses listed with every question you are to respond either YES (Y) or NO (N). In a given item **all, some, or none of the alternatives may be correct.**

340. Correct statements concerning the epidemiological data collected in the studies listed below include which of the following?

    (A) The Lipid Research Clinics Coronary Primary Preventions Trial (LRC-CPPT) used cholestyramine and found a significant decrease in fatal and nonfatal coronary heart disease events in the treated group

    (B) The Coronary Drug Project used nicotinic acid and showed no difference in coronary events in the treated group

    (C) The Familial Atherosclerosis Treatment Study (FATS) showed that angiographic evidence of atherosclerosis could be slowed, halted, or even regressed in the treatment group

    (D) The Helsinki Heart Study used gemfibrozil and showed that the treated group had less fatal and nonfatal coronary heart disease events

    (E) The United States National Heart, Lung, and Blood Institute (NHLBI) Type II Coronary Intervention Study showed no difference in the treatment and nontreatment groups for the progression of angiographic atherosclerosis

341. The Adult Treatment Panel II of the National Cholesterol Education Program (NCEP) has issued which of the following guidelines for the evaluation of hypercholesterolemia?

    (A) Measure total and high-density lipoprotein (HDL) cholesterol in all adults at age 20 and then every 5 years thereafter

    (B) Do a lipoprotein analysis on patients whose total cholesterol is less than 200 mg/dL and whose HDL is less than 35 mg/dL

    (C) Begin dietary therapy on patients whose low-density lipoprotein (LDL) is between 130 and 159 mg/dL with less than two risk factors

    (D) Begin treatment on all patients whose total cholesterol is greater than or equal to 240 mg/dL

    (E) Begin dietary therapy on patients whose LDL is greater than 160 mg/dL

342. True statements regarding atherosclerosis include which of the following?

    (A) The atherosclerotic plaque is composed of two basic components: intracellular and extracellular lipids and smooth muscle cells

    (B) Lesions of atherosclerosis primarily involve the media of the blood vessel

    (C) Fatty streaks are ubiquitous in all populations and do not necessarily progress to atherosclerotic lesions

    (D) Experimentally induced atherogenesis is initiated with migration of monocytes between endothelial cells, where they begin to accumulate lipid

    (E) While platelets contribute to thrombosis on established plaques, they do not contribute to the initiation of atherogenesis

343. Each of the following statements concerns the role of vascular endothelium in the modulation of atherosclerosis. True statements include

    (A) endothelial cells may transport plasma lipoproteins into the artery wall using vesicles

    (B) endothelial cells can produce endothelial derived growth factor, which leads to proliferation of smooth muscle and fibroblasts

    (C) endothelial cells proliferate only if their monolayer is injured and only at the margins of injury

    (D) experimentally, chronic hypercholesterolemia alone results in endothelial cell dysfunction that may culminate in an atherosclerotic lesion

    (E) experimentally, endothelial injury in the absence of hypercholesterolemia may lead to fibromusculoelastic lesions capable of regression

344. Correct statements regarding atherogenesis include which of the following?

(A) Lymphocytes are a frequent component of the atherosclerotic plaque

(B) Lipid-filled macrophages serve as an initial site to which platelets adhere and form mural thrombi in the evolution of the atherosclerotic plaque

(C) Experimentally, interference with normal platelet interaction has been shown to prevent the development of the atherosclerotic plaque

(D) Altered characteristics of flow in blood vessels may be responsible for the increased incidence of atherogenesis associated with hypertension

(E) Proliferation of smooth muscle in the mesangium of the kidney and increased thickness of capillary basement membrane in diabetics may be similar to proliferation of smooth muscle in atherogenesis

345. Correct statements regarding the development of intimal tears in coronary atherosclerotic plaques include which of the following?

(A) They are the major precipitating factor in coronary thrombi formation

(B) They invariably lead to acute total coronary occlusion

(C) They may lead to further plaque growth

(D) They may occur silently and not be clinically recognized

(E) They are caused by bleeding from transmedial vessels into the plaque

346. True statements regarding calcium channel blockers in the treatment of patients with stable angina pectoris include which of the following?

(A) Although chemically different, they act on the same receptor sites

(B) They decrease myocardial oxygen demand by decreasing afterload and reducing myocardial contractility

(C) They all decrease the heart rate

(D) They all have a negative inotropic effect

(E) They are generally better tolerated than beta blockers in elderly patients

347. Correct statement concerning right ventricular infarction include which of the following?

(A) Right ventricular free-wall infarction occurs in most patients with inferior wall infarction

(B) Electrocardiography (ECG) is of limited benefit in the diagnosis of right ventricular injury

(C) Right ventricular infarction should be treated aggressively with intravenous nitrates

(D) An elevated systolic pressure in both the right ventricle and pulmonary artery would be expected

(E) When right ventricular infarction is suspected, volume expansion is indicated

348. True statements regarding Q-wave and non-Q-wave infarction include which of the following?

(A) The incidence of Q-wave and non-Q-wave infarction is about equal

(B) The 1-month mortality of a Q-wave infarct and a non-Q-wave infarct is about equal

(C) The 2-year mortality of a Q-wave infarct and a non-Q-wave infarct is about equal

(D) Administration of diltiazem appears beneficial in patients with non-Q-wave infarcts but not in those with Q-wave infarcts

(E) Administration of beta blockers appears beneficial in patients with Q-wave infarcts but not in those with non-Q-wave infarcts

349. The major determinants of prognosis in the early evolving myocardial infarction period in the coronary care unit (CCU) include

(A) the location and size of the infarction on electrocardiogram (ECG)

(B) clinical evidence of congestive heart failure (CHF)

(C) the duration and severity of the chest pain

(D) the age of the patient

(E) the early occurrence of ventricular fibrillation not associated with evidence of heart failure

350. Mortality statistics in sudden cardiac death indicate that

(A) most patients who suffer sudden cardiac death have had an acute myocardial infarction

(B) the first year mortality in survivors of out-of-hospital sudden cardiac death where acute infarction has occurred is 25 percent

(C) the first year mortality in survivors of out-of-hospital sudden cardiac death not associated with acute infarction is around 5 percent

(D) sudden cardiac death occurs predominantly in patients with extensive coronary artery disease and left ventricular dysfunction

(E) one-third of the patients with ischemic heart disease present with sudden cardiac death as the initial and final event

351. Correct statements concerning the risk of coronary disease in patients with hypertension include which of the following?

(A) The incidence of coronary disease is low in populations where hypertension is associated with cholesterol levels less than 160 mg/dL

(B) Fixed hypertension increases the risk of coronary disease, but labile hypertension does not

(C) Isolated systolic hypertension of the elderly does not increase the incidence of coronary disease

(D) When hypertension is superimposed upon other risk factors, the coronary disease risk increases

(E) Antihypertensive medical therapy can actually worsen some risk factors such as hyperglycemia and lipid levels

352. Correct statements about modifiable risk factors for cardiovascular disease include which of the following?

(A) The coronary risk of former smokers decreases to that of the general population within several years of smoking cessation

(B) High-density lipoprotein (HDL) cholesterol is not affected by cigarette smoking

(C) Platelet aggregation is reduced after the cessation of smoking

(D) Early trials of antihypertensive therapy demonstrated no significant effect on myocardial infarction rates

(E) Treatment of mild diastolic hypertension does not reduce cardiovascular and all-cause mortality

353. In addition to being vasodilators, calcium channel blockers also have which of the following therapeutic effects?

(A) They have negative inotropic effects on the myocardium

(B) They depress cardiac contractibility and the height of the monophasic action potential

(C) Verapamil acts as an antiarrhythmic through interference with calcium conductance

(D) They have a relatively greater effect on arteries than veins

(E) They have a negative inotropic effect that is dose-dependent

354. Correct statements regarding hypotension associated with streptokinase infusion include which of the following?

(A) Hypotension is usually halted by cessation of the infusion

(B) The more rapid the infusion, the more likely a hypotensive reaction will occur

(C) Hypotension during an infusion is usually associated with anaphylaxis

(D) To avoid hypotension, the intravenous infusion should not exceed 500 units/kg/min

(E) Hypotension is usually associated with a mechanical complication of a myocardial infarction

355. Correct statements regarding heparin therapy include which of the following?

    (A) Heparin accelerates the formation of molecular complex between antithrombin III and several serine proteases

    (B) The main anticoagulant effect of heparin appears to be through the inhibition of thrombin-induced activation of factors V and VIII

    (C) Although intravenous heparin is commonly used in the treatment of unstable angina, its value for the prevention of myocardial infarction or recurrent ischemia has not been documented

    (D) Thrombocytopenia is a more frequent complication with bovine heparin than porcine heparin

    (E) The value of subcutaneous heparin in the reduction of mural thrombus following acute anterior myocardial infarction has not been proven

356. Complications of a streptokinase infusion include which of the following?

    (A) Hypotension
    (B) Anaphylactic reaction
    (C) Fever
    (D) Bleeding
    (E) Hemorrhagic stroke

357. Characteristics of coronary lesions that would indicate a greater than 85 percent success rate with coronary angioplasty include

    (A) discrete lesions less than 10 mm in length
    (B) total occlusions less than 3 months old
    (C) lesions in a segment angulated less than 45 degrees
    (D) minimal thrombus
    (E) little or no calcification

358. In comparison with routine balloon angioplasty, laser balloon angioplasty appears to be potentially superior for

    (A) ostial lesions
    (B) severely angulated lesions
    (C) heavily calcified lesions
    (D) chronic total occlusions
    (E) diffuse lesions

359. True statements regarding repeat coronary artery bypass surgery include

    (A) the operative risk of reoperation is about the same as the initial procedure
    (B) approximately 3 to 5 percent of patients require reoperation in the first 5 years after surgery
    (C) at reoperation saphenous vein grafts older than 5 years should be replaced even if there is no critical stenosis
    (D) approximately 10 percent of patients will require reoperation at 15 years after surgery
    (E) 5-year survival is approximately 90 percent after reoperation

DIRECTIONS: The group of questions below consists of four lettered headings followed by a set of numbered items. For each numbered item select

A	if the item is associated with	(A) **only**
B	if the item is associated with	(B) **only**
C	if the item is associated with	**both** (A) and (B)
D	if the item is associated with	**neither** (A) nor (B)

Each lettered heading may be used **once, more than once, or not at all.**

Questions 360–363

(A) Elevated LDL
(B) Elevated VLDL
(C) Both
(D) Neither

360. Frederickson type IIa hyperlipidemia

361. Frederickson type IIb hyperlipidemia

362. Frederickson type III hyperlipidemia

363. Frederickson type IV hyperlipidemia

VII. Coronary Heart Disease

Answers

281. The answer is B. *(pp 982–983)* Normal and elevated levels of triglycerides have been established. Levels less than 250 mg/dL are acceptable; levels between 250 and 500 mg/dL are borderline; and levels greater than 500 mg/dL are evidence of definite hypertriglyceridemia. Hypertriglyceridemia is often secondary to conditions that predispose to atherosclerosis such as obesity; excessive alcohol intake; diabetes mellitus; chronic renal failure; nephrotic syndrome; and the use of beta-blocking agents, estrogens, and corticosteroids. It is also seen as a component of familial combined hyperlipidemia, familial hypertriglyceridemia, and Frederickson's type V hyperlipidemia. Extremely high levels of triglycerides are associated with the development of pancreatitis.

282. The answer is E. *(pp 1003–1006)* The process of atherosclerosis begins with the development of flat lipid-rich lesions called fatty streaks. These early fatty streaks appear to consist almost entirely of macrophages. As the lesions expand they appear to contain smooth muscle cells that have migrated into the intima as well. These lesions become mixed macrophage–smooth muscle cell lesions in which both cells are lipid laden. Macrophages have been shown to release mitogens as potent as those derived from platelets. Macrophages release platelet-derived growth factor, interleukin 1, transforming growth factor-alpha, transforming growth factor-beta, and possibly fibroblast growth factor. It appears that the macrophage is the principal source of growth factor responsible for progression of the atherosclerotic lesion. Exposure of arterial smooth muscle cells to platelet-derived growth factor results in increased binding of LDL to these cells owing to the formation of an increased number of LDL receptors at the cell surface. This allows the cells to use exogenous sources of cholesterol for cell multiplication. The metabolic pathway of arachidonic acid leads to the formation of both thromboxane A_2 and prostacycline. Thromboxane A_2 is a powerful vasoconstrictor of smooth muscle and stimulates platelet aggregation. Aspirin and indomethacin inhibit thromboxane synthesis. Prostacycline is the principal product of cyclooxygenase activity in the walls of arteries and veins and is a potent vasodilator and inhibitor of platelet aggregation. Eicosapentaenoic acid is not completely metabolized by platelets and produces an inert form of thromboxane, thromboxane A_3. This fatty acid also forms an analogue of prostacycline in the endothelial cells that is as potent a vasodilator as prostacycline GI_2 and as effective in inhibiting platelet aggregation. Thus, this fatty acid may be protective against atherogenesis.

283. The answer is C. *(pp 999–1006)* Endothelial cells are quiescent as long as they are in contact with other endothelial cells or are contact-inhibited. If the cells are disrupted, they are stimulated to synthesize new DNA to proliferate and restore their continuity. Endothelial cells in culture are capable of producing collagen, prostacycline, factor VIII, and angiotensin converting enzyme. Factor VIII is required for platelet adherence and release, an important mechanism in the role of the development of the atherosclerotic plaque. Prostacycline on the other hand is a potent vasodilatory agent; it is also a potent inhibitor of platelet aggregation and protective against the development of atherogenesis. Prostacycline is synthesized by endothelial cells and smooth muscle cells. The principal mitogenic component present in whole blood serum and missing in cell-free plasma-derived serum is platelet-derived growth factor, which is responsible for the proliferation of smooth muscle cells. Smooth muscle and many other cells possess high-affinity LDL receptors. These receptors bind LDL, and the cell then internalizes the bound LDL and transports it to lysosomes, where it is degraded and free cholesterol is liberated for use by the cell. If the cell is exposed to excess LDL, there is a feedback inhibitory pathway in the cell that inhibits the synthesis of LDL receptors. Excess cholesterol within the cell inhibits cholesterol synthesis by the rate-limiting intracellular enzyme HMG-CoA reductase. LDL in hyperlipemic animals promotes endothelial injury and, indirectly, proliferation of smooth muscle cells and the production of new components of connective tissue. Thus, high LDL levels injure the endothelium and lead to proliferation of smooth muscle cells and formation of the atherosclerotic plaque.

284. The answer is D. *(pp 1010–1013)* The morphologic features of coronary atherosclerotic plaques can be quite variable. The plaque may be concentric and is more likely to be a fixed stenosis due to the effect of the diffuse internal thickening. An eccentric stenosis may have a retained area of normal vessel wall opposite the plaque, thus permitting tonal variations in the medial muscle that can further alter the shape of the lumen. The relative proportion of lipid and connective tissue that are contained in plaque can be quite variable with as much as 70 percent of soft plaque made up of extracellular cholesterol. These soft plaques have the highest risk of future thrombosis. The media behind coronary plaques undergo atrophy and may allow the plaque to bulge outward rather than inward initially, making it relatively imperceptible on a coronary arteriogram.

285. The answer is C. *(pp 1022–1023; Furchgott and Zawadzki, Nature 288:373–376, 1980)* Endothelial-dependent vasodilation is one of the most important functions of the normal endothelium. Furchgott and Zawadzki demonstrated the existence of an endothelial-derived humoral factor, which they termed endothelial-derived relaxing factor (EDRF), that caused the dilatation of blood vessels by diffusing to the underlying smooth muscle cells and increasing cyclic guanosine monophosphate (cGMP). Acetylcholine and other muscarinic cholinergic agonists cause dilatation with an intact endothelium and contraction when the endothelium is removed. Other vasodilators, such as serotonin, thrombin, flow, substance P, and adenine nucleotides, act through this mechanism. Early works suggest similarities of EDRF to nitric oxide (NO), one of which is the ease of degradation by oxygen-free radicals. Nitrous oxide (N_2O) is an anesthetic gas and has no relationship to EDRF.

286. The answer is E. *(p 1025)* Research within the past 10 years indicates that atherosclerosis creates a fundamental defect in endothelial function, primarily by affecting endothelial-dependent vasodilation. This is thought to be initiated through decreased activity of endothelial-derived relaxing factor (EDRF) and its corollary, nitric oxide (NO). There may be either decreased production of NO or normal or increased production of NO with increased degradation to inactive metabolites. However, EDRF is not hyperactive in atherosclerosis. The amino acid precursor of NO, arginine, causes a reversal of the endothelial-dependent vasodilator defect in an atherosclerotic animal model. Free-radical degradation of NO is thought to contribute to the contractile abnormality in atherosclerotic animal models and is reversed by superoxide dismutase, which is a free-radical scavenger. Nitrous oxide (N_2O) is an anesthetic agent and of a different molecular configuration than nitric oxide (NO).

287. The answer is C. *(pp 1076–1077)* Angina with a normal coronary arteriography usually occurs in women (70 percent) and is characterized by recurrent episodes of pain. Chest pain precipitating factors are reminiscent of ischemia but often with atypical features in regards to the duration of discomfort and the response to anginal agents. Exercise-induced ST-segment changes and thallium perfusion defects are commonly seen. The preponderance of evidence indicates that these patients have an abnormality in coronary vasomotor control at the microvascular level.

288. The answer is B. *(p 1066, Figure 58-1)*   After transient total occlusion of a coronary artery as may occur in unstable angina or after balloon inflation during angioplasty, there is a sequential hemodynamic response. Diastolic dysfunction occurs within seconds, followed in 10 sec or so by systolic dysfunction. Changes on the electrocardiogram (ECG) occur at about 20 sec, and angina, if present, occurs after about 25 sec. It is now apparent that patients may experience many ischemic episodes without progressing to angina.

289. The answer is D. *(p 1058)*   When a middle-aged man gives a history of classic effort-related angina, the predictive value of the history is approximately 90 percent. Although risk factors are helpful in identifying patients at high risk for the development of atherosclerotic coronary artery disease, the absence of risk factors by no means negates a suggestive history of angina pectoris. When the history of chest pain is more vague, the predictive accuracy may be only 70 to 80 percent. Moreover, the diagnostic accuracy of chest pain in middle-aged women is only about 50 percent.

290. The answer is D. *(p 1058)*   The exercise electrocardiogram (ECG) is often a helpful tool in both the diagnosis and determination of prognosis in patients with suspected coronary artery disease. However, in certain population groups where the incidence of coronary artery disease is quite low, there can be a high prevalence of false-positive responses. A positive ECG response in a young woman with atypical symptoms has a predictive accuracy of only about 50 percent, while in middle-aged men, the predictive accuracy is 70 to 80 percent.

291. The answer is C. *(p 1098)*   The angiographic appearance of both ergonovine-induced and spontaneous coronary artery spasm can be quite variable. Coronary vasospasm more commonly involves the right coronary artery but can involve any major coronary artery or bypass graft. It is usually localized to an atherosclerotic lesion. Spasm may appear as a localized constriction but also can be multifocal with several sites of spasm involving one artery or in different arteries. In some patients, the process may be diffuse, involving one or more arteries. Coronary spasm can induce both ST elevation and ST depression.

292. The answer is A. *(p 1100)*   Administration of ergonovine produces ischemic chest pain and ST-segment shifts in most patients with variant angina. It induces spasm in approximately 5 percent of patients with effort-related angina and is only rarely positive in patients with atypical chest pain. Coronary spasm can usually be induced with relatively low doses of ergonovine (0.05 to 0.15 mg). Once induced, coronary spasm should be promptly reversed with intracoronary nitroglycerin. Ergonovine is contraindicated in patients with recent myocardial infarction, unstable angina, left main disease, severe hypertension, and left ventricular dysfunction.

293. The answer is A. *(pp 1098–1099)*   Although Prinzmetal's original description of variant angina described episodes associated with ST-segment elevation, it has been shown that ST-segment depression occurs just as frequently with variant angina. Subendocardial ischemia, as reflected by ST-segment depression, may be in part due to subtotal coronary spasm or involvement of smaller branch vessels or may indicate the presence of significant collaterals. Vasospasm may be precipitated by exertion with the development of exercise-induced ST elevation. Variant angina frequently occurs at the same time of day, especially early in the morning. The episodes are intermittent and frequently characterized by periods of remission. About one-quarter of these patients have a history of migraine headaches.

294. The answer is E. *(pp 1099–1100)*   Administration of ergonovine, a vasoconstrictor, will produce coronary spasm in 90 percent of patients with active variant angina. A truly positive test requires reproduction of the patient's chest discomfort along with the demonstration of significant focal coronary spasm. In addition, there should be associated ST-segment elevation or depression. Once focal coronary spasm is demonstrated, it should be promptly relieved with sublingual intravenous or intracoronary nitroglycerin. Rarely does ergonovine produce refractory spasm or a positive result in patients with atypical pain in whom spasm is not suspected. High-grade, fixed obstruction with unstable angina pectoris is a contraindication to ergonovine administration although spasm on fixed lesions is not an uncommon clinical entity. Relative contraindications to ergonovine administration include recent myocardial infarction, uncontrolled angina, and uncontrolled arrhythmias. Absolute contraindications include severe hypertension, severe left ventricular dysfunction, severe aortic stenosis, and significant left main coronary artery occlusion. Ergonovine should generally be administered only in a catheterization laboratory or in a coronary care unit (CCU) in patients in whom coronary arteries are known to be arteriographically normal.

295. The answer is C. *(p 1090)*   Unstable angina is an acute manifestation of coronary artery disease and carries a significant risk of acute myocardial infarction and death within 3 months. The risk of acute myocardial infarction is approximately 10 to 20 percent, and the mortality rate is approximately 5 to 10 percent. In addition, there is a 20 to 25 percent incidence of recurrent severe ischemia occurring during hospitalization.

296. The answer is B. *(pp 1091–1092)*   The severity of the symptoms of angina seem to correlate with the prognosis in patients with unstable angina. Thus, patients who present with rest pain or prolonged episodes of ischemic chest pain have a worse prognosis than those presenting with new onset effort-related angina. The most powerful predictor of early cardiac events is whether recurrent angina occurs after hospitalization and implementation of intense medical therapy. Although exercise stress testing could be performed after a period of stabilization, it would be inappropriate in the acute phase of suspected unstable angina and, thus, is poorly studied.

297. The answer is D. *(pp 1093–1094)*   Both aspirin and heparin have been shown to significantly reduce the risk of fatal and nonfatal myocardial infarction in patients with unstable angina. Ticlopidine has also demonstrated a beneficial effect and may be used in patients who are intolerant of aspirin. The role of thrombolytic therapy in unstable angina remains unclear and at present is not recommended pending further studies.

298. The answer is B. *(p 1150)*   Complete rupture of the papillary muscle following acute myocardial infarction produces massive mitral regurgitation resulting in pulmonary edema and cardiogenic shock. Partial rupture of the papillary muscle may result in lesser degrees of mitral regurgitation, thereby permitting time for surgical correction. The posteromedial papillary muscle, which has a single blood supply, is much more susceptible to rupture than the anterolateral muscle, which has a dual blood supply from both the left anterior descending and left circumflex coronary arteries. Papillary muscle rupture may be more frequent in patients with a small infarction and well preserved left ventricular function since the shearing forces may be higher in this group of patients. In a patient with papillary muscle rupture and cardiogenic shock, the cardiac output may be so poor that a systolic murmur may not be heard. An oxygen stepup at the level of the right ventricle is diagnostic of a ruptured intraventricular septum rather than a ruptured papillary muscle. On Swan-Ganz catheterization, a large *v* wave in the pulmonary capillary wedge pressure tracing would be characteristic of papillary muscle rupture.

299. The answer is C. *(p 1151)*   External cardiac rupture, or cardiorrhexis, is much more common than rupture of the papillary muscle or ventricular septum and results in a hemopericardium with cardiac tamponade. The patient develops jugular venous distention as well as cardiogenic shock. Electromechanical dissociation (EMD) is a frequent accompanying event. Since most patients with external cardiac rupture have sustained a transmural infarction, the pericardial pain that is not improved by narcotics or steroids suggests impending myocardial rupture via the leak of blood through the transmural necrotic zone. Most patients unfortunately die suddenly without any preceding symptoms. The patient with myocardial rupture may experience sinus bradycardia or a slow junctional rhythm on the basis of vagal stimulation. Although pericardiocentesis may temporarily improve the effects of cardiac tamponade, only with immediate surgery and closure of the ruptured myocardium can the patient be saved. External cardiac rupture is seldom seen before the sixth decade of life and is associated with poor collateral circulation in the infarcted area, systemic arterial hypertension during the acute phase of infarction, and dilatation and thinning of the area of the infarction.

300. The answer is C. *(p 1109)*   Hibernating myocardium is a persistent contraction abnormality induced by a persistent and significant reduction in coronary blood flow; it can be reversed upon restoration of normal blood flow. Reduction of coronary blood flow to 20 percent of normal can produce loss of contractile function and is felt to be due to down regulation of myocardial contraction for purposes of myocardial survival. Distinguishing necrotic myocardium from hibernating myocardium is clinically important in evaluating patients who may benefit from coronary artery bypass surgery. Positron emission tomography (PET) may be useful in assessing potential myocardial viability.

301. The answer is B. *(p 1190)*   The most important prognostic determinant of prognosis in patients with stable angina pectoris is that of exercise tolerance. Patients with excellent exercise tolerance as assessed by exercise duration and the maximum heart rate achieved have a quite favorable prognosis with a short-term annual mortality of around 1 to 2 percent. Poor exercise tolerance as shown by the inability to complete stage II of the Bruce protocol portends an annual mortality of 6 to 10 percent.

302. The answer is B. *(pp 1192–1193)*   Numerous studies have shown that there is a substantial increase in the incidence of sudden death and myocardial infarction in patients with the onset of unstable angina pectoris, particularly patients with a history of stable angina or Prinzmetal's angina. The high-risk period appears to be 3 to 6 months following the onset of unstable symptoms with the incidence of sudden death or infarction reported as high as 19 percent in one series. Patients who experience ST-segment elevation during episodes or who respond poorly to maximal medical therapy have an even worse prognosis. Patients with isolated episodes of prolonged ischemic discomfort without evidence of infarction suffer the same mortality at 1 year as patients who have had a documented myocardial infarction.

303. The answer is C. *(pp 1196–1197)*   The first 12 months following a myocardial infarction is the most hazardous with mortality rates reported as high as 10 percent during this period. The most powerful predictors of outcome in the early postinfarction period are the degree of left ventricular dysfunction and objective evidence of ischemia during exercise stress testing. The occurrence of angina suggests another infarction and, therefore, is a poor prognostic sign. The degree of ST-segment elevation during the acute phase may give a gross estimate of the infarct size, but it is confounded by many variables and is not a very reliable measure.

304. The answer is D. *(pp 977, 1206–1209)*   Diets high in saturated fat and cholesterol elevate hepatocyte cholesterol concentration. This decreases the number of low-density lipoprotein (LDL) receptors and increases plasma LDL. Former smokers have a significantly lower risk of myocardial infarction and coronary death than do patients who continue to smoke, and coronary risk appears to approach that of nonsmokers within 2 to 10 years. Former smokers also have higher high-density lipoprotein (HDL) to LDL ratios and lower plasma fibrinogen levels. In patients with coronary disease and stable angina, active smoking induces changes in regional myocardial perfusion on nuclear scans. Several studies have shown that several antihypertensive therapies, when given to patients who continue to smoke, do not lead to a decrease in coronary events unlike their nonsmoking cohorts.

305. The answer is D. *(pp 1206–1207)*   In addition to recognized factors affecting coronary atherosclerosis, such as elevated lipids and hypertension, cigarette smoksing can affect the coronary arteries in many ways. The tone and reactivity of the vascular endothelium can be damaged by smoking, resulting in the release of thromboxane A_2 (TXA$_2$), enhanced vasopressin generation, increased α-adrenergic stimulation, and diminished prostacyclin (PGI$_2$) production. Circulating levels of catecholamines and free fatty acids are also increased, leading to increases in heart rate, blood pressure, and myocardial contractility with concomitant increases in vascular resistance, leading to increased myocardial oxygen demand. Patients who continue to smoke after myocardial infarction have the highest mortality. Increased platelet aggregation leads to a propensity to thrombosis with concomitant endothelial damage.

306. The answer is E. *(pp 1245–1246)*   Systolic compression of a large coronary artery due to intramyocardial bridging is a relatively rare arteriographic finding, occurring in less than 1 percent of patients studied for chest pain. It usually involves the left anterior descending coronary artery and is usually a benign incidental finding. There have been several case reports of patients with marked systolic compression (over 75 percent of diastolic diameter of a coronary artery) who had documented ischemic symptoms. These patients with refractory symptoms who have undergone coronary artery bypass or unroofing of the coronary segment have responded favorably.

307. The answer is C. *(p 1206; MRFIT, JAMA 248:1465–1477, 1982)*   In the Multiple Risk Factor Intervention Trial (MRFIT), the relationship of serum cholesterol to total mortality from all causes and from coronary heart disease were obtained in over 300,000 men over a follow-up of 6 years. Total mortality and coronary heart disease mortality rise dramatically at serum cholesterol levels greater than 200 mg/dL. Subjects with mean cholesterols of 167 mg/dL had the lowest coronary heart disease mortality, but below that level, total mortality seemed to rise. This is probably best explained by a cholesterol-lowering effect of cancer and does not appear to persist beyond 5 years of follow-up, probably because those patients with low cholesterol due to cancer have already died of their disease. The relationship between an increased total mortality and markedly low serum cholesterols has been observed in other studies as well.

308. The answer is B. *(pp 1243–1244)*   The most common pattern of anomalous aortic origin of a coronary artery is the left circumflex coronary artery arising from the right sinus of Valsalva or from the right proximal coronary artery; it does not appear to produce myocardial ischemia. When the left main coronary artery arises from the right sinus of Valsalva and courses between the aorta and pulmonary artery, there is an increased incidence of exercise-induced sudden death. In a similar fashion, ischemia may occur when the entire circulation branches from a single aortic ostium and must cross the base of the heart to the contralateral side where it is subjected to the potential risks of angulation, compression, and accelerated atherosclerosis. Anomalous origin of a coronary artery from the pulmonary artery usually presents in infancy and may produce recurrent angina or infarction, congestive heart failure (CHF), and mitral regurgitation. Atresia of the coronary ostium may be associated with myocardial ischemia or infarction in childhood.

309. The answer is D. *(p 1266)*   Bile acid sequestrants, such as cholestyramine, generally cause gastrointestinal side effects such as constipation and bloating. Bile acid sequestrants can elevate triglyceride levels in patients with moderate hypertriglyceridemia, especially those who consume alcohol. Bile sequestrants are contraindicated in severe hypertriglyceridemia because they raise triglyceride levels and because they can precipitate acute pancreatitis.

310. The answer is C. *(p 1267)*   Lovastatin, pravastatin, and simvastatin are all 3-hydroxy-3-methylglutaryl coenzyme A (HMG CoA) reductase inhibitors available in the United States. HMG CoA reductase inhibitors can produce indigestion in some patients. Mild elevation of liver transaminases may occur with institution of therapy, but the drug need not be discontinued unless the transaminase levels reach two to three times normal. HMG CoA reductase inhibitors can produce myopathy and rhabdomyolysis with renal failure when administered concomitantly to transplant patients taking cyclosporine to prevent rejection.

311. The answer is D. *(p 1284)*   Suicide attempts and accidental overdoses with beta blockers are being described with increasing frequency. Since β-adrenergic blockers are competitive pharmacological antagonists, their life-threatening effects (i.e., bradycardia and myocardial and ventilatory failure) can be overcome with the immediate infusion of a beta agonist, such as isoproterenol and dobutamine. In situations in which those drugs are ineffective, use of glucagon has been advocated. Glucagon activates the cyclic adenosine monophosphate (cAMP) mechanism independent of the beta receptor.

312. The answer is C. *(pp 1265–1269)*   Bile acid sequestrants have the property of binding bile acids in the intestinal tract and, therefore, preventing their absorption; examples include colestipol and cholestyramine. This results in an enhanced degradation of cholesterol into bile acids. The hepatic concentration of cholesterol falls, and this, in turn, stimulates the synthesis of low-density lipoprotein (LDL) receptors. Nicotinic acid (niacin) reduces both very low-density lipoprotein (VLDL) and LDL cholesterol and also raises the high-density lipoprotein (HDL) cholesterol level. These effects of niacin appear to be related to its action of inhibiting the hepatic secretion of VLDL.

Fibric acids, such as gemfibrozil and clofibrate, enhance the activity of lipoprotein lipase (LPL), partially inhibit the synthesis of VLDL triglycerides and cholesterol (with increased activity of LDL receptors), reduce the conversion of cholesterol into bile acids, and enhance the secretion of cholesterol into bile. These drugs are very effective in lowering plasma triglycerides. 3-Hydroxy-3-methylglutaryl coenzyme A (HMG CoA) reductase inhibitors act mainly in the liver by blocking cholesterol synthesis. This, in turn, stimulates the synthesis of LDL receptors, which leads to increased uptake of circulating VLDL remnants and LDL by the liver. The major indication is primary severe hypercholesterolemia. The primary action of probucol is to reduce the LDL cholesterol level. It clears LDL from the plasma and also lowers HDL cholesterol levels. The primary indication is moderate hypercholesterolemia.

313. The answer is C. *(p 1278)*   Propranolol and metoprolol are both lipid soluble and are almost completely absorbed in the small intestine. They are metabolized largely by the liver and tend to have relatively short plasma half-lives. Because of their lipid solubility, they are prone to affect the central nervous system (CNS) and to produce symptoms of depression, lethargy, and hallucinations. It is still not certain whether drugs that are less lipid soluble cause fewer of these adverse CNS reactions.

314. The answer is D. *(p 1385; Jones, Ann Surg 192(3):390–392, 1980)*   In a study by Jones and colleagues, the frequency of perioperative myocardial infarction was not statistically related to the extent of vessel disease, left ventricular dysfunction, or the incompleteness of revascularization. Poor distal reperfusion once grafting of the more proximal arteries has been performed seems to be associated with the highest incidence of perioperative infarctions.

315. The answer is E. *(pp 1295–1303)*   Studies have shown the efficacy of diltiazem, nifedipine, amlodipine, nicardipine, verapamil, and bepridil in the treatment of stable angina pectoris. Although 10 percent of patients with stable effort-related symptoms experience a severe exacerbation of angina with withdrawal of propranolol, no major reactions seem to occur with abrupt withdrawal of diltiazem, nifedipine, or verapamil. Both verapamil and diltiazem are effective in controlling the rate of atrial fibrillation but are rarely effective in converting acute and chronic atrial fibrillation to normal sinus rhythm. Verapamil and diltiazem terminate paroxysmal supraventricular tachycardia (PSVT) by slowing atrioventricular (AV) nodal conduction and increasing refractoriness but have minimal effect on the accessory pathway responsible for conducting the fibrillatory impulses in the Wolff-Parkinson-White syndrome. Bepridil has class I antiarrhythmic activity, but it is not approved for use in the United States. Oral verapamil is not effective in the treatment of ventricular ectopy. Intravenous calcium antagonists do not benefit patients with ventricular ectopy except in the case of myocardial infarction (perhaps an anti-ischemic effect).

316. The answer is A. *(p 1314)*   Although warfarin is found in the milk of nursing mothers, it appears in its inactive form and, therefore, is safe for breast-fed infants. In fat malabsorption states, vitamin K absorption is impaired, and the anticoagulation with warfarin is potentiated. Cholestyramine impairs the absorption of warfarin, thereby reducing the anticoagulant effect of the drug. Certain drugs such as phenylbutazone, trimethoprim-sulfamethoxazole, and amiodarone inhibit the clearance of warfarin and, therefore, can result in prolongation of the prothrombin time when the drugs are used concomitantly.

317. The answer is D. *(pp 1369, 2153)*   In patients who have both significant coronary artery disease and carotid vascular disease there has been controversy over which procedure should be done first or whether they should be done in combination. In general, patients with significant carotid occlusive disease but no cerebrovascular symptoms should have the coronary artery bypass procedure alone and elective carotid end-arterectomy at a later date. If the patient has active cerebrovascular symptoms (TIAs or nondisabling stroke within the last 3 months), then carotid endarterectomy should be performed in conjunction with coronary artery bypass surgery. The rationale behind this approach is that the morbidity and mortality of the two procedures done together are considerably higher than done alone. In addition, patients with significant carotid stenosis have a low rate of stroke due to hemodynamic changes during coronary artery bypass surgery. Indeed, most preoperative strokes are embolic in origin.

318. **The answer is A.** *(pp 1384–1385)* Neurologic deficits secondary to air embolism are usually transient and resolve completely at a variable rate during the postoperative period. Heparin is not indicated. On the other hand, embolization of particulate matter is usually more devastating and has less chance of resolution. The frequency of neurologic events increases as the age and general debilitation of bypass candidates increases. Little data on the effect of steroids on air embolism are available.

319. **The answer is D (4).** *(p 977)* Low-density lipoprotein (LDL) receptors bind and internalize LDL for the synthesis of cellular membranes and steroid hormones. The concentration of LDL receptors is in part dependent on age; high levels are seen early in life and decrease with age. High levels of LDL both in the blood and internally tend to down-regulate the receptors while low levels of cholesterol up-regulate the receptors. Most cell surfaces contain LDL receptors, the number of which determine blood levels of LDL.

320. **The answer is A (1, 2, 3).** *(p 984)* Certain levels of apolipoprotein provide additional evidence for the development of coronary atherosclerosis. A positive correlation with the premature development of coronary atherosclerosis is found with the presence of apolipoprotein B (apo B) and lipoprotein[a] (Lp[a]). A negative association with coronary atherosclerosis has been seen with the presence of apolipoprotein A-1 (apo A-1). Lp[a] has structural similarity to plasminogen and may, therefore, compete with plasminogen in the fibrinolytic pathway. This competition may lead to a decrease in the breakdown of fibrin.

321. **The answer is E (all).** *(p 1015)* Angiographic, angioscopic, and necropsy studies have all demonstrated that the development of unstable angina pectoris is due to the development of nonocclusive thrombi at the site of a fissured plaque. Platelet emboli may occur, producing small areas of myocardial necrosis in the distal myocardium. In addition, there may be varying degrees of vasomotor tone, further contributing to the dynamic occlusive process found in patients with unstable angina. Eventually the thrombotic lesion may progress to acute infarction or regress to allow plaque healing.

322. **The answer is E (all).** *(p 1027)* Increased numbers of inflammatory cells and their activation may be related directly to plaque instability, fracture, or fissuring, and thrombus formation. Activation of lymphocytes and macrophages may release oxygen-free radicals, form hydrogen peroxide (H_2O_2), and influence the secretion of degradative enzymes such as collagenase and haluronidase. These enzymes may degrade connective tissue and compromise the structural integrity of the plaque.

323. **The answer is C (2, 4).** *(pp 1027–1028, Figure 56-5)* The events that precipitate activation of an atherosclerotic plaque seem to be centered around activation of the macrophage. This activation may result in cytokine production, which increases adhesion molecule expression and further recruitment of mononuclear cells and lymphocytes. In addition, the activated macrophages produce procoagulant factors and growth factors. They may also secrete proteolytic agents such as collagenase, elastase, and free radicals that lead to tissue damage and disruption. Macrophages are also thought to contribute angiogenic factors that increase the neovascularization of the plaque. This neovascularization tends to destabilize the plaque rather than stabilize it.

324. The answer is B (1, 3). *(pp 1022–1024, Table 56-1)* The endothelium plays a central role in controlling the biology of the vessel wall, and healthy, functional endothelium is crucial to the prevention of disease. The most important normal function is endothelial-dependent vasodilation. This appears to be mediated via an endothelial-derived relaxing factor (EDRF) that causes the dilatation of blood vessels by diffusing to the underlying smooth muscle cells and increasing cyclic guanosine monophosphate (cGMP). In addition, the healthy endothelium creates a natural anti-inflammatory state by controlling the localization of circulating leukocytes. The endothelial surface is a prototypic nonthrombogenic surface as it produces agents that inhibit platelet aggregation, clot formation, and produces thrombolytic agents such as tissue plasminogen activator (tPA). Lastly, a normal endothelium is primarily growth-inhibitory. In a dysfunctional endothelium, such as in atherosclerosis, these functions are reversed. In this state, endothelium becomes prothrombotic, has a decreased vasodilatation and increased vasoconstriction responses, promotes growth of smooth muscle cells in the vascular wall, and becomes proinflammatory.

325. The answer is C (2, 4). *(p 1066)* The circadian rhythm of coronary ischemia has been well recognized. The amount of exertion required to provoke angina may be considerably less in some patients in the early morning hours. In addition, the evidence of acute myocardial infarction is much higher in the mornings. This diurnal variation of coronary ischemia is related to variations in catecholamine secretion, which are highest in the morning, and to a sensitivity to coronary vasoconstrictors, which also appears to be highest in the morning.

326. The answer is B (1, 3). *(p 1073)* The decision of whether to refer a patient for coronary revascularization involves many factors. Although there are many individual variables that must be considered, there are general guidelines that are useful. The variables employed include the severity of symptoms, the degree of ischemia on exercise stress testing, the status of left ventricular function, and the anatomical distribution of the coronary artery disease. Even patients with mild symptoms, little ischemia on exercise stress testing, but with left main disease or three-vessel disease with associated left ventricular dysfunction have significantly improved longevity with coronary artery bypass surgery as opposed to medical therapy. Patients with double-vessel disease with proximal left anterior descending stenosis also have enhanced longevity with coronary artery bypass surgery as compared to medical therapy.

327. The answer is B (1, 3). *(p 1100)* Sublingual nitrates, as well as calcium antagonists, are effective in preventing episodes of angina due to coronary vasospasm. Beta blockers may be useful in some patients with no significant coronary atherosclerotic obstruction; however, in patients with no significant obstruction, unopposed α-adrenergic vasoconstriction with concomitant blockade of β-adrenergic vasodilatation may lead to exacerbation of symptoms. Coronary artery bypass grafting alone has not been successful in the treatment of vasospastic angina as spasm in a nongrafted vessel or distal to the site of anastomosis may occur. Total denervation of the heart has also failed to prevent coronary vasospasm.

328. The answer is A (1, 2, 3). *(p 1130)* Thrombolytic therapy is clearly indicated in those patients presenting with ST-segment elevation and symptoms of prolonged MI whose onset has occurred within 6 h. Large, randomized trials have also demonstrated a definite benefit in those patients with LBBB and symptoms of acute MI. Although advanced age was a concern in the past, the benefits appear to outweigh the risks of thrombolytic therapy in the elderly. Large, randomized trials have for the most part demonstrated some benefit in the administration of thrombolytic therapy even 6 to 12 h after the beginning of ischemic pain in high-risk infarctions.

329. The answer is E (all). *(p 1225)* Prior to discharge following an acute myocardial infarction, physicians perform an exercise test to identify patients at increased risk for early reinfarction or sudden cardiac death. The intensity of the work load is preset using the following criteria: achievement of a work load to 3 to 3.5 METs (1 MET = 3.5 mL O_2 per kilogram of body weight per minute); achievement of a heart rate of 120 to

140 beats per minute; achievement of 60 percent of the age-predicted heart rate; or the presence of exercise-induced symptoms.

330. The answer is A (1, 2, 3). *(p 1255)* Several infectious diseases are known to affect the coronary arteries. For example, syphilis causes an ostial stenosis of the coronary arteries in 25 percent of patients with tertiary disease. Angina and myocardial infarction have ensued. Salmonellosis, typhus, and leprosy have also been associated with coronary arteritis. In 20 percent of patients with Kawasaki's disease, vasculitis of the vasa vasorum leads to coronary arteritis, coronary aneurysms, stenosis, and occlusion. However, although some studies suggest a retrovirus as the etiologic agent, the etiology is presently considered immunologic.

331. The answer is E (all). *(p 1247)* Coronary arterial aneurysms may be isolated or multiple; their etiology may be congenital or acquired. Congenital coronary artery aneurysms most commonly involve the right coronary artery and may lead to thromboses and subsequent infarction in a young person. Atherosclerotic coronary aneurysms account for most coronary aneurysms (50 percent) and are thought to be due to the destruction of the media. External trauma or internal trauma (e.g., from angioplasty or atherectomy) may damage the media and cause coronary aneurysms.

332. The answer is B (1, 3). *(pp 1275–1276)* Beta blockers as a group tend to have similar bioavailability and long half-lives, which allow single daily dosing. Atenolol and nadolol are water-soluble agents, which are incompletely absorbed through the gastrointestinal tract and eliminated unchanged by the kidney. Because of this renal elimination and consequent drug accumulation in renal failure, caution must be used when prescribing these particular beta blockers to patients with renal failure.

333. The answer is A (1, 2, 3). *(pp 1300–1301)* Diltiazem, nifedipine, and verapamil have all been used in the treatment of ischemic heart disease and chronic hypertension. Nifedipine has been the most popular calcium antagonist in the treatment of acute hypertension, but intravenous nicardipine has been recently approved for use in hypertensive crises. Diltiazem, nifedipine, and verapamil have all been effective in the treatment of silent myocardial ischemia either alone or in combination with nitrates. Verapamil and nifedipine improve left ventricular filling characteristics in patients with hypertrophic cardiomyopathy. Verapamil can improve exercise capacity and symptoms in patients with hypertrophic cardiomyopathy, even those refractory to beta blockers. Studies show a reduction in the size of myocardial necrosis with nifedipine, verapamil, and diltiazem in experimental coronary occlusion. However, the clinical trials of calcium antagonists in acute myocardial infarction have shown a small excess mortality in the treated group. A group of patients with non–Q-wave infarction treated with diltiazem had a lower reinfarction rate, but overall mortality was not affected.

334. The answer is A (1, 2, 3). *(pp 1316–1317)* Aspirin inhibits cyclooxygenase by acetylating the serine residue at the active site of the enzyme. This inhibition is irreversible and, therefore, lasts for the life of the platelet. Aspirin is rapidly absorbed in the stomach and upper small intestine. Platelet inhibition occurs within 60 min of oral administration. High doses of aspirin do not appear more efficacious than low doses in their effect on platelet inhibition. Low-dose aspirin inhibits the synthesis of both thromboxane A_2 (TXA_2) and prostacyclin (PGI_2). Although aspirin inhibits the secondary wave of aggregation induced by adenosine diphosphate (ADP), epinephrine, and low-dose collagen, a full aggregation response can be caused by thrombin and high concentrations of collagen even in the presence of aspirin.

335. The answer is C (2, 4). *(p 1321)* Ticlopidine is approved for clinical use by the Food and Drug Administration (FDA). It does not inhibit prostaglandin synthesis or cyclic adenosine monophosphate (cAMP) degradation. Ticlopidine may act on the platelet membrane to alter its reactivity and may block the interaction of fibrinogen and von Willebrand factor with platelets. It inhibits adenosine diphosphate (ADP)–induced platelet aggregation. It is important to note that optimal efficacy of the medication is reached only after several days of therapy. Most clinical trials have used 250 mg twice daily. Ticlopidine is effective in a variety of clinical disorders that include unstable angina, abrupt thrombotic occlusion in patients undergoing coronary angioplasty, transient ischemic attacks (TIAs), and strokes. The most important side effects are diarrhea (20 percent), rash (12 percent), and neutropenia (less than 1 percent).

336. The answer is C (2, 4). *(p 1330)*   Purified urokinase preparations are nonantigenic and nonpyrogenic. The incidence of bleeding episodes as compared to streptokinase administration is similar. Urokinase activates plasminogen directly. It has no specific affinity for fibrin and activates fibrin-bound and circulating plasminogen relatively indiscriminately. Circulating plasminogen activation and depletion of α_2-antiplasmin may occur, leading to systemic activation of the fibrinolytic system with low levels of fibrinogen.

337. The answer is E (all). *(p 1340)*   Despite significant technical improvements and operator experience, coronary angioplasty carries some risk to the patient. Certain predictors of abrupt vessel closure have been identified and include female sex, long lesions, bifurcated or angulated lesions, heavily calcified lesions, and the presence of thrombus. Despite years of active research, restenosis remains in the 30 to 50 percent range and is a particularly vexing problem with proximal left anterior descending lesions, ostial right coronary lesions, proximal or mid-vein graft lesions, and with chronic total occlusions.

338. The answer is E (all). *(pp 1367–1368)*   The selection of patients for consideration for coronary artery bypass surgery is based on the arteriographic findings, which indicate the amount of myocardium at risk. Large, randomized trials and retrospective analysis have established improvement in long-term survival in patients with left main stem disease, severe three-vessel disease, and double-vessel disease with proximal left anterior descending obstruction.

339. The answer is B (1, 3). *(p 1374)*   Ten or more years after surgery, the patency rate of the left internal mammary artery graft to the left anterior descending is 90 percent or greater. This translates into a significant increase in 10-year survival when this procedure is used in conjunction with saphenous vein grafts as opposed to saphenous vein grafts only. Saphenous vein bypass patency is approximately 80 percent at 5 years, but drops off to 40 to 60 percent at 10 years after surgery.

340. The answers are: A-Y, B-N, C-Y, D-Y, E-N. *(p 973, LRC-CPPT, JAMA 251:351–364, 1984; LRC-CPPT, JAMA 251:365–374, 1984; Frick, N Engl J Med 317:1237–1245, 1987; Canner, J Am Coll Cardiol 8:1245–1255, 1986; Brown, N Engl J Med 323:1289–1298, 1990; Brensike, Circulation 69:313–324, 1984)*   It is now well accepted that hypercholesterolemia should be treated. The Lipid Research Clinics Coronary Primary Prevention Trial (LRC-CPPT) used cholestyramine, the Helsinki Heart Study used gemfibrozil, and the Coronary Drug Project used niacin. All of these studies showed a decrease in fatal and nonfatal coronary heart disease events in the treated population. Angiographic atherosclerosis has been studied in the Familial Atherosclerosis Treatment Study (FATS) and the United States National Heart, Lung, and Blood Institute (NHLBI) Type II Coronary Intervention Study. These studies all showed that the progression of atherosclerosis could be slowed, halted, and even reversed with active treatment.

341. The answers are: A-Y, B-N, C-N, D-N, E-Y. *(pp 979–980; Second Report of NCEP, JAMA 209:3015–3023, 1993)*   The guidelines for treatment of hypercholesterolemia have been established by the Adult Treatment Panel II of the National Cholesterol Education Program (NCEP). These guidelines provide recommendations for the screening and initial treatment of asymptomatic patients without definite evidence of coronary heart disease. All adults at age 20 and every 5 years thereafter should have either a fasting or nonfasting assessment of total cholesterol and high-density lipoprotein (HDL). A lipoprotein analysis is recommended when the total cholesterol is more than or equal to 240 mg/dL and the HDL is less than or equal to 35 mg/dL. Treatment recommendations are based on a fasting determination of low-density lipoprotein (LDL). If the LDL is between 130 and 159 mg/dL and less than two risk factors are present (i.e., men 45 years of age or over, women 55 years of age or over, a positive family history, smoking, hypertension, HDL levels less than 35 mg/dL, or diabetes), then the LDL should be repeated annually. If more than two risk factors are present, dietary treatment should begin. If the LDL is greater than 160 mg/dL, then dietary treatment should also be initiated.

342. The answers are: A-N, B-N, C-Y, D-Y, E-N. *(pp 989–993)* Atherosclerotic lesions contain components of three cellular phenomena. These are (1) proliferation of smooth muscle cells, (2) formation of a connective tissue matrix of elastic fibers, collagen, and proteoglycans that is produced by proliferation of smooth muscle, and (3) accumulation of intracellular and extracellular lipid. High-cholesterol diets in animals induce monocytes to attach to the endothelium of arteries. These monocytes work their way through the endothelium and localize in the subendothelium, where they accumulate lipid and create the fatty streak. Smooth muscle cells collect subintimally in this area and stretch the endothelium thin so that breaks occur in the intima and expose lipid-filled macrophages. Platelets attach to the exposed macrophages and form mural thrombi. This platelet-macrophage interaction is thought to be basic to the initiation of atherogenesis since it stimulates the further proliferation of smooth muscle cells and the formation of the fibrous plaque. The fibrous plaque becomes vascularized and accumulates a lipid-filled core, which can calcify and hemorrhage. The intima of this advanced lesion can ulcerate and lead to further platelet aggregation and thrombosis. Atherosclerosis primarily involves the intimal layer of the blood vessel, but as the atherosclerotic lesion progresses the media may atrophy with a decreasing number of smooth muscle cells. It is interesting that the fatty streak does not inevitably lead to atherosclerosis as it is found in groups who do not develop atherosclerosis. Clearly, other factors affect the progression of this lesion.

343. The answers are: A-Y, B-Y, C-Y, D-Y, E-Y. *(pp 999–1002)* Endothelial cells provide a thromboresistant and selective-permeability barrier to the arterial wall. Endothelial cells can transport lipoproteins into the arterial wall using pinocytotic vesicles. Smaller molecules like HDL may be transported into the arterial wall in this way, but larger lipoprotein molecules like VLDL must be altered to be transported. Disruption of the endothelial cell barrier allowing interaction between circulating platelets and subendothelial components appears to be the initiating event in atherosclerosis. Animal evidence suggests that hypercholesterolemia without mechanical injury may lead to endothelial cell dysfunction that allows exposure to foam cells. Platelets then interact with these foam cells and underlying connective tissue creating smooth muscle migration and replication to form the fibromusculoelastic lesion. Experimentally, this fibromusculoelastic lesion will progress to a typical atherosclerotic lesion in animals on a high-cholesterol diet but may regress entirely in animals restricted in intake of saturated fat. The endothelial cell monolayer does not replicate unless it is interrupted by injury. The endothelial cells then replicate only in the area of injury in an attempt to preserve this monolayer. The endothelial cells may produce collagen, factor VIII, and angiotensin converting enzyme. They also produce endothelial-derived growth factor, which stimulates proliferation of fibroblasts and smooth muscle cells. This factor may have important functions in initiating the atherosclerotic lesion.

344. The answers are: A-Y, B-Y, C-Y, D-Y, E-Y. *(pp 999–1004)* The cap of the fibrous plaque covers a deeper layer of macrophages that are often intermixed with variable numbers of T lymphocytes. The presence of lymphocytes in the lesions raises the possibility that the immune response may be important in the genesis or progression of the lesion and that some lesions may represent an autoimmune response. Fatty streaks form at branches and bifurcations, accumulating increasing numbers of macrophages and smooth muscle cells. Breaks occur between the endothelial cells, exposing lipid-filled macrophages that serve as sites to which platelets adhere and form mural thrombi. These areas later demonstrate proliferative smooth muscle lesions. Factor VIII is required for platelet adherence and release. In swine with absent factor VIII (von Willebrand's factor), high-lipid diets induce intimal infiltrates of lipid but no smooth muscle proliferative lesions. Swine with factor VIII develop extensive proliferative lesions of atherosclerosis when fed high-lipid diets. This demonstrates the importance of platelet interactions at sites of endothelial alteration preceding the formation of lesions of atherosclerosis. The means by which hypertension induces atherosclerosis is not clear. Increased renin levels may include cellular changes that lead to atherosclerosis. Altered characteristics of flow including eddy currents and back flow of blood at selected anatomic sites within the arterial tree may result in focally altered endothelium and the development of atherosclerotic lesions. The reason for an increased incidence of atherosclerosis in diabetes is not clear. There appears to be a decrease in HDL levels. The mechanisms of smooth muscle proliferation in the mesangium of the kidney and the increased thickness of capillary basement membrane in diabetics may be related to smooth muscle proliferation in atherosclerosis.

345. The answers are: A-Y, B-N, C-Y, D-Y, E-N. *(pp 1014–1015)*   The process of tearing or fissuring of an atherosclerotic plaque allows blood to dissect into the plaque itself exposing it to the intensely thrombogenic lipid core. The thrombus may build up in the lumen, leading to total occlusion, or the plaque may reseal and heal by smooth muscle proliferation, leading to further plaque growth. It appears that subclinical plaque fissuring and intraplaque thrombosis are important factors in disease progression. The mechanism of intimal tears has been shown to be due to the development of mechanically weak cap tissue of a plaque due to reduced collagen content.

346. The answers are: A-N, B-Y, C-N, D-Y, E-Y. *(p 1071)*   Calcium channel blockers are a chemically diverse group of drugs that inhibit the flow of calcium (Ca^{2+}) into myocytes and smooth muscle cells. Different calcium channel blockers appear to react with different receptors and also have variable effects on different vascular beds and the myocardium. Diltiazem and verapamil tend to reduce heart rate and can slow atrioventricular (AV) conduction. All calcium channel blockers have a negative inotropic effect, especially verapamil. Nifedipine and nicardipine produce more arterial dilatation and may be associated with a reflex increase in heart rate.

347. The answers are: A-Y, B-N, C-N, D-N, E-Y. *(pp 1115–1116, 1137)*   Isolated right ventricular infarction is unusual as there is usually an accompanying inferoposterior left ventricular infarction. Some evidence of right ventricular infarction may be seen in two-thirds of patients in whom there is an inferoposterior infarction. The clinical picture of jugular venous distention, hypotension, occasional evidence of right ventricular third (S_3) and fourth (S_4) heart sounds and clear fields by roentgenogram and physical examination are characteristic of right ventricular infarction; the electrocardiogram (ECG) may be confirmatory with evidence of transient ST-segment elevation greater than 1 mm in lead V_{4R} in the absence of a left bundle branch block (LBBB), or another cause of an anteriorly directed ST vector (such as acute anterior infarction) may be confirmatory. Radionuclide ventriculography in acute right ventricular infarction shows evidence of right ventricular dilatation, a diminished right ventricular ejection fraction, and lesser evidence of left ventricular dysfunction. There may be evidence of inferoposterior damage of a mild nature in the left ventriculogram. Systolic pressures in the right ventricle and pulmonary arteries are normal. The left ventricular filling pressure may be normal or minimally elevated, whereas the right atrial pressure and the right ventricular distal pressure are disproportionately elevated. Right ventricular infarction should be treated with volume expansion, which increases the right-sided cardiac output, whereas measures that tend to decrease filling of the right ventricle, such as diuretics or nitrates, may aggravate the systemic arterial hypotension, which may accompany right ventricular infarction.

348. The answers are: A-Y, B-N, C-Y, D-Y, E-Y. *(p 1113)*   Both Q-wave and non-Q-wave infarctions are initiated by occlusion of a coronary artery by a thrombus superimposed on a ruptured or fissured plaque. However, in non-Q-wave infarction, early spontaneous reperfusion occurs. The early complication rate and mortality are much less for patients with non-Q-wave infarction. However, the long-term prognosis is about the same owing to the risk of reinfarction in patients with non-Q-wave infarction.

349. The answers are: A-Y, B-Y, C-N, D-Y, E-N. *(pp 1191–1195)*   The most important determinants of survival in patients with acute myocardial infarction after arrival at the hospital are the infarct size and the degree of left ventricular dysfunction. Patients with anterior transmural infarctions or with antecedent infarctions have more associated left ventricular dysfunction and, thus, a worse prognosis. Increasing age also adversely affects prognosis with some series showing patients over the age of 70 with transmural infarction having a mortality rate of 25 percent. Primary ventricular fibrillation occurring early after myocardial infarction and not associated with congestive heart failure (CHF) does not significantly worsen the prognosis if the fibrillation is reversed rapidly.

350. The answers are: A-N, B-N, C-N, D-Y, E-Y. *(p 1199; Cobb, Proceedings of the First US-USSR Symposium on Sudden Death)* Most patients who suffer sudden cardiac death have extensive coronary artery disease, but only 20 percent of these patients have had an acute infarction. There is also a significantly higher risk of recurrent sudden cardiac death after resuscitation in patients who have not had a previous acute infarction with a 1-year mortality of approximately 25 percent. In contrast, patients who experienced out-of-hospital sudden cardiac death in which acute myocardial infarction occurred had a 4 percent 1-year mortality rate after resuscitation in the Seattle study.

351. The answers are: A-Y, B-N, C-N, D-Y, E-Y. *(p 1207)* Hypertension is an independent risk factor for coronary disease. Patients who have hypertension and other risk factors have an even higher risk of developing coronary disease. Interestingly, a patient with hypertension and a low serum cholesterol does not seem to have an increased risk of coronary disease. Labile and fixed hypertension both increase the risk of coronary disease. Elevated systolic blood pressures in elderly persons have been shown to be another independent risk factor for cardiovascular disease. The ideal choice of an antihypertensive regimen depends on coexisting medical conditions such as diabetes or cholesterol abnormalities. Certain medicines such as beta blockers and thiazide diuretics can adversely affect lipid profiles.

352. The answers are: A-Y, B-N, C-Y, D-Y, E-N. *(p 1208)* Changes in diet and life-style and certain pharmacological therapies can modify risk factors for heart disease. Cessation of cigarette smoking decreases coronary risk by 50 percent within the first year. The coronary risk is the same as nonsmokers within 2 to 10 years. Emphasis placed by the physician on the importance of discontinuation of cigarette smoking is critically important. High-density lipoprotein (HDL) cholesterol levels can improve by up to 10 percent within 1 month of the discontinuation of cigarette smoking, and platelet aggregation decreases. The lack of any significant effect in early trials of antihypertensive therapy has been attributed to the pharmacological agents used in those studies. Thiazide diuretics can elevate triglycerides and cholesterol, and beta blockers can increase triglycerides. Both may also have an effect on insulin sensitivity and glucose intolerance. Decreased use of thiazides and increased use of calcium blockers or angiotensin-converting enzyme (ACE) inhibitors may decrease the incidence of cardiac events. Even mild diastolic hypertension (blood pressure of 95 mmHg) increases the risk of coronary disease, and therapy that effectively reduces the diastolic blood pressure has been shown to reduce cardiovascular mortality.

353. The answers are: A-Y, B-N, C-Y, D-Y, E-Y. *(pp 1291–1293)* Calcium antagonists, like nitroglycerin and papaverine, are coronary vasodilators; however, they have negative inotropic effects that are dose-dependent. In the dog papillary muscle, nifedipine is the most potent depressant (on a weight basis) as compared with verapamil (15 times) and diltiazem (40 times). Since the excitation-contraction of vascular smooth muscle is more sensitive than that of myocardial cells, the vasodilation of relatively low doses overshadows the negative inotropic effect. Unlike beta blockers, calcium antagonists suppress myocardial contractibility without affecting the height or contour of the monophasic action potential. The calcium antagonists have a greater effect on arteries than veins and, in therapeutic doses, do not affect venous capacitance (unlike nitrates). It appears that the antiarrhythmic and negative inotropic effects are mediated via interference with calcium conductance.

354. The answers are: A-Y, B-Y, C-N, D-Y, E-N. *(p 1328)* Hypotension, a common side effect of streptokinase infusion, occurs in 10 percent of cases and is more likely when the infusion is rapid. To avoid hypotension, the intravenous infusion should not exceed 500 units/kg/min. Hypotension is usually reversed with cessation of the infusion. If hypotension persists despite stopping the infusion, other causes of hypotension should be considered.

355. The answers are: A-Y, B-Y, C-N, D-Y, E-N. *(pp 1309–1313, Table 68-2)*   The main anticoagulant effect of heparin appears to be through the inhibition of thrombin-induced activation of factors V and VIII. It acts through the natural coagulation inhibitor, antithrombin III, which forms complexes with several serine proteases. The value of intravenous heparin in patients with unstable angina for the prevention of myocardial infarction and subcutaneous heparin in patients with myocardial infarction to prevent mural thrombi has been documented. Thrombocytopenia, a complication of heparin therapy, is more common with bovine than porcine heparin.

356. The answers are: A-Y, B-Y, C-Y, D-Y, E-Y. *(p 1328)*   Streptokinase infusions are associated with a number of complications. Transient hypotension occurs in about 10 percent of patients. Although shivering, pyrexia, and rash may occur in up to 10 percent of patients during or shortly after the infusion, major allergic reactions are rare. Bleeding is the most common complication. Minor bleeding occurs in 3 to 4 percent of patients, and major bleeding (requiring a transfusion) occurs in 0.4 to 1 percent of patients. Cerebral bleeding occurs in 0.1 to 0.2 percent of patients, and ischemic stroke occurs in 0.8 percent of patients.

357. The answers are: A-Y, B-N, C-Y, D-N, E-Y. *(pp 1349, 1356)*   Recent ACC/AHA classifications of coronary lesions identify certain characteristics that would indicate the probability of success with coronary angioplasty; type A, high success (>85 percent); type B, moderate success (60 to 85 percent); and type C, low success (<60 percent). Characteristics of type A lesions are that they are discrete, concentric, noncalcified, and in a nonangulated segment with no thrombus present. Chronic total occlusions of less than 3 months' duration can be opened with a moderate success rate of 60 to 85 percent. The success rate with older total occlusions is less than 60 percent.

358. The answers are: A-Y, B-N, C-N, D-Y, E-Y. *(p 1364)*   Laser balloon angioplasty along with other recently developed mechanical interventional devices has been used successfully in certain situations where the results of routine balloon angioplasty are suboptimal or poor. Laser balloon angioplasty appears useful with ostial lesions, old total occlusions, and diffusely diseased long lesions. The reported complication and restenosis rates appear to be similar to those of routine balloon angioplasty. With improved techniques, the risk of perforation has lessened.

359. The answers are: A-N, B-Y, C-Y, D-N, E-Y. *(p 1377)*   The potential need for repeat coronary artery bypass surgery increases with time from the initial operation. At 10 years, the incidence is about 15 percent; it increases to 30 percent at 15 years. In centers with experienced personnel, the risk for second operations is 2 to 5 percent and the complication rate is approximately twice that of the initial procedure. The mortality risk of a third coronary bypass procedure appears to be approximately 9 percent.

360–363. The answers are: 360-A, 361-C, 362-D, 363-B. *(p 982)*   Frederickson's classification of hyperlipidemia is useful to assess lipoprotein abnormalities. The phenotypes of type IIa, IIb, and IV are seen in familial combined hyperlipoproteinemia. Type IIa shows an elevation of low-density lipoprotein (LDL) cholesterol only; in type IIb, both LDL and very low-density lipoprotein (VLDL) cholesterol are elevated; and in type IV, only VLDL is elevated. In type III, the intermediate-density lipoprotein (IDL) is elevated with resulting high cholesterol and triglyceride levels.

VIII. Systemic Arterial Hypertension

DIRECTIONS: Each question below contains five suggested responses. Select the **one best** response to each question.

364. Which of the following statements best characterizes patients with hypertension secondary to fibrous dysplasia?

(A) The onset of symptoms occurs typically in the fifth decade

(B) A positive family history of hypertension is more likely than in essential hypertension

(C) Women are more often afflicted than men

(D) Obesity is common

(E) Severe retinopathy (grade III or IV) is evident on fundoscopic examination

365. True statements regarding patients with systemic arterial hypertension include all the following EXCEPT

(A) in general, total body water is normal

(B) total body sodium (Na$^+$) is significantly increased

(C) most patients demonstrate an inverse relationship between total peripheral resistance and the magnitude of intravascular volume

(D) epidemiological studies support a direct correlation between dietary sodium intake and the prevalence of hypertension

(E) there is a high prevalence of hypertension in patients with either hyperthyroidism or hypothyroidism

366. Which of the following statements best describes blood pressure measurements?

(A) An inaccurately low blood pressure may be measured if the cuff is too small

(B) Blood pressure measurements can underestimate true intra-arterial pressure in elderly patients with "pipe stem" arteries due to extensive peripheral atherosclerosis

(C) Blood pressure differences of 20 to 30 mmHg are often found when blood pressure is measured in both arms, even in the absence of advanced atherosclerosis

(D) The normal blood pressure response to standing is a slight decrease in systolic and a slight increase in diastolic pressure with little change in mean arterial pressure

(E) Orthostatic hypertension has been associated with abnormally low norepinephrine levels

367. All the following statements concerning hypertensive cardiovascular disease are correct EXCEPT

(A) hypertension is the most common cause of left ventricular hypertrophy

(B) a syndrome similar to syndrome X has been noted in hypertensive patients, especially those with left ventricular hypertrophy

(C) left ventricular hypertrophy is associated with an increased risk of complex ventricular arrhythmias, coronary heart disease, and sudden death

(D) the sensitivity of the Romhilt-Estes electrocardiographic (ECG) criteria for left ventricular hypertrophy is greater than 80 percent

(E) evidence of left ventricular hypertrophy by echocardiography can be found in 30 to 40 percent of hypertensive patients whose ECG is normal

368. Sodium nitroprusside is indicated for all the following hypertensive emergencies EXCEPT

(A) eclampsia

(B) hypertensive encephalopathy

(C) acute intracranial hemorrhage

(D) dissecting aneurysm

(E) acute left ventricular failure

369. The preferred drug given as monotherapy in managing the hypertension associated with preeclampsia is

(A) hydralazine

(B) methyldopa

(C) minoxidil

(D) prazosin

(E) phentolamine

DIRECTIONS: Each question below contains four suggested responses of which **one or more** is correct. Select

A	if	**1, 2, and 3**	are correct
B	if	**1 and 3**	are correct
C	if	**2 and 4**	are correct
D	if	**4**	is correct
E	if	**1, 2, 3, and 4**	are correct

370. True statements regarding systemic arterial hypertension include which of the following?

(1) In untreated patients, hyperuricemia is directly related to a decrease in renal blood flow

(2) Mildly hypertensive patients (diastolic 90 to 94 mmHg) have an increased incidence of death coincident with antihypertensive therapy

(3) For any degree of arterial pressure, black patients have lesser renal blood flow and higher renal vascular resistance

(4) Renal changes usually follow the development of echocardiographically demonstrable left ventricular hypertrophy

371. Correct statements regarding malignant or accelerated hypertension include which of the following?

(1) Over 97 percent of patients die within 1 year if not treated

(2) There is an onion-skinned appearance of the arterioles throughout the body

(3) The arterioles are prone to severe spasm

(4) Microangiopathic hemolytic anemia can occur

372. Left ventricular hypertrophy, a complication of systemic arterial hypertension, is characterized by which of the following statements?

(1) It is the major cardiac alteration of hypertensive disease

(2) One of the earliest cardiac changes is impaired diastolic function

(3) It is an independent risk factor for sudden death

(4) Age and race but not gender are contributing factors to its development

373. Hemodynamic alterations in systemic arterial hypertension include

(1) an increased total body venous capacity

(2) an increased vascular smooth muscle tone

(3) contraction of intravascular volume in the very early stages

(4) an increased vascular resistance

374. Correct statements regarding target organ damage from hypertension include which of the following?

(1) The severity of retinopathy noted on fundoscopic examination does not correlate with prognosis in untreated patients

(2) Though hypertension is the most important risk factor for stroke, the incidence of stroke does not increase with increasing blood pressure

(3) Microalbuminuria is defined as a urinary albumin excretion of 15 to 200 μg/min, which is detected on the clinical dipstick test for proteinuria

(4) Focal seizures and other focal neurologic signs can occur in patients who appear clinically to have hypertensive encephalopathy

375. Clinical characteristics typical of patients with essential hypertension as compared to patients with surgically cured atherosclerotic renovascular hypertension include

(1) an early age of onset

(2) a high percentage of black patients

(3) a high incidence of obesity

(4) an abnormal creatinine (greater than 1.4 mg/dL)

SUMMARY OF DIRECTIONS

A	B	C	D	E
1, 2, 3 only	1, 3 only	2, 4 only	4 only	All are correct

376. Correct statements regarding the variability of blood pressure measurements include which of the following?

 (1) Blood pressure variability increases with age
 (2) Blood pressure variability is more striking for systolic than for diastolic blood pressure
 (3) "White coat" hypertension describes blood pressure that is elevated in the physician's office but not during usual daytime activities
 (4) Blood pressure is lowest in the early morning hours and highest at night

377. Cardiac findings that are likely to be found in the trained athlete include

 (1) electrocardiographic (ECG) findings of increased vagal tone (i.e., sinus bradycardia, first- or second-degree atrial ventricular block, or junctional rhythm)
 (2) diastolic dysfunction on Doppler echocardiography
 (3) an elevated left ventricular mass index (LVMI) on echocardiography
 (4) left ventricular hypertrophy on echocardiography of 13 mm or more

378. Findings typical of patients with pheochromocytoma include

 (1) headaches, sweating, and palpitations
 (2) elevated urinary excretion of metanephrine, vanillylmandelic acid (VMA), and total catecholamines
 (3) elevated plasma catecholamine levels in over 90 percent of patients
 (4) reduction in plasma norepinephrine following a clonidine suppression test

379. Side effects of thiazide and related sulfonamide diuretics include

 (1) increased low-density lipoprotein (LDL) cholesterol
 (2) hypercalcemia
 (3) hyperuricemia
 (4) insulin resistance

380. Selective α_1-adrenergic blockers have which of the following characteristics?

 (1) They are contraindicated in elderly patients because of orthostatic hypotension
 (2) They may reduce insulin resistance
 (3) They usually worsen the obstructive symptoms of prostatic hyperplasia
 (4) They have a beneficial effect on serum lipids

381. Correct epidemiological data regarding systemic arterial hypertension in special patient populations include which of the following?

 (1) In the United States, hypertension is accompanied by a higher mortality rate in blacks than in whites
 (2) Black hypertensive patients respond better to beta blockers or angiotensin-converting enzyme (ACE) inhibitors than to diuretics or calcium antagonists
 (3) For comparable levels of blood pressure, blacks have evidence of renal disease more often than whites
 (4) The prevalence of hypertension (140 mmHg systolic and 90 mmHg diastolic) in a population of blacks ages 65 to 74 years is around 30 percent

382. Medications that have been shown to reverse left ventricular hypertrophy associated with systemic arterial hypertension include

 (1) β-adrenergic blockers
 (2) angiotensin-converting enzyme (ACE) inhibitors
 (3) calcium antagonists
 (4) central alpha$_2$ agonists

383. Angiotensin-converting enzyme (ACE) inhibitors can cause an abrupt increase in serum creatinine when administered to patients with which of the following clinical presentations?

(1) Hypovolemia
(2) Congestive heart failure (CHF)
(3) Hypotension
(4) Renal artery stenosis

VIII. Systemic Arterial Hypertension

Answers

364. The answer is C. *(p 1412)* Several features help to differentiate the hypertension of fibrous dysplasia from other types of hypertension. Patients with fibrous dysplasia are likely to present with hypertension before 35 years of age. Patients are likely to be women and white. Indeed, in some studies, 80 percent of patients with fibrous dysplasia were women, and 90 percent were white. Patients with fibrous dysplasia are likely to be thin and have abdominal bruits. They are not likely to have severe retinopathy, cardiomegaly, or an abnormal creatinine of greater than 1.5 mg/dL.

365. The answer is B. *(pp 1393–1394)* In general, total body water is normal in hypertension. Although epidemiological studies reliably show a correlation between dietary sodium (Na^+) intake and the prevalence of hypertension, there is little evidence to indicate that total body Na^+ is increased. Most patients with essential hypertension demonstrate an inverse relationship between the height of arterial pressure or total peripheral resistance and the magnitude of intravascular volume. Other forms of hypertension in general demonstrate a similar inverse relationship, including patients with renal artery disease and pheochromocytoma. Certain states of hormonal alterations have been associated with hypertension. For example, there is high prevalence of hypertension in patients with either hyperthyroidism or hypothyroidism. The incidence of hypertension is also increased among patients with hypercalcemic diseases.

366. The answer is D. *(pp 1403–1404)* False elevations of blood pressure occur often if regular-sized blood pressure cuffs are used in adult patients whose midarm circumference exceeds 33 cm. Auscultatory measurements can also overestimate intra-arterial pressure in some elderly patients, presumably because of "pipe stem" arteries due to extensive peripheral arteriosclerosis. Blood pressure should be measured initially in both arms, and all subsequent determinations should be performed in the arm with the highest pressure. Differences greater than 10 mmHg are unusual in the absence of advanced arteriosclerosis. The normal blood pressure response to standing is a slight decrease in systolic and slight increase in diastolic pressure with little change in mean arterial pressure. The usual criteria for orthostatic hypotension is a standing reduction in systolic pressure of 20 mmHg or more or a mean arterial pressure of 10 percent or more. Orthostatic hypertension (i.e., an increase in diastolic pressure exceeding 8 to 10 mmHg upon standing) is associated with elevated norepinephrine levels and evidence of increased neurogenic tone.

367. The answer is D. *(pp 1408–1409)* Hypertension is the most common cause of left ventricular hypertrophy. Left ventricular hypertrophy is an important clinical finding because it is associated with an increased risk of complex ventricular arrhythmias, coronary heart disease, and sudden death. Echocardiography is also important because it may demonstrate changes in left ventricular hypertrophy during treatment for hypertension. The electrocardiogram (ECG) is also able to diagnose left ventricular hypertrophy; however, the sensitivity of the ECG is somewhat low, and even when the Romhilt-Estes criteria are applied, the sensitivity in some studies is only 58 percent with false-positive rates of 3 percent (when compared to hearts hypertrophied at autopsy). Echocardiography can diagnose left ventricular hypertrophy in 30 to 40 percent of patients whose ECG is normal. Patients with hypertension and left ventricular hypertrophy may be susceptible to myocardial ischemia even in the absence of coronary atherosclerosis at catheterization. This may reflect impaired coronary blood flow in these patients. This syndrome is often compared to syndrome X (i.e., anginalike chest discomfort with normal coronary angiography and no evidence of vasospasm).

368. The answer is A. *(p 1444)* Sodium nitroprusside is recommended for most hypertensive emergencies, including hypertensive encephalopathy, acute intracranial hemorrhage, acute cerebral infarction, acute left ventricular failure, malignant hypertension, and dissecting aneurysm. It is not recommended for the treatment of eclampsia, acute myocardial ischemia, and post–coronary bypass hypertension. The drug of choice for eclampsia is intravenous methyldopa.

369. The answer is B. *(p 1437)* Hydralazine and minoxidil are direct vasodilators with a poorly understood mechanism of action. They cause reflex tachycardia and fluid retention. Methyldopa is a centrally acting alpha$_2$-adrenoreceptor agonist and, when given as monotherapy, is the preferred drug in managing the hypertension associated with preeclampsia. Prazosin is a selective α_1-adrenergic blocker, and phentolamine is a nonselective α_1-adrenergic blocker.

370. The answer is E (all). *(pp 1396–1398)* With untreated hypertension, there is an association with hyperuricemia that is independent of abnormal purine metabolism or a history of gout. The height of serum uric acid levels in untreated patients is directly related to a decrease in renal blood flow and an increase in renal vascular resistance. The J-shaped mortality curve considers the possibility that mildly hypertensive patients may have an increased incidence of death coincident with antihypertensive therapy. Impaired regulatory flow response and impaired coronary perfusion have been implicated in this process. Regardless of the degree of hypertension, blacks have a lower renal blood flow and higher vascular resistance compared to whites. Left ventricular hypertrophy as determined by echocardiography precedes renal arteriolar thickening and fibrinoid deposition in the glomeruli and proteinuria.

371. The answer is E (all). *(pp 1397–1398)* In malignant and accelerated hypertension, the clinical course is rapidly progressive with over 97 percent of patients dying within 1 year if not treated. Pathologically, there is an onion-skinned appearance of the arterioles throughout the body with round cell infiltration in the media of the vessel wall, deposition of protein and complement within the muscle layer, and severe arteriolar spasm. There is diminished peripheral blood flow, especially to the kidney, provoking hyperreninemia, hyperaldosteronism, and microangiopathic hemolytic anemia.

372. The answer is A (1, 2, 3). *(pp 1395–1397)* Left ventricular hypertrophy is the major cardiac change associated with hypertension; it is an independent risk factor for sudden death. Patients with left ventricular hypertrophy have an increased prevalence of ventricular tachycardia; thus, sudden death may be produced by lethal ventricular arrhythmias even if significant coronary artery disease is not present. Contributing factors for the development for left ventricular hypertrophy in arterial hypertension include age, race, and gender of the patient, the presence of coexisting diseases, and humoral substances. One of the earliest cardiac changes related to the development of left ventricular hypertrophy is impaired diastolic function, manifested by a fourth heart sound (S$_4$) in conjunction with a left arterial abnormality on the electrocardiogram (ECG).

373. The answer is C (2, 4). *(pp 1391–1393)* Patients with systemic arterial hypertension have an increased arterial pressure associated with increased luminal narrowing that raises the total peripheral resistance and reduces the total body venous capacity. Increased vascular resistance can be mediated through enhanced adrenergic input of humoral agents, local vasoactive peptides, or ions. Early in hypertension, the venoconstriction is not associated with contraction in intravascular volume; therefore, venoconstriction redistributes volume to the cardiopulmonary area from the periphery. With progression of the vascular disease and more intense vasoconstriction, intravascular volume contracts progressively.

374. The answer is D (4). *(pp 1408–1411)* Fundoscopic examination assesses the prognosis and severity of hypertension. On fundoscopic examination, retinopathy is classified as type I (constriction), II (sclerosis and arteriovenous nicking), III (hemorrhages and exudates), and IV (papilledema). In untreated retinopathy, there were 5-year survival rates in each of the four categories of 85, 50, 13, and 0 percent, respectively. Hypertension is the most important risk factor for the development of hemorrhagic or atheroembolic stroke. The incidence of stroke increases with further elevations in blood pressure. Focal seizures and other focal neurologic signs can occur in patients who have hypertensive encephalopathy. These focal seizures or signs are often associated with structural lesions such as cerebral hemorrhage or infarctions. Patients who present with focal neurologic signs should undergo further diagnostic evaluation with computerized tomography (CT) and magnetic resonance imaging (MRI). Microalbuminuria is not detected on the usual clinical dipstick test for protein. In addition to microalbuminuria, glomerular hyperfiltration can be an early marker of hypertensive nephropathy. "Lacunar" infarcts are microhemorrhages, or occlusions, of small vessels, which can result in small areas of infarctions, most often in the putamen, thalamus, caudate nucleus, pons, or posterior limb of the internal capsule.

375. The answer is A (1, 2, 3). *(p 1413)* Several clinical characteristics are helpful in distinguishing patients with essential hypertension and patients with atherosclerotic renovascular hypertension. Patients with essential hypertension are more likely to be young and black. There is no difference with regard to sex or a positive family history of hypertension between these two groups. Patients with atherosclerotic renovascular hypertension are more likely to have grade III or IV fundoscopic changes and abdominal bruits and are less likely to be obese. The laboratory examinations of serum potassium (K+) and serum creatinine are not helpful in differentiating these hypertensive patients. Similarly, cardiomegaly found on roentgenogram is not helpful in differentiating these two groups.

376. The answer is A (1, 2, 3). *(p 1404)* The variability of blood pressure increases with age and with the level of blood pressure. It is more striking with systolic than with diastolic pressure. Blood pressure follows a circadian rhythm and is highest in the early morning hours and lowest at night. The phenomenon of "white coat" hypertension describes blood pressure that is elevated when measured by the physician in the office but is normal during usual daytime activities. To account for blood pressure variability, a minimum of two measurements on each of three different days is recommended for a diagnosis of hypertension in uncomplicated cases of mild-to-moderate elevation of blood pressure.

377. The answer is B (1, 3). *(pp 1404–1408)* The trained athlete's electrocardiogram (ECG) may show evidence of increased vagal tone (i.e., sinus bradycardia, first- or second-degree atrial ventricular block, or junctional rhythm). Other changes include high-amplitude R waves, elevation of the ST segments, and inversion of the T waves. There are several echocardiographic findings in the trained athlete, including increased left ventricular mass index (LVMI) and increased left ventricular end-diastolic internal dimension and volume. Echocardiographic findings not usually present in the trained athlete are diastolic dysfunction and left ventricular hypertrophy of 13 mm or more. Because of the incidence of sudden death in athletes with undiagnosed hypertrophic cardiomyopathy, care must be taken when evaluating an athlete who presents for evaluation of elevated blood pressure. In addition, elevations in systolic blood pressure may be the first clue to Marfan's syndrome with aortic insufficiency.

378. The answer is A (1, 2, 3). *(pp 1418–1419)* The classic symptom triad of pheochromocytoma includes headaches, sweating, and palpitations. In addition, hypertension may be difficult to control and often associated with orthostatic hypotension. Patients may manifest inappropriate sinus tachycardia and have recurrent arrhythmias. There is often an association with neurofibromatosis, café au lait spots, von Hippel–Lindau disease, Sturge-Weber syndrome, and tuberous sclerosis. In addition, the family history may be positive for pheochromocytoma, medullary thyroid carcinoma, or hyperthyroidism. The most common screening tests for pheochromocytoma are urinary excretion of total catecholamines, metanephrine, and vanillylmandelic acid (VMA). Most studies indicate that the excretion of metanephrine is the most sensitive of the urinary screening tests. In addition, plasma catecholamine levels (usually both norepinephrine and epinephrine) are elevated in most patients. A useful test to differentiate pheochromocytoma from essential hypertension is the clonidine suppression test. A dose of 0.3 mg of clonidine is given, and plasma catecholamine levels are drawn immediately before and 3 hours later. Blood pressure and heart rate are reduced similarly in hypertensive pheochromocytoma and nonpheochromocytoma patients. However, plasma norepinephrine (and to a lesser extent epinephrine) is essentially unchanged in patients with pheochromocytoma but is reduced markedly in patients with essential hypertension. This is because the central action of clonidine does not block the peripheral production of catecholamines.

379. The answer is E (all). *(p 1430)* Side effects of thiazide and related sulfonamide diuretics can include hypocalcemia, hypomagnesemia, hyperuricemia, insulin resistance, glucose intolerance, hypercholesterolemia, increased low-density lipoprotein (LDL) cholesterol, hypertriglyceridemia, sexual dysfunction, weakness, leukopenia, and allergic skin rash. Hypercalcemia can also occur with thiazide diuretics while the reverse is expected with loop diuretics since the latter cause an increase in urinary calcium (Ca^{2+}) excretion.

380. The answer is C (2, 4). *(p 1436)* Selective α_1-adrenergic blockers (e.g., prazosin, terazosin, and doxazosin) and nonselective α_1-adrenergic blockers (e.g., phentolamine and phenoxybenzamine) are the only antihypertensive agents that have beneficial effects on the lipid profile. This includes a reduction in total cholesterol triglycerides and an increase in high-density lipoprotein (HDL) cholesterol. Selective α_1-adrenergic blockers also have a beneficial effect on glucose metabolism since they reduce insulin resistance. These medications are not contraindicated in the elderly but should be used cautiously because of an orthostatic hypotensive "first-dose" response. It has also been reported that α_1-adrenergic blockers reduce obstructive symptoms of prostatic hypertrophy.

381. The answer is B (1, 3). *(p 1440; Working Group on Hypertension in the Elderly, JAMA 256:70–74, 1986)* In the United States, hypertension occurs more frequently in blacks than in whites; it also tends to be more severe and is accompanied by a higher mortality. For comparable levels of blood pressure, blacks have evidence of left ventricular hypertrophy by echocardiogram and evidence of renal disease more often than whites. In general, black hypertensive patients respond better to diuretics or calcium antagonists than beta blockers or angiotensin-converting enzyme (ACE) inhibitors, although many exceptions exist. The National Health and Nutrition Examination Survey (NHANES II) showed that the prevalence of hypertension, using the definition of 140 mmHg systolic and 90 mmHg diastolic, was 63 percent for whites and 76 percent for blacks in the 65- to 74-year-old age-group.

382. The answer is E (all). *(p 1441)* All the major classes of antihypertensive agents eventually reduce left ventricular mass with the possible exception of the direct vasodilator agents such as hydralazine or minoxidil. The central alpha$_2$ agonists, β-adrenergic blockers, angiotensin-converting enzyme (ACE) inhibitors and calcium antagonists apparently reduce the left ventricular mass sooner than the diuretics.

383. The answer is E (all). *(pp 1433–1435)* Angiotensin-converting enzyme (ACE) inhibitors tend to dilate the postglomerular arteriole selectively, thus reducing intraglomerular pressure without reducing the glomerular filtration rate (GFR). However, in patients with bilateral or unilateral renal artery stenosis, preexisting renal insufficiency, congestive heart failure (CHF), hypovolemia, or hypertension, where the GFR is maintained by angiotensin II–mediated constriction of the postglomerular (efferent) arteriole, ACE inhibitors can cause an abrupt increase in serum creatinine concentration and even acute renal failure.

IX. Valvular Heart Disease

DIRECTIONS: Each question below contains five suggested responses. Select the **one best** response to each question.

384. All the following are major Jones Criteria (1992) for the diagnosis of acute rheumatic fever EXCEPT

(A) carditis
(B) polyarthralgia
(C) chorea
(D) erythema marginatum
(E) subcutaneous nodules

385. Which of the following statements regarding the surgical treatment for aortic stenosis is true?

(A) Successful aortic valve replacement does not significantly alter the subsequent risk of sudden death
(B) In the evaluation of patients for aortic valve replacement, all men and women over the age of 35 years should undergo coronary arteriography
(C) When mechanical or ultrasonic debridement of the aortic valve is successfully performed, the results generally last well over 15 years
(D) If complete coronary revascularization is performed, the operative risk is not significantly different than that of aortic valve replacement alone
(E) The probability of freedom from valve reoperation at 10 years in patients with cryopreserved homografts is about 90 percent

386. All the following clinical manifestations are commonly found in acute aortic regurgitation EXCEPT

(A) bounding peripheral and capillary pulses
(B) soft first heart sound (S_1)
(C) a third heart sound (S_3)
(D) near normal left ventricular impulse
(E) normal to slightly decreased aortic diastolic pressure

387. In aortic valve replacement, a high-risk group can be identified when

(A) an Austin Flint murmur is heard
(B) the pulse pressure exceeds 50 percent of the peak systolic pressure
(C) a third heart sound (S_3) is present
(D) left ventricular end-systolic dimension is greater than 55 mm
(E) there is premature closure of the mitral valve before onset of the QRS complex

388. The most common valvular lesion resulting from external blunt trauma as in an automobile accident is

(A) tricuspid stenosis
(B) tricuspid regurgitation
(C) aortic stenosis
(D) aortic regurgitation
(E) mitral regurgitation

389. Which one of the following statements regarding tricuspid valve disease is true?

  (A) Atrial myxomas involve only the left side of the heart
  (B) The most frequent symptoms in tricuspid stenosis are syncope and chest pain
  (C) Elevation of the mean right atrial pressure above 10 mmHg produces peripheral edema
  (D) Tricuspid stenosis is the dominant valve lesion seen in Ebstein's anomaly
  (E) Tricuspid stenosis aggravates the symptoms of mitral stenosis

390. Malignant carcinoid tumor with metastases most frequently involves which of the following valves?

  (A) Aortic and mitral valves
  (B) Aortic and tricuspid valves
  (C) Aortic and pulmonic valves
  (D) Tricuspid and pulmonic valves
  (E) Tricuspid and mitral valves

391. All the following statements concerning the role of papillary muscles in mitral regurgitation (postmyocardial infarction) are true EXCEPT

  (A) the anterior set of papillary muscles is involved more frequently than the posteromedial set in the development of mitral regurgitation
  (B) the severity of mitral regurgitation depends on whether an entire set or only isolated heads of a muscle are involved
  (C) in most cases, the blood supply to the posteromedial papillary muscle arises from the left anterior descending coronary artery
  (D) papillary muscle function may be impaired due to an adjacent wall motion abnormality
  (E) ischemia without infarction can lead to transient mitral regurgitation

392. All the following statements regarding mitral stenosis are true EXCEPT

  (A) ninety percent of patients with mitral stenosis recall a history of acute rheumatic fever
  (B) rheumatic fever is the most common cause of mitral stenosis
  (C) calcification of the mitral annulus rarely causes symptomatic mitral stenosis
  (D) obstruction to diastolic flow is due to the funnel-shaped structure of the mitral valve and fused chordae tendineae
  (E) mitral annular calcification may present as conduction system disease (heart block)

393. Which of the following statements concerning tissue degeneration with valvular regurgitation in patients with artificial heart valves is true?

  (A) This complication occurs most frequently in the first 2 years after implantation due to structural problems
  (B) Aortic valves are more frequently affected than mitral valves
  (C) The elderly are more often affected than young patients
  (D) Surgical correction of paravalvular leaks can usually be accomplished by additional suturing rather than replacing the entire valve
  (E) All surgical leaks should be surgically corrected, even if not hemodynamically significant

DIRECTIONS: Each question below contains four suggested responses of which **one or more** is correct. Select

A	if	**1, 2, and 3**	are correct
B	if	**1 and 3**	are correct
C	if	**2 and 4**	are correct
D	if	**4**	is correct
E	if	**1, 2, 3, and 4**	are correct

394. The carditis of acute rheumatic fever may cause inflammation of the

  (1) epicardium
  (2) pericardium
  (3) endocardium
  (4) aortic arch

395. Correct statements concerning the association of streptococcal infection and the development of rheumatic fever include which of the following?

  (1) To initiate the rheumatic process, group A streptococci must infect the upper respiratory tract
  (2) Although not as common, streptococcal A pyoderma or impetigo may initiate the process
  (3) A relatively small percentage of individuals who sustain a group A infection are at risk
  (4) Group A streptococcal pharyngitis is exclusively a disease of children younger than 15 years of age

396. The arthritis of acute rheumatic fever

  (1) affects the large joints
  (2) is always symmetrical
  (3) is migratory
  (4) may lead to chronic arthritis

397. Conditions associated with a diastolic rumble include

  (1) left atrial myxoma
  (2) ventricular septal defect
  (3) atrial septal defect
  (4) aortic regurgitation

398. The treatment of acute aortic regurgitation should include

  (1) oral hydralazine as it delays the time from the initial evaluation to aortic valve replacement
  (2) postponement of valve replacement in asymptomatic patients with considerable cardiac enlargement and normal left ventricular systolic function
  (3) an intra-aortic balloon pump when severe hypotension is present
  (4) the homograft valve, which is especially resistant to postoperative infection when used for endocarditis

399. Correct statements concerning the diagnosis and treatment of tricuspid regurgitation include which of the following?

  (1) Right ventriculography is the gold standard in estimating the degree of regurgitation
  (2) Right ventricular systolic pressure can be estimated by Doppler echocardiography
  (3) Replacing the mitral valve in patients with severe rheumatic mitral regurgitation and severe secondary tricuspid regurgitation invariably reduces the degree of tricuspid regurgitation
  (4) Tricuspid annuloplasty is preferred over valve replacement in the surgical treatment of severe secondary tricuspid regurgitation

400. Causes of mitral stenosis include

  (1) rheumatic valvulitis
  (2) bacterial vegetations
  (3) congenital stenosis
  (4) myxomatous degeneration

401. Presenting symptoms of mitral stenosis may include

    (1)   hemoptysis
    (2)   seizures
    (3)   hoarseness
    (4)   palpitations

402. Findings more typical of acute than chronic mitral regurgitation include

    (1)   fatigue and dyspnea on exertion
    (2)   pressure overload on the left atrium and pulmonary veins with normal left ventricular dimensions
    (3)   holosystolic apical murmur
    (4)   large v wave on pulmonary capillary wedge pressure tracing

403. Myocardial infarction may lead to mitral regurgitation in which of the following ways?

    (1)   Dilatation of the left ventricle
    (2)   Rupture of a papillary muscle
    (3)   Dysfunction of a nonruptured papillary muscle
    (4)   Perforation of mitral valve leaflets

404. Optimum management of clinically significant mitral regurgitation may include

    (1)   enalapril
    (2)   norepinephrine
    (3)   furosemide
    (4)   epinephrine

405. Echocardiographic evidence of mitral valve prolapse may be seen in patients with

    (1)   hypertrophic cardiomyopathy
    (2)   rheumatic heart disease
    (3)   coronary artery disease
    (4)   myxomatous degeneration of the mitral valve

406. Valve lesions that are very commonly associated include which of the following?

    (1)   Aortic stenosis with tricuspid stenosis
    (2)   Tricuspid valve prolapse with mitral valve prolapse
    (3)   Aortic regurgitation and pulmonic regurgitation
    (4)   Tricuspid stenosis with mitral stenosis

407. Multivalvular disease may be caused by

    (1)   rheumatic fever
    (2)   myxomatous degeneration
    (3)   endocarditis
    (4)   calcification of valves in elderly patients

408. True statements regarding rheumatic multivalvular disease include which of the following?

    (1)   Rheumatic fever is a very common cause of combined disease of the mitral and aortic valves
    (2)   In combined aortic and mitral stenosis, the aortic systolic murmur may be faint on physical examination
    (3)   The inflammatory process of rheumatic fever often results in fusion of the valve leaflets
    (4)   The tricuspid valve is commonly involved in rheumatic multivalvular disease

409. Systemic embolism from mechanical heart valves has which of the following characteristics?

    (1)   It occurs at a rate of 1 to 3 percent a year
    (2)   It is more common with valves in the aortic than in the mitral position
    (3)   Major episodes cause death or permanent neurologic defects at a rate of approximately 1 percent a year
    (4)   Thrombi are demonstrable on the valve by echocardiography

410. During aortic valve replacement surgery, it may be necessary to insert a prosthesis that is larger than the native aortic valve annulus. Surgical techniques that have been developed to allow the use of larger prostheses include

    (1)   tilting the prosthetic valve without enlarging the aortic root
    (2)   extension of the aortotomy through the annular ring into the region of the noncoronary cusp and enlargement of the aorta with pericardial patch
    (3)   the Konno procedure
    (4)   the DeVega annuloplasty

SUMMARY OF DIRECTIONS

A	B	C	D	E
1, 2, 3 only	1, 3 only	2, 4 only	4 only	All are correct

411. Absolute contraindications to percutaneous mitral balloon valvotomy (PMV) in patients with significant mitral stenosis include

(1) long-standing atrial fibrillation
(2) mitral regurgitation of 2+ or more
(3) mitral valve leaflet calcification
(4) recent thromboembolic event

412. The operative risk of valve replacement surgery and more complex valvular replacement procedures has been well defined. Correct statements concerning this operative risk include which of the following?

(1) The operative risk in an isolated aortic replacement is greater for preoperative aortic regurgitation than stenosis
(2) The operative risk in an isolated mitral valve replacement is adversely affected by significant pulmonary hypertension
(3) The operative risk in isolated mitral valve replacement is 3 to 8 percent
(4) The operative risk in multiple valve replacement is 5 to 15 percent

DIRECTIONS: Each question below contains five suggested responses. For **each** of the **five** responses listed with every question you are to respond either YES (Y) or NO (N). In a given item **all, some, or none of the alternatives may be correct.**

413. The clinical manifestations of aortic stenosis are best described by which of the following statements?

(A) The most frequent symptom of aortic stenosis is angina pectoris

(B) Average survival after the onset of syncope is 8 to 9 years

(C) After symptoms of heart failure develop, survival has been estimated at 2 years

(D) An anacrotic notch in the carotid artery pulse indicates concomitant significant aortic regurgitation

(E) Less than 10 percent of individuals with aortic stenosis have a diastolic blow of accompanying aortic regurgitation

414. Correct statements regarding aortic stenosis include which of the following?

(A) Measurement of mean valvular gradient gives the best estimate of the severity of aortic stenosis

(B) Aortic cusp separation of less than 8 mm as measured in the long axis by two-dimensional echocardiogram is suggestive of severe aortic stenosis

(C) Symptomatic aortic stenosis is a relative contraindication to exercise testing

(D) A bicuspid aortic valve is two times more common in women than men

(E) The incidence of bicuspid aortic stenosis has been estimated at 4 in 1000 live births

415. Laboratory findings usually observed in patients with chronic aortic regurgitation include

(A) increased left ventricular voltage on electrocardiogram (ECG)

(B) calcification of the aortic valve on chest roentgenogram

(C) elongation of the left ventricular apex inferiorly and posteriorly

(D) delayed closure of the mitral valve on echocardiography

(E) diastolic fluttering of the anterior leaflet of the mitral valve

416. Correct statements regarding mitral valve repair include which of the following?

(A) It carries a lower operative mortality compared to mitral valve replacement

(B) It carries a higher incidence of reoperation compared to mitral valve replacement

(C) Preservation of the mitral valve–papillary muscle apparatus probably helps maintain ventricular function

(D) Optimal ventricular function is usually regained even when mitral repair is performed at the time of advanced left ventricular dysfunction

(E) Active infection of the mitral valve precludes attempts to save the valve

IX. Valvular Heart Disease

Answers

384. The answer is B. *(pp 1453–1454, Table 78-1)* The current Jones Criteria (1992) are intended only for the diagnosis of initial attacks of acute rheumatic fever; therefore, previous rheumatic fever and rheumatic heart disease are not included as manifestations. True polyarthritis rather than arthralgia is a major manifestation of acute rheumatic fever. Arthralgia is a minor manifestation along with fever, elevated levels of acute phase reactants (such as erythrocyte sedimentation rate and C-reactive protein), and a prolonged PR interval on the electrocardiogram (ECG). The finding of two major or of one major and two minor criteria indicates a high probability of rheumatic fever if supported by evidence of a preceding group A beta-hemolytic streptococcal upper respiratory infection. The absence of evidence for this preceding infection should make the diagnosis suspect. Evidence of a preceding streptococcal infection may be obtained by means of a positive throat culture for group A streptococci or a history of scarlet fever. Other reliable laboratory confirmation may be obtained by elevation of the streptococcal antibody titers such as antistreptolysin O (ASO) titer, antistreptokinase, and antideoxyribonuclease B titer (anti-DNase B).

385. The answer is E. *(pp 1463–1466)* It is estimated that approximately 50 percent of patients diagnosed clinically as having severe aortic stenosis will die within 5 years of the time of diagnosis. This risk is significantly lowered if successful aortic valve replacement is performed. In the evaluation of patients for aortic valve replacement, all men over age 35 and all postmenopausal women should undergo coronary arteriography. In general, results of either mechanical or ultrasonic debridement of the aortic valve are not long-lasting. Complete coronary revascularization should be performed together with aortic valve replacement whenever indicated; however, the risk is significantly increased over that of aortic valve replacement alone. In patients with cryopreserved homografts, the probability of freedom from valve reoperation at 10 years is 90 percent.

386. The answer is A. *(pp 1471–1472)* A number of clinical findings contrast acute and chronic aortic regurgitation. In acute aortic regurgitation, the classic peripheral manifestations of chronic aortic regurgitation may be absent or significantly reduced. The systolic blood pressure may not rise (and in fact may be decreased) because of a fall in the forward stroke output. The aortic diastolic pressure is normal or slightly decreased since it cannot fall below the left ventricular diastolic pressure, which is usually markedly elevated in acute aortic regurgitation. The classic picture of bounding peripheral and capillary pulses is usually absent. A ventricular third heart sound (S_3) gallop is common. Since the mitral valve tends to close prematurely, the first heart sound (S_1) tends to be soft or absent. The left ventricle does not dilate acutely; thus, the left ventricular impulse is not displaced or sustained.

387. The answer is D. *(pp 1473–1474)* Echocardiographic studies before and after aortic valve replacement indicate that a left ventricular and systolic dimension greater than 55 mm usually identifies a high-risk surgical group. In aortic regurgitation, a third heart sound (S$_3$) gallop is frequently heard and reflects the early diastolic filling. A rumbling diastolic murmur may be heard at the apex. Premature closure at the mitral valve usually suggests more severe regurgitation. None of these factors, however, identify a high-risk group for surgery. A wide pulse pressure suggests chronic aortic regurgitation in which left ventricular diastolic pressure is *not* severely elevated.

388. The answer is B. *(p 1520)* The most common valvular lesion following external blunt trauma as in an automobile accident is traumatic tricuspid regurgitation, the main cause of which is rupture of the papillary muscle or chordae. Laceration of leaflet tissue is less common. Rupture of tricuspid papillary muscles has also been described following external cardiopulmonary resuscitation. There is extensive variability in how well traumatic tricuspid regurgitation is tolerated. Prolonged survival (up to 39 years) has been reported. In general, rupture of a papillary muscle is not as well tolerated as rupture of chordae.

389. The answer is C. *(pp 1519–1521)* Tricuspid valve disease may take multiple forms ranging from rheumatic tricuspid stenosis to carcinoid syndrome. The etiologies may also include endocardial fibroelastosis, endomyocardial fibrosis, and systemic lupus erythematosus. Mechanical obstruction of the valve can occur with a right atrial myxoma, tumor metastasis, and thrombi in the right atrium. The right atrium is the second most common location for isolated cardiac myxomas. This occurs in roughly 15 to 20 percent of myxomas. The most frequent symptoms in tricuspid stenosis are dyspnea and fatigue. When mitral stenosis coexists, the development of significant tricuspid stenosis can diminish the symptoms of dyspnea, orthopnea, and paroxysmal nocturnal dyspnea by preventing the increase in pulmonary congestion and pulmonary hypertension. Mild elevations of the right atrial pressure to values of 10 mmHg may lead to marked venous hypertension with concomitant changes, such as jugular venous distention, ascites, and peripheral edema. Ebstein's malformation is a condition that involves an abnormal attachment of the septal tricuspid valve leaflet that leads to significant tricuspid regurgitation in most cases.

390. The answer is D. *(pp 1519–1521)* In approximately 10 percent of patients with malignant carcinoid tumor (usually originating in the ileum) with extensive metastases, the tricuspid and pulmonary valves are affected. The involvement of the tricuspid valve usually results in regurgitation, although tricuspid stenosis may result. The carcinoid syndrome with cardiac involvement of the pulmonic valve can create slight pulmonic stenosis and associated regurgitation. Symptoms of the carcinoid syndrome also include facial flushing, increased intestinal activity, diarrhea, and bronchospasm.

391. The answer is A. *(pp 1492–1493)* Mitral regurgitation post–myocardial infarction can be due to a number of factors. Those factors include rupture of a portion of the entire papillary muscle, infarction, leading to dysfunction of the papillary muscle, or ischemia of the papillary muscle. An adjacent wall motion abnormality may impair papillary muscle function further. Rupture of the papillary muscle involves the posteromedial set of muscles more commonly than the anterior set by a ratio of 4 to 1. Severity of mitral regurgitation resulting from rupture of the papillary muscle depends on whether an entire set or only isolated heads are involved.

392. The answer is A. *(pp 1483–1484)* Only 50 percent of patients with recognized mitral stenosis recall a history of acute rheumatic fever; however, the most common cause of mitral stenosis remains rheumatic fever and, in the temperate zones around the world, severe mitral stenosis can occur in children and adolescents. Although mitral annulus calcification is a rare cause of mitral stenosis, it is likely to present as a chest roentgenogram phenomenon (massive calcification noted on the posteroanterior and lateral chest roentgenograms). It presents as a very mild murmur of mitral regurgitation or as heart block due to involvement of the conduction system. Due to the nature of the contraction and scarring of the mitral valve and chordae tendineae seen in rheumatic mitral valve disease, a funnel-shaped structure is formed, which leads into the body of the left ventricular cavity.

393. The answer is D. *(pp 1541–1542)* Tissue degeneration with valvular regurgitation is the most frequent hemodynamic form of artificial valve disease. This complication is rare in the first 3 years after implantation, but it occurs at the rate of about 2 to 3 percent per year after 3 years of implantation. After 10 years, the rate is about 5 percent per year. It occurs more commonly in younger patients and in patients with valves in the mitral position, not the aortic position. Small paravalvular regurgitant leaks do not usually require surgical correction. When repair is necessary, additional suturing is usually sufficient.

394. The answer is A (1, 2, 3). *(p 1453)* Acute rheumatic fever produces a pancarditis that affects the pericardium, epicardium, myocardium, and endocardium. The aortic arch is not affected. On clinical grounds, extremely fulminant cases of carditis may be difficult to differentiate from a viral myocarditis. A frequent finding in acute rheumatic fever carditis is mitral insufficiency due to acute inflammation of the valve itself. Isolated aortic insufficiency is rare.

395. The answer is B (1, 3). *(p 1451)* The association between group A beta-hemolytic streptococci and acute rheumatic fever has been recognized for many years. Only group A streptococcal upper respiratory infections initiate the process that leads to rheumatic fever. Streptococcal infections of the skin or extrapharyngeal sites, such as pyoderma or impetigo, will not initiate the process. Less than 3 percent of patients with true streptococcal infection of the upper respiratory tract develop acute rheumatic fever, and recent data suggest that this attack rate may even be less. The highest incidence of group A streptococcal pharyngitis occurs in children between the ages of 5 and 15, but it is not uncommon for outbreaks of streptococcal pharyngitis and rheumatic fever to occur in adults such as military recruits.

396. The answer is B (1, 3). *(p 1453)* The arthritis associated with acute rheumatic fever is always an exquisitely painful migratory polyarthritis. The migratory nature of this arthritis is an important clinical manifestation. The arthritis may or may not be symmetrical. Involvement of a single joint is rare. The arthritis generally affects the large joints such as the ankles, knees, elbows, shoulders, and wrists. Occasionally, the small joints of the hands and feet may be affected. However, when this occurs other diagnoses should be considered. The arthritis of rheumatic fever does not lead to chronic joint involvement.

397. The answer is E (all). *(p 1486)* The diastolic rumble in mitral stenosis is due to obstruction of the mitral valve. A diastolic rumble may also develop across the mitral valve due to an increased flow rate across the valve that occurs in conditions such as atrial septal defect, ventricular septal defect, or a patent ductus arteriosus. A diastolic murmur is also heard in aortic regurgitation as the aortic jet impinges on the anterior leaflet of the mitral valve, producing the classic Austin Flint rumble across the mitral valve. In patients with left atrial myxoma, the myxoma may obstruct the valve and lead to a diastolic murmur. Other causes of diastolic mitral valve murmurs include the Cary Coombs murmur of acute rheumatic fever and the diastolic murmur of cor triatriatum. Therefore, not all diastolic murmurs are due to mitral stenosis.

398. The answer is C (2, 4). *(pp 1474–1475)* Studies using oral hydralazine have shown that it improved cardiac performance and may also delay the progression of left ventricular dilatation in asymptomatic cases. However, there are no data that demonstrate either a reduced mortality or a delay in the time from initial evaluation to aortic valve replacement with hydralazine. Valve replacement should be considered in patients with significant aortic regurgitation who develop decreasing systolic function, systolic dimensions of the left ventricle greater than 55 mm on echocardiography, or progressive symptoms. In the presence of wide open aortic regurgitation an intra-aortic balloon pump is contraindicated since it aggravates the situation. The homograft valve, which is resistant to postoperative infection when used with endocarditis, is especially useful in younger patients who wish for a relatively morbidity-free existence.

399. The answer is C (2, 4). *(pp 1519–1526)* Common etiologies of tricuspid regurgitation include infectious endocarditis, myocardial infarction, trauma, congenital abnormalities, and tricuspid valve prolapse. Tricuspid regurgitation is secondary to left-sided heart failure and pulmonary hypertension as well as right-sided heart failure that leads to right ventricular dilatation and papillary muscle misalignment. Assessing the degree of tricuspid regurgitation with right ventriculography is difficult as the catheter overrides the tricuspid valve and ventricular irritability can induce regurgitation. Doppler echocardiography can estimate the severity of tricuspid regurgitation, and color Doppler can delineate the patterns and sites of regurgitation. Many patients with significant mitral valve disease develop moderate-to-severe tricuspid regurgitation. Replacement of the mitral valve often leads to an amelioration of the tricuspid regurgitation. The risk of annuloplasty in combination with either aortic or mitral valve surgery is about 10 percent. Ring annuloplasty probably provides the best long-term results. When tricuspid valve replacement is necessary, the 30-day operative risk increases 15 to 20 percent. In general, the early and late results of tricuspid annuloplasty have been superior to valve replacement, and therefore, the trend of surgical practice has been to avoid valve replacement when possible. There is an important incidence of thrombosis with a tricuspid prosthesis, and the long-term functional results have been less favorable than those of aortic and mitral valve replacements.

400. The answer is A (1, 2, 3). *(p 1483)* Mitral stenosis most commonly results from recurrent rheumatic endocarditis; however, resistance to diastolic flow across the mitral valve may result from other causes, such as congenital stenosis, thrombus formation, atrial myxoma, bacterial vegetations, and calcification in the valve and in the annulus. With rheumatic mitral stenosis, there is leaflet and chordae tendineae scarring and contraction. There are often adhesions and fusion of the commissures between the two leaflets. This scarring and contraction process along with shortening of the chordae causes the adherent leaflets to be held in a downward position. The entire process culminates in formation of a funnel-shaped structure of the leaflets. The inlet to the funnel is at the level of the left atrial floor and is wider than the apex, which is in the ventricular cavity.

401. The answer is E (all). *(p 1484)* Mitral stenosis may present with a number of complaints, which are typically secondary to elevations in the left atrial pressure and pulmonary capillary wedge pressure. Other complaints are secondary to the markedly enlarged left atrium and the local compression that it may produce. Patients may also present with complications resulting from arrhythmias, such as emboli from the enlarged left atrium in patients with atrial fibrillation. Common presenting complaints include dyspnea, fatigue, palpitations, and hemoptysis. Less common complaints include hoarseness, chest pain, seizures, or a cerebrovascular accident from an embolus. The most prominent complaint in mitral stenosis is dyspnea due to pulmonary venous engorgement.

402. The answer is C (2, 4). *(pp 1497–1498)* Presentations of acute and chronic mitral regurgitation differ in a number of ways. In acute mitral regurgitation with a normal or slightly low left atrial compliance, mitral regurgitation leads to marked elevation in the left atrial, pulmonary, and venous pressures. Because of the small size of the left atrium and its normal compliance, a very large v wave may be seen on the pulmonary capillary wedge pressure tracing. Acute mitral regurgitation, therefore, produces a pressure overload on the left atrium and pulmonary veins with normal left ventricular dimensions initially. In chronic mitral regurgitation, the volume overload on the left heart causes a dilated left ventricle and chronic mitral regurgitation, leading to a dilated left atrium with markedly low left atrial compliance. Because of the low compliance, there is typically not a large v wave on the pulmonary capillary wedge pressure tracing. The physiology of chronic mitral regurgitation is one of left ventricular volume overload, left ventricular dilatation and eccentric hypertrophy, and left atrial enlargement. The presenting symptoms for acute mitral regurgitation typically include acute pulmonary edema, whereas patients with chronic mitral regurgitation initially present with no symptoms and finally develop fatigue and dyspnea. A holosystolic murmur may be heard in both but is more commonly heard in patients with chronic mitral regurgitation.

403. The answer is A (1, 2, 3). *(p 1492)* Myocardial infarction may lead to mitral regurgitation in a number of ways. With a large infarction, mitral regurgitation may result from dilatation of the left ventricle and papillary muscle misalignment. With occlusion of either a single circumflex artery or a right coronary artery branch, infarction of a papillary muscle may result in severe mitral regurgitation. While coronary occlusion may not rupture the muscle, the infarcted muscle may lead to papillary muscle misalignment, which, in turn, may cause mitral regurgitation. Perforation of the mitral valve leaflets in patients with myocardial infarction is not seen, but perforated valve leaflets in patients with bacterial endocarditis may occur. Chordal rupture in patients with bacterial endocarditis of the mitral valve may also occur.

404. The answer is B (1, 3). *(p 1500)* The aim of therapy of mitral regurgitation is to diminish the left ventricular afterload since the left atrium serves as a low-pressure sink during ejection. This is best achieved with vasodilator therapy, including nitroprusside, hydralazine, or angiotensin-converting enzyme (ACE) inhibitors such as enalapril. In patients with heart failure, preload reduction with furosemide is also part of the management of these patients. Because the ejection fraction in these patients is typically normal, the ejection phase indices need not be improved with inotropic support unless the patient has end-stage disease. Therefore, increasing the inotropic state in the stable patient with mitral regurgitation merely increases the regurgitation into the left atrium. Furthermore, drugs that increase the systemic afterload, such as phenylephrine hydrochloride or norepinephrine worsen symptoms by increasing the regurgitant volume into the left atrium.

405. The answer is E (all). *(pp 1503–1504)* In primary mitral valve prolapse, there is marked proliferation of the spongiosa layer, which results in interchordal hooding due to the leaflet redundancy. Secondary mitral valve prolapse has multiple etiologies. Echocardiographic mitral valve prolapse, including mitral regurgitation, has been reported in acute coronary occlusion both in experimental animal models and in human clinical settings. Relative displacement of the ischemic papillary muscles is invoked. Rheumatic mitral valve involvement may result in echocardiographic prolapse, usually the anterior leaflet. Histologically, proliferation of the spongiosa is absent. Posterior mitral valve leaflet prolapse has been described in hypertrophic cardiomyopathy as a result of a disproportionately small left ventricular cavity and altered papillary muscle alignment.

406. The answer is C (2, 4). *(p 1531)* Myxomatous degeneration of the mitral, aortic, and tricuspid valves has been seen in combination. Myxomatous degeneration of the tricuspid valve is rarely seen without mitral valve prolapse. Furthermore, in patients with rheumatic tricuspid stenosis, there is always concomitant mitral stenosis present. Tricuspid valve prolapse is one of the causes of primary tricuspid regurgitation. In patients with normal right and normal pulmonary artery pressures, it is uncommon for patients to require tricuspid valve replacement or annuloplasty. One of the clues to the presence of tricuspid stenosis in patients with mitral stenosis is that peripheral edema may not respond to administration of digitalis.

407. The answer is E (all). *(pp 1531–1532)* Multivalvular disease indicates obstruction or incompetence of multiple cardiac valves. Rheumatic fever is an important cause of combined disease of the mitral and aortic valves. The tricuspid valve is not often involved in the rheumatic process but is commonly affected by right ventricular failure resulting from left ventricular decompensation. Other conditions that impair both the aortic and mitral valves include rheumatic fever, myxomatous degeneration with prolapse, calcification in the aged and endocarditis. Calcification involves both the aortic and mitral valves. Stenosis of the aortic valve is most common, whereas mitral calcification creates regurgitation but rarely stenosis. Myxomatous degeneration can cause valvular prolapse of the aortic and the mitral valve. Unusual aneurysms of the aortic sinuses and ascending aorta can develop in Marfan's syndrome, while changes of a dilated annulus, atrioventricular (AV) valve prolapse, ruptured chordae, and annular calcification involve the mitral valve.

408. The answer is A (1, 2, 3). *(pp 1531–1532)* Rheumatic fever is an important cause of combined disease of the mitral and aortic valves. The tricuspid valve is rarely involved in the primary rheumatic process but may be impaired by secondary changes in the right ventricle. Combined aortic and mitral valve disease is very common in rheumatic fever. In some studies, involvement of these two valves approaches 99 percent. The cardinal pathological findings in the inflammatory process of rheumatic fever is cusp fusion. This is distinctly different from valvular calcification in the aged. The physical examination in multivalvular disease is difficult as one murmur may obscure another. This is often seen when the murmur of aortic stenosis is faint with coexistent severe mitral stenosis.

409. The answer is B (1, 3). *(pp 1542–1543)* Systemic embolism is the most important complication of mechanical heart valves. It occurs at a rate of about 1 to 2 percent a year in valves in the aortic position and about 2 to 3 percent a year in valves in the mitral position. Many embolic episodes are minor and transient, but major episodes such as those causing death and permanent neurological deficits occur at a rate of approximately 1 percent a year. Major bleeding episodes in patients taking long-term anticoagulation occur at a rate of about 1 to 3 percent a year. Long-term anticoagulation with warfarin is required to prolong the international normalized ratio (INR) to 2.5 to 3.5, which corresponds to a prolongation of the prothrombin time to approximately 1.5 to 2 times normal.

410. The answer is A (1, 2, 3). *(p 1549)* Three techniques have been developed that allow placement of a prosthesis that is larger than the native aortic annulus. The first is to simply tilt the prosthesis so that it is above the annulus. This allows a valve with a larger diameter than the annulus to be used. A second technique involves extension of the aortotomy down into the region of the noncoronary cusp, allowing enlargement of the aortic annulus. The defect in the aortic wall is then repaired with a patch of pericardium or dacron. A third method, the Konno or Raston procedure, involves extending the aortotomy into the interventricular septum, creating a ventricular septal defect, which is repaired with a dacron patch. This procedure is a more radical procedure than the other methods and accommodates the insertion of a prosthetic valve three to four times the size of the native annulus. A DeVega annuloplasty is designed to decrease the circumference of the tricuspid annulus in tricuspid valve repair.

411. The answer is C (2, 4). *(pp 1568–1571, Tables 86-1 and 86-2)* Since the mechanism of successful percutaneous mitral balloon valvotomy (PMV) is the actual splitting of fused mitral commissures by the balloon, the best results may be anticipated in patients with mobile valves, no subvalvular disease, and no calcification. However, mild-to-moderate degrees of calcification may be acceptable, especially if the combined echocardiographic score is less than 8. Severe calcification of the valve is a strong contraindication for PMV. Additional ideal factors for PMV include young age, a short history of mitral stenosis, and normal sinus rhythm. Recent atrial fibrillation is not a contraindication for PMV, and even long-standing atrial fibrillation, although an unfavorable factor, is not an absolute contraindication. Absolute contraindications to PMV are left atrial thrombus, a thromboembolic event within 3 months, mitral regurgitation of 2+ or more, left ventricular thrombus, and associated surgical coronary or other valvular disease.

412. The answer is E (all). *(p 1553)* Aortic valve replacement performed in institutions where surgical volume is adequate involves minimal operative risk. The usual operative risk is 2 to 5 percent, and the major preoperative determinants that increase this risk include advanced age of the patient, coexisting atherosclerotic coronary vascular disease, and a decline in left ventricular systolic function. Isolated mitral valve replacement has an attendant operative risk of 3 to 8 percent. Preoperative determinants of increased mortality include the aforementioned criteria plus a steady increase in risk as the level of pulmonary hypertension increases. When multiple valvular replacements are performed during a single operation, the operative risk increases to 5 to 15 percent. In these patients, increased operative mortality has been associated with tricuspid valve disease and hemodynamically significant coronary artery disease. Tricuspid valve replacement is unusual and mechanical prostheses have not functioned successfully in this position.

413. The answers are: A-Y, B-N, C-Y, D-N, E-N. *(pp 1459–1461)* Angina pectoris symptoms develop in about 50 to 70 percent of patients with aortic stenosis. Life expectancy after the onset of exertional chest discomfort averages about 5 years. After the onset of syncope, the average survival has been estimated at 3 to 4 years, while survival after the onset of symptoms of congestive heart failure (CHF) has been estimated at 2 years. On physical examination, an anacrotic notch in the arterial pulse indicates severe aortic stenosis. A high-pitched diastolic blow heard in up to 50 percent of patients with aortic stenosis denotes accompanying aortic regurgitation.

414. The answers are: A-N, B-Y, C-Y, D-N, E-Y. *(pp 1461–1462)* When the cardiac output becomes significantly reduced in patients with aortic stenosis, the gradient across the aortic valve can decline dramatically even though the valve area is severely stenotic. Therefore, it is important to always calculate the aortic valve area when estimating the severity of the aortic stenosis. Bicuspid aortic stenosis predominates in men over women at a ratio of 4 to 1. Diminished aortic cusp separation suggests either significant obstruction at a valvular level or diminished cardiac output. In either case, this echocardiographic finding in a patient with aortic stenosis suggests severe disease. Overexertion can be fatal in patients with critical aortic stenosis.

415. The answers are: A-Y, B-N, C-Y, D-N, E-Y. *(p 1472)* The electrocardiogram (ECG) in patients with chronic aortic regurgitation usually shows increased left ventricular voltage, and in late stages, atrioventricular (AV) conduction abnormalities can develop. On the chest roentgenogram, dilatation of the left ventricle is the most common abnormality seen. When calcification of the aortic valve is noted, it suggests concomitant aortic stenosis. Diastolic fluttering of the anterior leaflet of the mitral valve can be seen on echocardiography, and because the aortic regurgitant flow can impinge on the anterior leaflet of the mitral valve, there is usually premature closure of the mitral valve leaflet.

416. The answers are: A-Y, B-N, C-Y, D-N, E-Y. *(pp 1558–1564)* Mitral valve repair carries a lower operative mortality than mitral valve replacement. The need for reoperation is also lower. Patients who undergo mitral valve repair and who have advanced left ventricular dysfunction have a higher morbidity and mortality. If optimal left ventricular function results are to be obtained by correcting mitral regurgitation, surgery should be performed before deterioration of left ventricular function or the development of pulmonary hypertension. Preservation of the mitral valve–papillary muscle apparatus probably improves results in patients with mitral valve repair by maintaining ventricular function. Unfortunately, an active infection of the mitral valve prevents the valve from being repaired, necessitating replacement.

X. Myocardial, Pericardial, and Endocardial Disease

DIRECTIONS: Each question below contains five suggested responses. Select the **one best** response to each question.

417. An unusual finding on electrocardiogram (ECG) in a patient with myocarditis is

(A) sinus tachycardia
(B) diffuse ST-segment and T-wave changes
(C) increased QRS voltage
(D) complete atrioventricular (AV) block
(E) left bundle branch block (LBBB)

418. Which of the following statements concerning the clinical picture of hemochromatosis is true?

(A) It is a progressive overload of lead, leading to cirrhosis, diabetes, hyperpigmentation, and cardiac dysfunction
(B) Sudden death is the most common result in genetic hemochromatosis
(C) The electrocardiogram (ECG) is often abnormal and may show high voltage and nonspecific ST-segment and T-wave changes
(D) Severe myocardial fibrosis is usually found
(E) Phlebotomy or deferoxamine can normalize or improve left ventricular function

419. Which of the following statements best describes the β-adrenergic pathway in idiopathic dilated cardiomyopathy?

(A) There is decreased activation of the adrenergic nervous system in chronic heart failure
(B) Beta$_1$ receptors are up-regulated
(C) The inotropic response to calcium (Ca^{2+}) administration is unchanged
(D) The response to exogenous beta agonists are unchanged
(E) The beta$_2$-agonist responsiveness is unchanged

420. Which of the following statements concerning left ventricular outflow obstruction in hypertrophic cardiomyopathy is true?

(A) It is due to diastolic anterior motion of the mitral valve and middiastolic contact with the ventricular septum
(B) It can be worsened by beta-blocking drugs due to decreased myocardial contractility
(C) It can be increased by squatting and a secondary increase in atrial pressure
(D) It can be increased by the Valsalva maneuver
(E) It can be decreased by exercise

421. A morphological characteristic of most patients with hypertrophic cardiomyopathy is

(A) an enlarged left ventricular cavity
(B) a concentric pattern of left ventricular hypertrophy
(C) normal-sized atria
(D) a fibrous plaque on the endocardium of the left ventricle
(E) normal mitral valve leaflets

422. All the following features are common to both restrictive cardiomyopathy and constrictive pericarditis in the catheterization laboratory EXCEPT

(A) an elevated right atrial pressure with a steep *y* descent
(B) an elevated right ventricular systolic pressure with a sharp dip and plateau in diastole
(C) pulmonary hypertension
(D) a left ventricular filling pressure that is appreciably higher than right ventricular filling pressure
(E) an elevated pulmonary wedge pressure

423. Infective endocarditis due to a virulent primary pathogen, which evolves over days to weeks with hectic progress, early complications, and a diagnosis usually made within less than 2 weeks is best described by the term

(A) subacute bacterial endocarditis (SBE)
(B) acute bacterial endocarditis (ABE)
(C) native valve endocarditis (NVE)
(D) early prosthetic valve endocarditis (PVE)
(E) nonbacterial thrombotic endocarditis (NBTE)

424. A relatively low risk for infective endocarditis is found in patients with

(A) a prosthetic heart valve
(B) a ventricular septal defect
(C) syphilitic aortitis
(D) a patent ductus arteriosus
(E) coarctation of the aorta

425. Compared to patients who do not abuse drugs, infective endocarditis in parenteral drug abusers may involve

(A) *Pseudomonas* species as the most common bacterial etiology
(B) *Candida* species as the most common fungal agent
(C) a similar incidence of right-sided valvular involvement
(D) a frequent incidence of pulmonary valve involvement
(E) rare instances of infection limited to the left side

426. A prompt search for colonic cancer should be initiated in patients who develop bacteremia or endocarditis caused by

(A) *Streptococcus sanguis*
(B) *Streptococcus faecalis*
(C) *Streptococcus bovis*
(D) *Escherichia coli*
(E) *Neisseria gonorrhoeae*

427. Urgent or early valve replacement surgery in the absence of congestive heart failure (CHF) or recurrent emboli should be considered in patients with

(A) acute staphylococcal endocarditis of the aortic valve related to parenteral drug abuse
(B) acute staphylococcal endocarditis of the tricuspid valve related to parenteral drug abuse
(C) penicillin-sensitive streptococcus endocarditis of the aortic valve
(D) fungal endocarditis of an aortic valve prosthesis
(E) enterococcal endocarditis of the aortic valve

DIRECTIONS: Each question below contains four suggested responses of which **one or more** is correct. Select

A	if	**1, 2, and 3**	are correct
B	if	**1 and 3**	are correct
C	if	**2 and 4**	are correct
D	if	**4**	is correct
E	if	**1, 2, 3, and 4**	are correct

428. Correct statements regarding the clinical manifestations of myocarditis include which of the following?

(1) The most commonly identified cause is Coxsackie B virus infection
(2) Patients often present with a syndrome suggestive of left ventricular dysfunction and dilated cardiomyopathy
(3) An elevated erythrocyte sedimentation rate is found in most patients
(4) Creatine kinase MB release occurs in most patients

429. The diagnosis of myocarditis by endomyocardial biopsy may be limited by the

(1) timing of the biopsy
(2) number of samples obtained by biopsy
(3) rigidity of the diagnostic criteria
(4) ability of biopsy to obtain only left ventricular tissue

430. True statements regarding carcinoid tumors include which of the following?

(1) The carcinoid syndrome is characterized by flushing, telangiectasias, diarrhea, and bronchoconstriction
(2) Carcinoid heart disease occurs in nearly all patients with classic carcinoid syndrome
(3) Cardiac lesions of the carcinoid syndrome usually involve the right heart, primarily the tricuspid and pulmonic valves
(4) Carcinoid tumors usually secrete large amounts of 5-hydroxyindoleacetic acid, which accounts for the findings in the carcinoid syndrome

431. Correct statements regarding the pathology of idiopathic dilated cardiomyopathy include which of the following?

(1) The weight of the heart is increased
(2) Left ventricular wall thickness is usually increased
(3) Microscopy reveals marked myocyte hypertrophy despite the dilated nature of the disease
(4) The degree of fibrosis appears more severe than the extent of systolic or diastolic dysfunction

432. Characteristics that appear to correlate with prognosis in idiopathic dilated cardiomyopathy include the

(1) severity of left ventricular dysfunction
(2) cardiac index
(3) filling pressures
(4) pulmonary artery pressures

433. Correct statements regarding ventricular arrhythmias and sudden death in patients with idiopathic dilated cardiomyopathy (IDC) include which of the following?

(1) The incidence of sudden death is increased in patients with ventricular arrhythmias in the setting of IDC
(2) Inducible polymorphic ventricular tachycardia on electrophysiological study correlates with the risk of sudden death
(3) Inducible unimorphic ventricular tachycardia on electrophysiological study predicts the later occurrence of spontaneous ventricular tachycardia
(4) Inducible ventricular fibrillation on electrophysiological study correlates with the risk of sudden death

SUMMARY OF DIRECTIONS

A	B	C	D	E
1, 2, 3 only	1, 3 only	2, 4 only	4 only	All are correct

434. Which of the following pharmacological agents improve survival in heart failure?

(1) Angiotensin-converting enzyme (ACE) inhibitors
(2) Diuretics
(3) Hydralazine and isosorbide dinitrate
(4) Nifedipine

435. The use of digitalis in patients with idiopathic dilated cardiomyopathy has which of the following effects?

(1) It improves ejection fraction
(2) It improves exercise tolerance
(3) It improves clinical symptoms
(4) It controls ventricular rate in atrial fibrillation

436. The potential benefits of β-adrenergic blockade in idiopathic dilated cardiomyopathy include

(1) a reduction in heart rate
(2) a reduction in afterload via a reduction in renin
(3) an improved ventricular diastolic function
(4) a reduction in sudden death

437. Diastolic dysfunction in hypertrophic cardiomyopathy has which of the following characteristics?

(1) It is present in most patients
(2) It is presumed to be responsible for symptoms of fatigue, exertional dyspnea, and angina
(3) It may occur in the absence of symptoms
(4) It causes an increase in the contribution of early diastole to overall left ventricular filling

438. Important pathophysiological components of hypertrophic cardiomyopathy include

(1) left ventricular outflow obstruction
(2) diastolic dysfunction
(3) myocardial ischemia
(4) arrhythmias

439. Histological features of hypertrophic cardiomyopathy include

(1) cardiac muscle cell disorganization
(2) myocardial scarring
(3) abnormalities of the small intramural coronary arteries
(4) enlargement of the left ventricular cavity

440. Correct statements regarding myocardial ischemia in hypertrophic cardiomyopathy include which of the following?

(1) There is excessive myocardial oxygen demand that exceeds the capacity of the coronary system to deliver oxygen
(2) There is compromise of coronary blood flow to the myocardium due to the presence of coronary atherosclerosis in most patients
(3) There is prolonged diastolic relaxation resulting in elevated myocardial wall tension
(4) There is dilatation of coronary microvessels

441. Correct statements regarding genetic factors in hypertrophic cardiomyopathy include which of the following?

(1) It follows an autosomal pattern of inheritance involving chromosome 14
(2) The occurrence of sudden death should prompt an evaluation in surviving relatives
(3) Hypertrophic cardiomyopathy is the leading cause of sudden death in young competitive athletes
(4) Hypertrophic cardiomyopathy may be excluded in children by a screening echocardiogram

442. A reasonable definition of restrictive cardiomyopathy should include

  (1) a clinical picture that simulates constrictive pericarditis
  (2) increased jugular venous pressure with prominent x and y descents
  (3) pulmonary congestion
  (4) an enlarged heart

443. Which of the following abnormalities on electrocardiogram (ECG) may help differentiate restrictive cardiomyopathy from constrictive pericarditis?

  (1) Left bundle branch block (LBBB)
  (2) Right bundle branch block (RBBB)
  (3) Left ventricular hypertrophy
  (4) Right ventricular hypertrophy

444. Correct statements regarding the treatment of restrictive cardiomyopathy include which of the following?

  (1) Benefit may be obtained from diuretics when filling pressures are high and there is systemic and pulmonary congestion
  (2) Calcium channel blocking agents may improve diastolic compliance
  (3) Relatively high levels of filling pressure are required to sustain ventricular filling
  (4) Digitalis is usually beneficial even when systolic pump function and contractility are normal

445. Neoplasms that commonly metastasize to the pericardium include

  (1) carcinoma of the esophagus
  (2) carcinoma of the lung
  (3) carcinoma of the stomach
  (4) malignant melanoma

446. The diagnosis of acute pericarditis is more likely than the diagnosis of acute transmural myocardial infarction when the electrocardiogram (ECG) reveals

  (1) a diffuse, upwardly concave ST-segment elevation greater than 5 mm
  (2) reciprocal ST-segment depression in leads aV_R and V_1
  (3) associated T-wave inversion and a simultaneous ST-segment elevation
  (4) diffuse PR-segment depression except for leads aV_R and V_1

447. Hemodynamic patterns that are predominant in both restrictive cardiomyopathy and constrictive pericarditis include

  (1) a prominent right atrial y descent
  (2) a jugular venous diastolic collapse wave
  (3) a right ventricular early diastolic dip and late diastolic plateau
  (4) a left ventricular end-diastolic pressure greater than the right ventricular end-diastolic pressure

448. Constrictive pericarditis may occur as a result of

  (1) tuberculosis
  (2) open heart surgery
  (3) rheumatoid arthritis
  (4) mulibrey nanism

449. Most cases of fungal endocarditis are caused by species of

  (1) *Nocardia*
  (2) *Aspergillus*
  (3) *Sporothrix*
  (4) *Candida*

450. Visceral pericardiectomy in combination with parietal pericardiectomy is the surgical treatment of choice for

  (1) postpericardiotomy syndrome
  (2) recurrent pericardial effusion
  (3) Dressler's syndrome
  (4) recurrent constrictive pericarditis

SUMMARY OF DIRECTIONS

A	B	C	D	E
1, 2, 3 only	1, 3 only	2, 4 only	4 only	All are correct

451. In isolated, severe aortic valve regurgitation complicated by endocarditis, vegetations would be likely to form on the

(1) aortic surface of the aortic valve leaflets
(2) ventricular surface of the aortic valve leaflets
(3) coronary ostia just above the aortic valve
(4) chordae tendineae of the anterior leaflet of the mitral valve

452. Physical findings that may be seen in both subacute bacterial endocarditis (SBE) and acute bacterial endocarditis (ABE) include

(1) petechiae
(2) Osler's nodes
(3) Janeway's lesions
(4) clubbing of the fingers

453. In combination with positive blood culture results, major echocardiographic criteria that may indicate infective endocarditis include

(1) oscillating intracardiac target on valve or supporting structure in the absence of an alternative anatomic explanation
(2) new dehiscence of a prosthetic valve
(3) evidence of an abscess on the valve, supporting structure, or endocardium
(4) a new left ventricular wall motion abnormality

454. In cases where the specific organism has not yet been identified, appropriate broad-spectrum antibiotic therapy for subacute bacterial endocarditis in a patient not allergic to penicillin should include intravenous

(1) ampicillin
(2) nafcillin
(3) gentamicin
(4) chloramphenicol

455. There is a greater than 50 percent chance of significant transient bacteremia in dental procedures such as

(1) extraction of one or more teeth
(2) simple fillings outside the gum line
(3) cleaning and scaling teeth
(4) adjustment of orthodontic appliances

DIRECTIONS: The group of questions below consists of four lettered headings followed by a set of numbered items. For each numbered item select

A	if the item is associated with	(A) **only**
B	if the item is associated with	(B) **only**
C	if the item is associated with	**both** (A) and (B)
D	if the item is associated with	**neither** (A) nor (B)

Each lettered heading may be used **once, more than once, or not at all.**

Questions 456–459

(A) Cardiac tamponade
(B) Constrictive pericarditis
(C) Both
(D) Neither

456. Bimodal venous return

457. Increased intrapericardial pressure

458. Prominent systolic collapse wave

459. Pulsus paradoxus

X. Myocardial, Pericardial, and Endocardial Disease

Answers

417. The answer is C. *(p 1594)* Common abnormalities on electrocardiogram (ECG) in patients with myocarditis include sinus tachycardia, diffuse ST-segment and T-wave changes, left bundle branch block (LBBB), complete atrioventricular block, and a myocardial infarction. Arrhythmias include supraventricular arrhythmias, ventricular tachycardia, complete heart block (with Stokes-Adams attacks), and sudden death (presumably due to either complete heart block or ventricular tachycardia). There is some overlap between pericarditis and myocarditis, which may make interpretation of the ECG difficult. Prolongation of the QTC interval and low voltage of the QRS have been noted.

418. The answer is E. *(pp 1600–1601)* Hemochromatosis is the progressive overload of iron in tissues, which results in cirrhosis, diabetes, hyperpigmentation, and cardiac dysfunction. Congestive heart failure (CHF) is the leading cause of death in genetic hemochromatosis. The electrocardiogram (ECG) may show low voltage and nonspecific ST-segment and T-wave changes. Although the iron deposition causes fibrosis in most patients, the fibrosis tends to be mild. Treatment of genetic hemochromatosis involves removal of excessive body iron and supportive treatment. After iron removal by either phlebotomy or deferoxamine, cardiac dysfunction may normalize, and left ventricular function may improve.

419. The answer is C. *(pp 1610–1611)* There is activation of the adrenergic nervous system in chronic heart failure. There is a 30 percent reduction in beta$_2$-agonist responsiveness. Beta$_1$ receptors are down-regulated. Although there is a reduction in the responsiveness to exogenous beta agonist, the inotropic response to calcium (Ca^{2+}) administration is unchanged.

420. The answer is D. *(pp 1626–1627)* Left ventricular outflow obstruction in hypertrophic cardiomyopathy is a dynamic obstruction. It is caused by systolic anterior motion of the mitral valve and midsystolic contact with the ventricular septum. Interventions or circumstances that decrease myocardial contractility (beta-blocking drugs) or increase ventricular volume or arterial pressure (squatting or vasoconstrictor agents) reduce or abolish the obstruction. Interventions or circumstances that increase contractility (exercise or isoproterenol) or that decrease arterial pressure or ventricular volume (Valsalva maneuver or administration of an agent producing hypotension) increase the degree of obstruction.

421. The answer is D. *(pp 1622–1625)* The left ventricular cavity is usually small or normal in size in hypertrophic cardiomyopathy. Thus, the increased left ventricular mass is due to an increase in ventricular wall thickness. Although a symmetric (concentric) pattern of left ventricular hypertrophy may occasionally be seen, hypertrophy is almost always asymmetric. Usually, the septum shows the greatest magnitude of hypertrophy. Other findings include enlargement of the atria, thickening of the mitral valve leaflets, and areas of fibrosis in the ventricular wall. Approximately 75 percent of hearts show a characteristic fibrous plaque on the mural endocardium of the left ventricle in apposition to the anterior mitral leaflet; presumably, this results from systolic (as well as diastolic) contact between the mitral valve and the septum.

422. The answer is D. *(pp 1639–1642)* The differentiation between restrictive cardiomyopathy and constrictive pericarditis is often difficult. Features common to both conditions include (1) an elevated right atrial pressure with a steep *y* descent; (2) an elevated right ventricular systolic pressure with a sharp dip and a plateau in diastole; (3) pulmonary hypertension; and (4) an elevated wedge pressure. However, a left ventricular filling pressure that is appreciably higher than right ventricular filling pressure strongly favors the diagnosis of restrictive cardiomyopathy. In difficult cases where the differentiation between restrictive cardiomyopathy and constrictive pericarditis is not possible, endomyocardial biopsy may furnish the accurate diagnosis.

423. The answer is B. *(p 1681)* The term infective endocarditis refers to a microbial infection of the endothelial lining of the heart, which usually develops on heart valves but occasionally appears elsewhere on the endocardium. Although sometimes confusing, the terms subacute and acute bacterial endocarditis (SBE and ABE) remain in common use and still have descriptive value. SBE is caused by organisms of low virulence such as *Streptococcus viridans,* which evolves over several weeks or months and has a limited ability to infect other tissues. On the other hand, ABE is a virulent infection occurring over a short period of time and is caused by primary aggressive pathogens such as *Staphylococcus aureus,* which have the potential to cause invasive infections in other areas of the body. Native valve endocarditis (NVE) affects a heart valve that was either normal or previously damaged by congenital or acquired disease. Infection of an artificial heart valve is termed prosthetic valve endocarditis (PVE). Early PVE occurs within the first 2 months after surgery and late PVE thereafter. It is possible for SBE or ABE to be either NVE or PVE as long as the endocarditis affects heart valves. A previous term for noninfective endocarditis referred to sterile vegetations within the heart. A newer descriptive term is nonbacterial thrombotic endocarditis (NBTE), which highlights the thrombotic nature of these sterile lesions rather than an infective or inflammatory nature.

424. The answer is C. *(pp 1682–1686, Table 94-2)* In spite of wide variation with individual studies, the relative propensity of various cardiac lesions to become infected may be estimated by combining large published series of cases. Two opposite ends of the spectrum may be represented. A relatively high-risk group includes patients with prosthetic heart valves, previous infective endocarditis, aortic valve disease, mitral regurgitation, patent ductus arteriosus, ventricular septal defect, coarctation of the aorta, and Marfan's syndrome. A very low- or negligible-risk group includes patients with mitral valve prolapse without regurgitation, atrial septal defects of the secundum type, arteriosclerotic plaques, coronary artery disease, syphilitic aortitis, cardiac pacemakers, and surgically corrected cardiac lesions without prosthetic implants more than 6 months postoperatively.

425. The answer is B. *(pp 1683–1684, Table 94-3)* Strains of *Staphylococcus aureus* cause more cases of endocarditis (approximately 50 percent) among parenteral drug abusers than any other bacterial species. By comparison, infections with the species of *Pseudomonas* occur in only 15 percent of drug abusers but are notably more common than in nonaddicts. Parenteral drug abusers have an incidence of fungal endocarditis occurring approximately 5 percent of the time, and when it occurs, the most common pathogen is *Candida.* The incidence of right-sided valvular infections is greater in intravenous drug abusers than any other endocarditis group. Nevertheless, infection limited to the left side still occurs in approximately 50 percent of the abuser group. The tricuspid valve is nearly always affected when right-sided infections occur. Ironically, pulmonic valve infection is unusual, even in abusers of parenteral drugs.

426. The answer is C.   *(pp 1686–1687)*   *Streptococcus viridans* accounts for most cases of subacute bacterial endocarditis. *Streptococcus sanguis* is a member of this strain. The nonenterococcal group D species, *Streptococcus bovis* accounts for about one-fifth of streptococcal D cases. Gastrointestinal lesions, especially colonic polyps and cancers, are commonly present in patients who develop *Strep. bovis* bacteremia or endocarditis. Identification of this species should prompt an early investigation for colonic disease, whether or not the patient has gastrointestinal symptoms. Strains of *Streptococcus faecalis* cause about 10 percent of streptococcal cases. They are usually found in association with infections of the genitourinary tract in women of childbearing age and old men with prostate enlargement. *Escherichia coli* is a gram-negative bacillus that accounts for a very small number of cases of native valve endocarditis. Although associated with the gastrointestinal tract, this is not a hallmark of colonic lesions. *Neisseria gonorrhoeae* is a rare cause of endocarditis since the introduction of penicillin.

427. The answer is D.   *(pp 1701–1702)*   Appropriate timing of valve replacement surgery is crucial in patients with varieties of endocarditis. In the absence of major complications such as congestive heart failure (CHF) or recurrent emboli, trying to effect an antimicrobial sterilization is an important first step before considering valve surgery. Penicillin-sensitive streptococcal endocarditis almost always can be cured with antibiotic therapy alone. Similarly, young drug addicts with acute staphylococcal endocarditis have a good prognosis with appropriate antibiotic therapy, particularly if the aortic valve is involved. Even if the aortic valve is involved, in the initial absence of CHF or recurrent emboli, a strong course of antibiotic therapy is indicated. On the other hand, acute staphylococcal endocarditis in a nonparenteral drug abuser usually has a poor prognosis with medical therapy alone. This situation is particularly ominous if the aortic valve is involved. Successful treatment of fungal prosthetic valve endocarditis by antifungal agents alone is negligible, even in the absence of CHF. This is such a critical situation that early surgical intervention for total eradication of the organism is warranted.

428. The answer is A (1, 2, 3).   *(pp 1591–1594, Table 88-1)*   Many infectious agents have been associated with myocarditis, the most common being Coxsackie B virus infection. In most cases, myocarditis is clinically silent, but the most obvious symptom is an antecedent viral syndrome. Left ventricular dysfunction in a syndrome compatible with dilated cardiomyopathy identifies a significant proportion of patients. An elevated erythrocyte sedimentation rate occurs in most patients, and an elevated white blood cell count is found in approximately 25 percent of patients. Creatine kinase MB release is found in a small percentage of patients (approximately 12 percent).

429. The answer is A (1, 2, 3).   *(pp 1595–1596; Aretz, Am J Cardiovasc Pathol 1:3–14, 1986)*   Endomyocardial biopsy must be performed as quickly as possible to maximize the diagnostic yield. A sample is technically adequate only when four to six fragments are available for interpretation. If the sample is too sparse or myocyte injury is not demonstrated, then a repeat biopsy may be indicated. The criteria for the diagnosis of active myocarditis are variable. The working standard is the Dallas criteria, which define active myocarditis as "an inflammatory infiltrate of the myocardium with necrosis or degeneration of adjacent myocytes not typical of the ischemic damage associated with coronary artery disease." Indeed, myocarditis may be focal or patchy, thereby limiting the technique of endomyocardial biopsy. Endomyocardial biopsy is usually performed in the right heart, and therefore, tissue is obtained from the right side of the ventricular septum. Left ventricular tissue is usually not obtained in the routine endomyocardial biopsy.

430. The answer is B (1, 3).   *(pp 1598–1599)*   Carcinoid tumors usually arise from the gastrointestinal tract and secrete large amounts of serotonin. Serotonin is later metabolized to 5-hydroxyindoleacetic acid. Characteristics of the carcinoid syndrome include flushing, telangiectasias, diarrhea, and bronchoconstriction. Approximately half of all patients with classic carcinoid syndrome experience carcinoid heart disease. Carcinoid heart disease tends to involve the right side of the heart, causing dysfunction of the tricuspid and pulmonic valves. Usually this is tricuspid regurgitation rather than tricuspid stenosis. The primarily right-sided cardiac involvement suggests that a blood-borne product of the tumor is responsible for the cardiac disease.

431. The answer is B (1, 3). *(pp 1609–1610)* In idiopathic dilated cardiomyopathy, the weight of the heart is increased. Although the weight is increased, left ventricular wall thickness is usually not increased because of the marked dilatation of the ventricular cavities. Scarring does occur, even in the absence of significant narrowing of the epicardial coronary arteries. In most cases, the degree of fibrosis is not extensive enough to cause changes in systolic or diastolic function. The characteristic findings on microscopy are marked myocyte hypertrophy and very large bizarre-shaped nuclei.

432. The answer is E (all). *(pp 1611–1613)* Left ventricular enlargement correlates with poor prognosis in some studies of idiopathic dilated cardiomyopathy. The severity of left ventricular dysfunction appears to be a better predictor of prognosis. Cardiac index has also been shown to correlate with clinical outcome. Higher filling pressures and pulmonary artery pressures have been observed in patients who die from idiopathic dilated cardiomyopathy as compared to pressures in survivors.

433. The answer is B (1, 3). *(p 1613)* Ventricular arrhythmias are very common in patients with idiopathic dilated cardiomyopathy. The incidence of sudden death in patients with ventricular arrhythmias in this setting may be increased. Electrophysiological studies yield important information about these patients. The induction of polymorphic ventricular tachycardia or ventricular fibrillation does not correlate with clinical or hemodynamic variables or with the risk of sudden death, but the induction of unimorphic ventricular tachycardia does predict the later occurrence of spontaneous unimorphic ventricular tachycardia.

434. The answer is B (1, 3). *(pp 1615–1616)* Vasodilator therapy improves pumping performance and reduces the work load of the heart. The angiotensin-converting enzyme (ACE) inhibitors and the combination of hydralazine and isosorbide dinitrate are two effective vasodilator regimens. Therapy with ACE inhibitors or the combination of hydralazine and isosorbide dinitrate also improves survival in heart failure. Though diuretics are effective in the treatment of heart failure, their ability to improve survival as single agents has not been proven. Similarly, calcium channel blockers may be effective in heart failure, but their ability to improve survival has not been well documented.

435. The answer is E (all). *(pp 1615–1616)* Digitalis is a widely used drug in the treatment of heart failure and atrial fibrillation. It is the drug of choice for controlling the ventricular rate in atrial fibrillation. In addition, it may be effective in controlling the ventricular response in atrial flutter. Digitalis has also been shown to improve exercise tolerance, ejection fraction, and clinical symptoms as compared with placebo.

436. The answer is E (all). *(pp 1616–1617)* Despite the wide use of medical treatment in idiopathic dilated cardiomyopathy, the mortality and morbidity remain high. One new investigational approach to treatment is the use of β-adrenergic blockade, the potential benefits of which include a reduction in sudden death, a reduction in heart rate, an improved ventricular diastolic function, and a reduction in afterload via indirect mechanisms such as a reduction in renin. Beta blockade has not been approved for the treatment of idiopathic dilated cardiomyopathy by the Food and Drug Administration (FDA); therefore, the use of beta blockers for this purpose cannot be recommended outside the context of controlled clinical trials.

437. The answer is A (1, 2, 3). *(p 1627)* The abnormalities in relaxation and filling of the left ventricle are the characteristic features known as diastolic dysfunction. In hypertrophic cardiomyopathy, these findings are present in about 80 percent of patients. Diastolic dysfunction is presumed to be responsible for symptoms of fatigue, exertional dyspnea, and angina pectoris. The rapid filling phase of diastole is significantly prolonged and associated with a decreased rate and volume of rapid filling compared with normal. Consequently, there is an apparently compensatory increase in the contribution of atrial systole to overall left ventricular filling. Diastolic dysfunction may occur in the absence of symptoms but in the presence of outflow obstruction.

438. The answer is E (all). *(pp 1626–1627)*   The symptoms of hypertrophic cardiomyopathy include pulmonary congestion, fatigue, chest pain, palpitations, and impaired consciousness. The pathophysiological components that have been identified at present include left ventricular outflow obstruction, diastolic dysfunction, myocardial ischemia, and arrhythmias.

439. The answer is A (1, 2, 3). *(p 1625)*   Certain histological features of the left ventricular myocardium are relevant components of the cardiomyopathic muscle and the underlying disease process in hypertrophic cardiomyopathy. These include cardiac muscle cell disorganization, myocardial scarring, and abnormalities of the small intramural coronary arteries. Usual dilatation of the left ventricular cavity is not a finding in hypertrophic cardiomyopathy.

440. The answer is B (1, 3). *(p 1627)*   Myocardial ischemia is abundantly evident in hypertrophic cardiomyopathy. Potential mechanisms responsible for myocardial ischemia include excessive myocardial oxygen demand that exceeds the capacity of the coronary system to deliver oxygen, compromise of the coronary blood flow to the myocardium due to abnormal intramural coronary arteries, and prolonged diastolic relaxation, resulting in elevated myocardial wall tension. Dilatation of coronary microvessels and advanced atherosclerosis have not been described in hypertrophic cardiomyopathy.

441. The answer is A (1, 2, 3). *(pp 1627–1628)*   Hypertrophic cardiomyopathy is genetically transmitted with an autosomal pattern of inheritance. This has been localized to chromosome 14. The occurrence of premature sudden cardiac death in a family should dictate a genetic and echocardiographic evaluation in surviving relatives. Hypertrophic cardiomyopathy appears to be the leading cause of sudden death in young competitive athletes; however, it has not been determined definitively whether or not children with hypertrophic cardiomyopathy identified by genetic analysis but without left ventricular hypertrophy should be disqualified from competitive athletics. Morphologic expression of hypertrophic cardiomyopathy may not be complete until adulthood, and the failure to demonstrate left ventricular hypertrophy by a single echocardiogram in childhood does not exclude the diagnosis.

442. The answer is A (1, 2, 3). *(pp 1637–1638)*   Restrictive cardiomyopathy is a systemic or idiopathic disorder of the myocardium with a clinical and hemodynamic picture that simulates constrictive pericarditis. There should be increased jugular venous pressure with prominent *x* and *y* descents, a small or normal-sized heart, pulmonary congestion, and the absence of ventricular hypertrophy or dilatation. Ventricular systolic function is normal, and no stenotic valvular lesion or outflow tract obstruction should exist.

443. The answer is E (all). *(p 1641)*   The electrocardiogram (ECG) is almost always abnormal in restrictive cardiomyopathy. Left bundle branch block (LBBB) and right bundle branch block (RBBB) strongly favor a diagnosis of restrictive cardiomyopathy. The same is true for left and right ventricular hypertrophy. Generalized low voltage is often seen when restrictive cardiomyopathy is secondary to amyloidosis, but it may be seen in constrictive pericarditis with effusion. In constrictive cardiomyopathy, sinus rhythm is often maintained until the late stages of the disorder, and atrioventricular (AV) conduction disturbances are rare.

444. The answer is A (1, 2, 3). *(p 1642)*   The medical treatment of restrictive cardiomyopathy is unsatisfactory. When filling pressures are extremely high and there is evidence of systemic or pulmonary congestion, significant benefit can be obtained from diuretics. Calcium channel blocking agents may be effective in increasing diastolic compliance. Vasodilation should be used very cautiously because it may decrease ventricular filling, which may result in a deterioration of the clinical picture. Digitalis and other positive inotropes are usually not indicated if systolic pump function and contractility are normal. In restrictive cardiomyopathy, a relatively high level of ventricular filling pressure must be maintained if ventricular filling is to be maintained. For these reasons, caution must be used when using drugs such as diuretics, vasodilators, and calcium channel blocking agents.

445. The answer is C (2, 4). *(p 1667)* The leading primary neoplasms that may metastasize to the pericardium include carcinoma of the lung, carcinoma of the breast, lymphoma, leukemia, and malignant melanoma. Although melanoma may involve the myocardium extensively, it rarely produces clinical findings except when the pericardium is involved. Rare metastatic neoplasms of the pericardium include carcinomas of the colon, esophagus, kidney, ovary, prostate, and stomach. Sarcomas rarely metastasize to the pericardium. A mesothelioma is the most common primary pericardial neoplasm. Lymphangioma, hemangioma, and teratoma are rare primary neoplasms that may affect the pericardium.

446. The answer is C (2, 4). *(pp 1650–1651)* There are four classical electrocardiographic (ECG) stages that have been described in the evolution of acute pericarditis. The first stage consists of diffuse ST-segment elevation with an associated PR-segment depression except for leads aV_R and V_1. Since these leads are mirror images to the rest of the chest and precordial leads, reciprocal ST-segment depression and corresponding PR elevation will be present rather than the converse. When ST-segment elevation occurs in acute pericarditis, the elevation is seldom greater than 5 mm in magnitude; such a degree of ST-elevation generally indicates transmural myocardial infarction. The second stage consists of a normalization phase, which may be followed by a third phase of diffuse T-wave inversion. The last stage consists of either permanent abnormal T waves or a normalization of T-wave inversion. The absence of Q waves, an upwardly concave ST-segment elevation, and the absence of associated T-wave inversion with ST-segment elevation are all consistent with acute pericarditis. When localized ST elevation with true reciprocal ST depression and significant T-wave inversion occur at the same time as the ST-segment elevation, this usually indicates acute transmural myocardial infarction.

447. The answer is A (1, 2, 3). *(pp 1640, 1662–1663)* Differentiation of constrictive pericarditis from a restrictive cardiomyopathy may be quite difficult. Cardiac catheterization assists in making this distinction. However, many hemodynamic pictures of constrictive pericarditis are matched by a restrictive cardiomyopathy. A prominent *y* descent in the right atrial tracing, which represents a diastolic collapse wave, and the right ventricular early diastolic dip and late diastolic plateau may be seen in both entities. However, when the left ventricular end-diastolic pressure is greater than the right ventricular end-diastolic pressure, this is usually indicative of restrictive cardiomyopathy rather than restrictive pericarditis. On some occasions, however, the distinction between the two compressive syndromes may be difficult and may only be resolved by an intramyocardial biopsy.

448. The answer is E (all). *(pp 1662–1665)* Although case reports of tuberculosis in the United States have progressively decreased over the past half century, tuberculosis is still a cause of chronic constrictive pericarditis. For the future, this incidence may increase in view of the development of resistant forms of the tuberculous bacillus. Conceptionally, pericardial constriction should not occur after open heart surgery when the anterior pericardium is left open upon closure of the chest wall. Nevertheless, pericardial constriction has been reported following cardiac surgery (0.2 percent in one series) and is thought to be secondary to fibrous thickening of the posterior pericardium with a fibrous type hemorrhagic shell over the anterior pericardium. Some type of pericardial involvement occurs in approximately 30 percent of patients with rheumatoid arthritis. When constrictive pericarditis develops in this situation, it is usually subacute and seldom calcified. Mulibrey nanism is an acronym for *mu*scle, *li*ver, *br*ain, and *ey*e. This refers to an autosomal recessive disorder characterized by a connective tissue disease that involves the listed tissues in addition to a definite component of pericardial constriction.

449. The answer is C (2, 4). *(p 1687)* Although many species of fungi potentially may infect the endocardium, *Candida* and *Aspergillus* are the two genera that account for most cases. *Candida* endocarditis of the native valve usually occurs in narcotic addicts or in patients receiving chronic parenteral hyperalimentation. *Aspergillus* often involves prosthetic valves. Fungal involvement of native heart valves in nonaddicts is rare.

450. The answer is D (4). *(pp 1677–1678)* The pericardium consists of two layers, the parietal membrane, which is the outside fibrous coat with an inner serosal layer, and the visceral membrane, which is reflected and contiguous with the epicardium. The space between these two layers is lubricated with a small amount of serosal fluid, which maintains a slight negative atmospheric pressure in a healthy pericardium. Recurrent constrictive pericarditis involves inflammation and fibrous adherence of both the parietal and visceral pericardium; thus, when surgery is required for resistant constrictive pericarditis, an extensive parietal in combination with a visceral pericardiectomy is the treatment of choice. A recurrent pericardial effusion resistant to medical therapy is effectively treated with just a parietal pericardiectomy as long as the visceral pericardium is not fibrotic. The postpericardiotomy syndrome and Dressler's syndrome are clinical manifestations of an inflammatory type of pericarditis; they are generally self-limited and respond to anti-inflammatory agents.

451. The answer is C (2, 4). *(pp 1688–1689, Figure 94-3; Rodbard, Circulation 27:18–28, 1963)* Rodbard developed the concept that endocarditis occurs where blood flows from a high-pressure source through an orifice into a low-pressure sink. Vegetations are, thus, more likely to develop beyond the orifice impediment within the area of low pressure as a result of Venturi effects and turbulence. Vegetations may also develop on jet lesions—that is, sites where endothelial roughening has occurred in response to a swift, turbulent bloodstream. In the case of pure, severe aortic insufficiency, vegetations would appear on the ventricular surface of the valve, reflecting a high-velocity regurgitant stream passing through an incompetent orifice to a low-pressure sink (left ventricle in diastole). A severe regurgitant stream from the aortic valve may cause a jet lesion on the chordae tendineae of the anterior leaflet of the mitral valve, creating a nidus for a potential vegetation.

452. The answer is A (1, 2, 3). *(pp 1692–1693)* On physical examination, petechiae are common in both subacute bacterial endocarditis (SBE) and acute bacterial endocarditis (ABE) but are rare in nonbacterial thrombotic endocarditis (NBTE). Petechiae may be due to microembolization, capillary fragility, or as in some cases of ABE, secondary to disseminated intravascular coagulopathy. Splinter hemorrhages are found in about 20 percent of patients with SBE. Osler's nodes occur in 10 to 20 percent of patients with SBE and in fewer than 10 percent of patients with ABE. These are painful, tender erythematous nodules in the skin of the extremities, usually in the pulp of the fingers. Janeway's lesions are small, flat, nontender red spots, irregular in outline, and less than 5 mm in diameter found on the palms and soles of a few patients with SBE and ABE. Unlike petechiae, they are not hemorrhagic, and they blanch on pressure. Clubbing of the fingers previously was common in SBE but is now found in less than 10 percent of cases. It is not seen in ABE since the pathogenesis is probably a result of a little understood reaction to a subacute indolent organism.

453. The answer is A (1, 2, 3). *(pp 1695–1696; von Reyn, Ann Intern Med 95:505–518, 1981)* Clinical criteria for the diagnosis of infective endocarditis based on modified definitions first proposed by von Reyn and colleagues should include two major criteria, or one major and three minor criteria, or five minor criteria. One of the major criteria is defined as positive blood culture results that identify typical microorganisms for infective endocarditis, and persistently positive cultures in one or more blood samples drawn more than 12 hours apart, or all of three or a majority of four or more separate blood cultures with the first and last drawn at least 1 hour apart. If coupled with the second major criteria of echocardiographic findings, the clinical criteria for infective endocarditis may be met. Positive specific major echocardiographic results include: (1) oscillating intracardiac target on valve or supporting structures, in the path of regurgitant jets, or on iatrogenic devices in the absence of an alternative anatomic explanation; or (2) abscess; or (3) new dehiscence of a prosthetic valve or new valvular regurgitation. The worsening or changing of a preexistent murmur is not sufficient criteria. A new wall motion abnormality of the left ventricle is not echocardiographic evidence for endocarditis. Six minor criteria include a variety of clinical presentations and a sector of echocardiographic findings, which are less specific for infective endocarditis than those listed above.

454. The answer is B (1, 3). *(pp 1699–1701, Table 94-7)* Pending specific organism identification, subacute bacterial endocarditis requires broad-spectrum therapy that covers most streptococci (including *Streptococcus faecalis*) and gram-negative bacilli. In patients with normal renal function who are not sensitive to penicillin, the following regimen is appropriate: ampicillin 2.0 g intravenously every 4 hours plus gentamicin, 1.5 mg/kg intravenously every 8 hours. If acute bacterial endocarditis is suspected, nafcillin 2.0 g intravenously every 4 hours should be added to the regimen to cover *Staphylococcus aureus*. Although it covers certain anaerobic bacteria, chloramphenicol is a bacteriostatic agent with a limited spectrum and significant side effects, which preclude its use as a broad-spectrum agent in endocarditis.

455. The answer is B (1, 3). *(pp 1703–1704, Table 94-8)* The incidence of transient bacteremia after extraction of one or more teeth is 82 percent and after periodontal surgery is 88 percent. When a dentist cleans and scales the teeth, gum injury is always involved, and susceptible patients should receive a prophylactic antibiotic regimen. Based on present information, prophylaxis is probably not necessary for minor dental procedures that do not involve the gums, such as simple fillings outside the gum line and adjustment of orthodontic appliances, as these procedures do not result in a significant bacteremia.

456–459. The answers are: 456-B, 457-A, 458-A, 459-C. *(pp 1654–1664)* Each of the pericardial compressive syndromes of cardiac tamponade and constrictive pericarditis, although similar, represents a distinct pathophysiological mechanism. Tamponade can be thought of as being an elastic form of compression in direct contradistinction to the rigid shell compression of pericardial constriction. Thus, in tamponade, the venous return is unimodal and confined to ventricular systole with a corresponding systolic collapse wave or prominent *x* descent. On the other hand, constrictive pericarditis preserves the normal bimodal cardiac filling, yet the overall cardiac volume is limited by the rigid pericardium. Since the heart cannot exceed the set volume attained near the end of the first third of diastole, during ejection there is little impediment to venous return, and the normal *x* descent is preserved. When the tricuspid valve opens in early diastole, compression is still insignificant at end systole; blood rushes in at a markedly increased rate, resulting in a significant diastolic collapse wave or *y* descent in the right atrial tracing. The *y* descent also corresponds to the early diastolic dip in the right ventricular and left ventricular wave form.

Pulsus paradoxus is a misnomer and refers to an exaggeration of the usual inspiratory decline in systolic arterial pressure and relates to a situation when the decline is greater than 10 mmHg. Pulsus paradoxus is a classical sign of cardiac tamponade and is present in over 90 percent of the cases. It is less common in constrictive pericarditis but may occur in approximately 50 percent of the cases.

The pathophysiological mechanism of cardiac tamponade is directly related to the increased intrapericardial pressure due to the dynamic fluid or elastic buildup. In constrictive pericarditis, however, this dynamic element is absent as the pericardium is fibrotic and serves as a mechanical impediment to cardiac filling. There is no fluid element or increased intrapericardial pressure except for the syndrome known as effusive-constrictive pericarditis where there is a residual fluid element in combination with some rigid construction. However, this is not considered pure constrictive pericarditis.

XI. Congenital Heart Disease

DIRECTIONS: Each question below contains five suggested responses. Select the **one best** response to each question.

460. The development of the heart prior to septation is characterized by all the following statements EXCEPT

(A) the growing bulboventricular tract normally bends to the right and anteriorly, resulting in a descending limb (embryonic ventricle) and an ascending limb (bulbus cordis)

(B) the atrioventricular (AV) valves, the ventricles, and the arterial roots are all derived from the bulboventricular loop

(C) the external shape of the heart and the basic configuration of a four-chambered organ is completed within the first month of embryonic life

(D) reversal of the cardiac loop results in congenitally corrected transposition of the great vessels

(E) the truncoaortic sac, the atria, and the sinus venosus arise from the bulboventricular loop and are, thus, intrapericardial structures

461. Embryonic valve formation is characterized by all the following statements EXCEPT

(A) the atrioventricular (AV) valves are thin and fibrous because they are derived predominantly from endocardial tissue

(B) tricuspid atresia results from fusion of endocardial cushion tissue that borders the AV canal

(C) the aortic and pulmonary valves are derived from the truncal and intercalated valve cushions

(D) absence of the aortic or pulmonary valve arises from a failure to form the arterial valve anlagen

(E) the bicuspid aortic valve results from either failure of development of an intercalated valve cushion or fusion of adjacent valve anlagen

462. The congenital defect LEAST likely to cause congestive heart failure (CHF) in the first week of life is

(A) severe valvular regurgitation
(B) aortic atresia
(C) ventricular septal defect
(D) critical aortic stenosis
(E) coarctation of the aorta

463. A newborn child with persistent fetal circulation manifests all the following clinical features EXCEPT

(A) severe hypoxia

(B) acidosis despite tachypnea

(C) a chest roentgenogram that shows diminished vascular flow

(D) a physical examination characterized by a parasternal heave, a loud second heart sound (S_2), and a systolic murmur

(E) a higher oxygen level in the umbilical artery than in the radial artery

464. Which of the following statements concerning the transition of the fetal circulation to the neonatal circulation is true?

(A) Umbilical arterial blood has a higher saturation than the umbilical venous blood

(B) Umbilical blood, like maternal venous blood, is usually 50 to 60 percent saturated

(C) Despite the extracardiac and intracardiac shunts, left ventricular and right ventricular output must remain equal

(D) The ductus arteriosus normally diverts more than 80 percent of the right ventricular output

(E) Less than 5 percent of the cardiac output crosses the foramen ovale since it is only a potential space not an actual conduit

465. A child who presents with an isolated large ventricular septal defect, evidence of a diminishing left-to-right shunt, absence of an atrial flow rumble, a systolic murmur that radiates to the left sternal border, a widely split second heart sound (S_2), and a progressive decrease in the intensity of the pulmonic component is most likely to have

(A) a septal defect closure

(B) pulmonary hypertension

(C) an erroneous initial diagnosis

(D) subpulmonic stenosis

(E) pulmonary emboli

466. All the following statements regarding valvular pulmonic stenosis with an intact ventricular septum are true EXCEPT

(A) cyanosis can occur with severe pulmonary valvular stenosis

(B) a gradient less than 50 mmHg across the pulmonic valve excludes severe pulmonary stenosis

(C) as obstruction across the valve increases, the intensity of P_2 decreases

(D) as obstruction across the valve increases, the peak intensity occurs later in systole

(E) the magnitude of right ventricular forces in the anterior precordial leads correlates well with the degree of obstruction

467. A 16-year-old cyanotic patient with Ebstein's anomaly is likely to have all the following clinical manifestations EXCEPT

(A) a chest roentgenogram revealing marked cardiomegaly and diminished pulmonary blood flow

(B) an echocardiogram revealing a large tricuspid valve with delayed closure as compared with the mitral valve

(C) a loud split first heart sound (S_1) with the murmur of tricuspid regurgitation

(D) right ventricular hypertrophy on the electrocardiogram (ECG)

(E) an intracardiac ECG that reveals a ventricular tracing in an area where the pressure is atrial in contour

468. Characteristics of patients with total anomalous pulmonary venous return include all the following EXCEPT

(A) the presence of either a patent foramen ovale or an atrial septal defect

(B) the presence of a common chamber superior to the left atrium and inferior to the tracheal bifurcation

(C) the absence of pulmonary obstruction if the conduit from the common pulmonary venous chamber terminates above the diaphragm

(D) a high frequency of pulmonary vein obstruction if the conduit from the common chamber terminates below the diaphragm

(E) an echo-free space behind the left atrium compatible with a pericardial effusion

469. All the following statements regarding sinus of Valsalva fistula are true EXCEPT

(A) the noncoronary cusp usually ruptures into the right ventricular outflow tract, whereas aneurysms of the right sinus of Valsalva rupture into the right atrium

(B) aneurysms of the right sinus of Valsalva are frequently associated with supracristal ventricular septal defects

(C) all defects should be repaired surgically because of the natural history

(D) at the time of presentation, blood cultures should be drawn to rule out endocarditis

(E) some patients present with a tearing mid-precordial pain in addition to congestive heart failure (CHF)

470. Pregnancy is likely to be tolerated *poorly* in all the following patients EXCEPT

(A) a 21-year-old woman with uncorrected tetralogy of Fallot

(B) a 20-year-old woman with Eisenmenger's syndrome secondary to a ventricular septal defect

(C) a 35-year-old woman with a 2:1 secundum atrial septal defect and normal pulmonary artery pressures

(D) a 20-year-old woman with asymptomatic Marfan's syndrome and an aortic root which is only minimally enlarged

(E) a 19-year-old woman with primary pulmonary hypertension

471. The following pairings of congenital abnormalities with expected complications are all correct EXCEPT

(A) transposition of the great vessels after the Mustard operation; right ventricular (RV) failure

(B) congenitally corrected transposition; Ebstein's anomaly of the mitral valve

(C) coarctation of the aorta; postoperative hypertension

(D) tetralogy of Fallot; stroke and cerebral abscess

(E) Ebstein's anomaly; arrhythmias and sudden death

472. Exercise should be limited in all the following patients with congenital disease EXCEPT

(A) postoperative exercise-induced ventricular tachycardia

(B) postoperative tetralogy of Fallot with good hemodynamic repair

(C) moderate-to-severe hypertrophic cardiomyopathy

(D) moderate-to-severe pulmonary vascular disease

(E) Marfan's syndrome with aortic root dilatation of 6 cm

DIRECTIONS: Each question below contains four suggested responses of which **one or more** is correct. Select

A	if	**1, 2, and 3**	are correct
B	if	**1 and 3**	are correct
C	if	**2 and 4**	are correct
D	if	**4**	is correct
E	if	**1, 2, 3, and 4**	are correct

473. The formation of seven septa account for the normal partitioning of the embryonic heart. Septa that form actively rather than passively include the

(1) septum of the atrioventricular (AV) canal
(2) septum secundum of the atrium
(3) conal septum
(4) muscular portion of the ventricular septum

474. Congenital abnormalities due to defects in septation include

(1) tetralogy of Fallot
(2) aorticopulmonary septal defect
(3) double-outlet right ventricle
(4) persistent atrioventricular (AV) canal

475. Correct associations of an embryonic aortic arch and the fully developed segment of the great vessels in the adult include which of the following pairs?

(1) Second aortic arch—common carotid and proximal internal carotid arteries
(2) Fourth left aortic arch—transverse aortic arch between left carotid and left subclavian
(3) Fifth aortic arch—ductus arteriosus and the descending aortic arch
(4) Truncus arteriosus—aortic and pulmonary roots

476. Disorders in which congenital cardiac abnormalities are associated with a recessive mode of inheritance include

(1) Holt-Oram syndrome
(2) familial atrial septal defect
(3) supravalvular aortic stenosis
(4) Ellis-van Creveld syndrome

477. Which of the following connective tissue disorders are correctly matched with their clinical manifestations?

(1) Marfan's syndrome—dilatation of the aorta and mitral valve prolapse
(2) Pseudoxanthoma elasticum—pulmonary artery stenosis and right heart failure
(3) Ehlers-Danlos syndrome—aortic rupture and sudden death
(4) Cutis laxa—coronary artery disease and myocardial infarction

478. Which of the following genetically transmitted syndromes are matched with the correct cardiac manifestations?

(1) X-linked muscular dystrophy—congestive heart failure (CHF)
(2) Emery-Dreifuss muscular dystrophy—dilated cardiomyopathy with atrial paralysis
(3) Myotonic dystrophy—conduction abnormalities
(4) Friedreich's ataxia—hypertrophic cardiomyopathy

479. In which of the following systemic disorders with known genetic transmission are the succeeding cardiac manifestations correct?

(1) Hurler's syndrome—congestive heart failure (CHF), aortic insufficiency, and mitral regurgitation
(2) Fabry's disease (angiokeratoma corporis diffusum)—hypertrophic cardiomyopathy, mitral valve dysfunction, and myocardial infarction
(3) Osteogenesis imperfecta—mitral valve prolapse and aortic dilatation
(4) Gaucher's disease—constrictive pericarditis and pulmonary hypertension

480. Cardiovascular disorders are associated with which of the following chromosomal abnormalities?

(1) Down's syndrome
(2) Edwards' syndrome
(3) Turner's syndrome
(4) DiGeorge syndrome

481. Syndromes associated with cardiomyopathy in which an autosomal dominant transmission is proven include

(1) phytanic acid storage disease
(2) hypertrophic obstructive cardiomyopathy
(3) type II glycogen storage (Pompe's) disease
(4) systemic amyloidosis

482. Correct statements regarding the pathophysiology of Ebstein's anomaly include which of the following?

(1) Since pulmonary artery pressures are normal, the dominant shunt is left-to-right
(2) The electrocardiogram (ECG) shows a deformed tricuspid valve with delayed closure
(3) The ECG shows right ventricular hypertrophy that is compatible with anatomic abnormalities on the right side
(4) An intracardiac ECG reveals an area in the right heart that is ventricular in origin but has pressure that is atrial in contour

483. Conditions associated with corrected transposition of the great arteries include

(1) pulmonary atresia or stenosis
(2) ventricular septal defect
(3) Ebstein's malformation of the left-sided tricuspid valve
(4) Ebstein's malformation of the right-sided tricuspid valve

484. Medical management of patients with tetralogy of Fallot may include

(1) endocarditis prophylaxis
(2) oral or intravenous propranolol
(3) erythropheresis
(4) prostaglandin administration

485. Abnormalities associated with corrected transposition of the great vessels include

(1) ventricular septal defect
(2) left-sided tricuspid valve
(3) pulmonary atresia or stenosis
(4) atrioventricular (AV) block

486. Complications of cyanotic heart disease include

(1) gout
(2) polycythemia
(3) cerebrovascular accidents
(4) brain abscess

487. Complications that are possible after surgery for congenital heart disease include

(1) complete heart block late after repair of tetralogy of Fallot
(2) a small left-to-right shunt following repair of atrioventricular (AV) canal
(3) pulmonary valve regurgitation following repair of tetralogy of Fallot
(4) idiopathic hypertension following repair of coarctation of the aorta

488. Which of the following aortic arch abnormalities are matched with the correct clinical manifestations?

(1) Right aortic arch and mirror-image branching—tetralogy of Fallot
(2) Double aortic arch—pulsatile mass in the supraclavicular area
(3) Pulmonary artery sling—tracheomalacia and tetralogy of Fallot
(4) Cervical aortic arch—respiratory obstruction and tetralogy of Fallot

489. Recommendations for an asymptomatic 20-year-old woman who has a secundum atrial septal defect include

(1)   surgery if the pulmonary systemic blood flow ratio ($\dot{Q}_p/\dot{Q}_s$) is greater than 1.7 to 1

(2)   a delay for surgical repair until after pregnancy because of the risk of endocarditis at the repair site

(3)   surgical closure if the pulmonary/systemic blood flow ratio ($\dot{Q}_p/\dot{Q}_s$) is 1.7 to 1 with moderate pulmonary hypertension, a systemic arterial oxygen saturation of 94 percent, and a total pulmonary resistance of 8 Wood units/m^2

(4)   no genetic counseling since atrial septal defects occur randomly rather than as genetic traits

490. Physicians examining patients with patent ductus arteriosus are likely to find

(1)   coarctation of the aorta and ventricular septal defect

(2)   a shunt whose magnitude can be determined by the cross-sectional area of the ductus

(3)   a history of maternal exposure to rubella in the first trimester

(4)   arterial oxygen saturation in the legs that exceeds that measured in the arms when pulmonary resistance equals or exceeds systemic resistance

491. Indications for closure of a patent ductus arteriosus include

(1)   uncontrollable congestive heart failure (CHF) in a newborn

(2)   persistence of the patent ductus arteriosus in a 6-year-old child

(3)   growth retardation and signs of a significant shunt in an infant

(4)   catheter passage across a patent ductus arteriosus with a calculated pulmonary vascular resistance of 960 dynes·sec·cm^{-5}

492. Which of the following criteria are indicative of severe valvular aortic stenosis in a 12-year-old child?

(1)   Paradoxical splitting of the second heart sound (S_2)

(2)   Left ventricular hypertrophy by voltage criteria

(3)   A pulse pressure of less than 20 mmHg

(4)   Absence of a palpable thrill with a normal pulse pressure

493. An 11-year-old child presents with evidence of left ventricular outflow obstruction. The presence of which of the following criteria would favor the diagnosis of subvalvular obstruction over a valvular obstruction?

(1)   An ejection click at the apex

(2)   Poststenotic dilatation of the aorta on chest roentgenogram

(3)   Left ventricular hypertrophy on the electrocardiogram (ECG)

(4)   An early diastolic murmur of aortic regurgitation

494. In a patient with a large atrial septal defect and normal pulmonary artery pressures, blood flows from left-to-right because the

(1)   right atrium is more distensible than the left atrium

(2)   tricuspid valve is more capacious than the mitral valve

(3)   right ventricle is thinner and more compliant than the left ventricle

(4)   pressure in the left atrium is higher than the right atrium

SUMMARY OF DIRECTIONS

A	B	C	D	E
1, 2, 3 only	1, 3 only	2, 4 only	4 only	All are correct

495. Patients who meet the criteria for closure of a ventricular septal defect include

(1) an asymptomatic 8-year-old child with a $\dot{Q}_p/\dot{Q}_s$ ratio of 2 to 1 and no pulmonary hypertension

(2) a 9-year-old child with mild dyspnea on exertion, cardiomegaly, a $\dot{Q}_p/\dot{Q}_s$ of 1.5 to 1 and no pulmonary hypertension

(3) an adult with a $\dot{Q}_p/\dot{Q}_s$ of 1.5 to 1 with mild symptoms and mild pulmonary hypertension

(4) a 2-year-old with a large septal defect and pulmonary hypertension with a pulmonary-systemic vascular resistance of 0.4 to 1.0

496. A physician examining a patient with a moderate ventricular septal defect (0.5 to 1.0 cm²/m²) could expect also to find

(1) a significant left-to-right shunt

(2) mild-to-moderate elevation of pulmonary artery pressures

(3) volume overload of the left heart

(4) equal pressures in the right and left ventricles

497. Patients at risk for the long-term development of congestive heart failure (CHF) include

(1) a child with a Mustard procedure done at 6 years of age for transposition of the great vessels

(2) an adult with congenitally corrected transposition of the great vessels

(3) a child with a Fontan procedure done at age 6 for tricuspid atresia

(4) an adult with tetralogy of Fallot corrected as a child

498. Pulmonary vascular obstructive disease is likely to develop in children with

(1) nonrestrictive ventricular septal defect with no pulmonary outflow tract obstruction

(2) Ebstein's anomaly with an atrial septal defect

(3) a patent ductus arteriosus and a $\dot{Q}_p/\dot{Q}_s$ of 3:1

(4) tetralogy of Fallot

DIRECTIONS: Each question below contains five suggested responses. For **each** of the **five** responses listed with every question you are to respond either YES (Y) or NO (N). In a given item **all, some, or none of the alternatives may be correct.**

499. Correct statements concerning genetic factors that predispose patients to atherosclerosis include which of the following?

(A) Increased levels of lipoprotein a (Lp[a]) are associated with a protective effect against atherosclerosis

(B) Apolipoproteins serve a structural role in the formation and stabilization of lipoproteins

(C) Hepatic high-density lipoprotein (HDL) contains apolipoproteins B (apo B), and small intestine HDL contains apolipoprotein E (apo E)

(D) HDL is synthesized predominantly in the liver and small intestine

(E) Lipoproteins consist of an esterified core of lipids surrounded by a lipid monolayer in which apolipoproteins are imbedded

500. An 8-year-old child presents with cyanotic heart disease characterized by a systolic thrill and a harsh midsystolic murmur at the left sternal border. The murmur ends before the second heart sound (S_2), which is single. The electrocardiogram (ECG) reveals normal sinus rhythm and right ventricular hypertrophy. The chest roentgenogram reveals a concave pulmonary segment and an apex elevated from the diaphragm. Correct statements about this patient include which of the following?

(A) Signs of congestive heart failure (CHF) would be unusual

(B) Drugs, maneuvers, or activities that increase myocardial contractility or decrease right ventricular volume increase the intracardiac gradient

(C) The echocardiogram reveals an overriding aorta with discontinuity of both anterior and posterior aortic walls with the subvalvular structures

(D) Cardiac catheterization reveals a normal right atrial pressure, equal pressures of the right and left ventricles, and normal pressure in the pulmonary artery

(E) Cardiac catheterization is unnecessary since the diagnosis is established; surgery should be the next step

XI. Congenital Heart Disease

Answers

460. The answer is E. *(pp 1713–1715)* The vascular system first appears in embryos at about 3 weeks of age but rapidly progresses to form a vascular plexus with subsequent formation of a parallel system of heart tubes. Fusion of the heart tubes allows for the formation of the single bulboventricular tube. The growing bulboventricular tract normally bends to the right and anteriorly with the descending limb in continuity with the embryonic atria forming the embryonic ventricle and the ascending limb of the loop becoming the bulbus cordis. With reversal of the loop to the left and anteriorly, all structures derived from the bulboventricular loop [i.e., the atrioventricular (AV) valves, the ventricles, and the arterial roots] show mirror image reversal. Since the extrapericardial structures (i.e., the atria, the sinus venosus, and the truncoaortic sac) remain correctly aligned, isolated congenitally corrected transposition with isolated ventricular inversion arises. The external shape and a rough four-chambered configuration is rapidly formed by the first month of embryonic life.

461. The answer is A. *(pp 1721–1722)* The atrioventricular (AV) valves partially arise from mesenchymal endocardial cushion tissue; however, most of the tissue contributing to the AV valve cusps arise from the muscular ventricular wall. By a process of diverticulation and undermining, a rim of ventricular muscle is formed at the AV orifice, which is attached to the papillary muscle by chordae tendineae. These rudimentary valves are thick at first and become thin during development. The aortic valves are derived from the truncal and intercalated valve cushions. Failure to develop the arterial valve anlagen results in the absence of the arterial valves, whereas tricuspid atresia results from fusion of the endocardial cushion tissue, which borders the AV canal. The bicuspid aortic valve results from either failure to form an intercalated valve cushion or, more commonly, fusion of adjacent valve anlagen during development.

462. The answer is C. *(p 1763)* Heart failure in the first 18 hours of life is usually due to lesions in which volume load is independent of pulmonary flow as in valvular regurgitation. Myocarditis, endocardial fibroelastosis, congenital heart block, and supraventricular tachycardia (SVT) can produce congestive heart failure (CHF) from the time of birth. Noncardiac abnormalities such as arteriovenous fistulae, sepsis, and depressed myocardial contractility due to hypoxia, hypoglycemia, or sepsis are also potential causes. Most full-term infants with significant heart failure in the first week have critical obstruction to arterial flow often unmasked by closure of the ductus arteriosus. Lesions that require a pulmonary vascular bed with low resistance to express their severity fully (e.g., ventricular septal defects and some forms of transposition of the great vessels) do not become evident until pulmonary resistance drops in the second week.

463. The answer is E. *(p 1763)* Persistent fetal circulation or persistent pulmonary hypertension leads to right-to-left shunting via the patent foramen ovale or a patent ductus arteriosus. The condition is characterized by severe hypoxia and acidotic serum. The newborn appears tachypneic, while the precordial examination reveals a parasternal heave, a loud second heart sound (S_2), and a systolic murmur. A greater oxygen level in the right radial artery than in the umbilical artery confirms right-to-left shunting via a persistent patent ductus arteriosus. The chest roentgenogram reveals diminished pulmonary blood flow without pulmonary parenchymal disease.

464. The answer is D. *(pp 1762–1763)* The placental circulation provides the fetus with all the necessary nutritional requirements, including oxygen. Since the fetal lungs are not expanded, a high flow bypassing them is of no detrimental consequence. Three vascular channels are of extreme importance in the fetal circulation. (1) The foramen ovale allows blood to pass from the right atrium to the left atrium, bypassing the fetal lungs. (2) The ductus arteriosus connects the pulmonary artery to the aorta distal to the left subclavian, bypassing uninflated lung tissue. (3) The ductus venosus shunts blood from the placenta through the umbilical cord to bypass the liver. The return of blood to the heart from the inferior vena cava equals 65 to 70 percent of the combined ventricular output. About 25 percent of the total ventricular output crosses over the foramen ovale to the left atrium joining roughly 5 to 10 percent of the combined ventricular output returning from the fetal lungs. Thus, the right ventricle pumps two-thirds of the combined ventricular output, whereas the left ventricle pumps only one-third. About 85 to 90 percent of the blood ejected by the right ventricle is directed through the patent ductus arteriosus. Umbilical venous blood has a P_{O_2} of about 30 to 35 mmHg and an oxygen saturation of 80 percent; umbilical arterial blood has a P_{O_2} of about 26 to 28 mmHg and an oxygen saturation of 55 to 60 percent. The calculated fetal pulmonary vascular resistance is quite high but falls progressively until term. After birth, pulmonary vascular resistance drops due to decreased kinking (with lung expansion) and decreased vasoconstriction (due to increased P_{O_2}). Adult resistance levels are reached by 6 to 8 weeks of age.

465. The answer is D. *(pp 1768–1773)* With septal defect closure, the systolic murmur becomes softer and shorter in duration. Splitting of the second heart sound (S_2) becomes easily audible with inspiration, and the pulmonic component becomes softer. Decreased flow due to pulmonary hypertension leads to a decreased intensity and duration of the systolic murmur with narrow splitting of S_2 and accentuation of the pulmonic component due to higher pulmonary pressures. The development of subpulmonic stenosis decreases flow across the outflow tract, increasing the turbulence. The systolic murmur radiates toward the left sternal border. With prolongation of right ventricular ejection, S_2 is widely split; with a decrease in pulmonary pressure, the intensity of P_2 decreases.

466. The answer is B. *(pp 1796–1799)* Cyanosis may occur in the presence of severe valvular pulmonic stenosis as a result of stretching of the patent foramen ovale with elevated right atrial pressures, leading to right-to-left shunting. The gradient across the pulmonic valve depends on the flow; therefore, in the presence of right ventricular dysfunction and a depressed cardiac output, a gradient of 30 mmHg may be significant. As the obstruction across the valve increases, the systolic murmur peaks later in systole due to the required force necessary to maintain ejection. With increasing obstruction, the antegrade flow decreases and therefore, the intensity of P_2 decreases. The magnitude of the anterior forces in V_1 and V_2 on the electrocardiogram (ECG) are a rough correlate of the degree of obstruction across the pulmonary outflow tract.

467. The answer is D. *(pp 1802–1803)* Ebstein's anomaly is characterized by a normally attached anterior leaflet of the tricuspid valve to the annulus with attachment of the posterior and septal leaflets to the ventricular wall below the annulus. Thus, the functional right ventricle is small. The tricuspid valve can be both restrictive to forward flow and regurgitant. Cyanosis results from the high right atrial pressure and the nearly universal presence of an atrial septal defect or patent foramen ovale. The roentgenographic and echocardiographic features listed in the question are classic for Ebstein's anomaly. The first heart sound (S_1) is loud and widely split, correlating with the delayed tricuspid closure seen echocardiographically. An intracardiac electrocardiogram (ECG) reveals an atrial pressure tracing but a ventricular electrocardiogram in the atrialized segment of the right ventricle.

468. The answer is E. *(pp 1804–1806)*   In total anomalous venous return, all the pulmonary vessels unite in a common chamber superior to the left atrium. This chamber may be visualized echocardiographically as a free space behind the left atrium. A pericardial effusion would be seen behind the left ventricle and would not extend behind the left atrium. The supradiaphragmatic communications are rarely complicated by venous obstruction, whereas subdiaphragmatic communications frequently have associated pulmonary venous obstruction, leading to an elevated pulmonary capillary wedge pressure and congestive heart failure (CHF). Interatrial communication is necessary to transport partially oxygenated blood to the left heart and sustain life until surgical correction can be performed.

469. The answer is A. *(pp 1784–1785)*   Sinus of Valsalva fistula is an unusual congenital weakness at the union of the aorta to the left ventricle. Defects in the posterior (noncoronary) sinus rupture into the right atrium, whereas those in the right sinus rupture into the right ventricular outflow tract. Supracristal ventricular septal defects are seen in half the cases of aneurysms of the right coronary sinus. Patients may present with slow rupture secondary to bacterial endocarditis or acutely with precordial tearing and congestive heart failure (CHF). Blood cultures should be drawn at the time of presentation because of the high incidence of endocarditis. With the development of a large shunt, CHF can progress rapidly. All defects should be repaired because of the natural history of this disease.

470. The answer is C. *(pp 1832–1833)*   It is estimated that congenital heart disease accounts for about 1 percent of natural deaths. There is a significant incidence of abortion and about a 10 to 15 percent incidence of offspring with congenital heart disease in mothers with congenital heart disease. There is a 30 to 40 percent increase in blood volume, a drop in systemic vascular resistance, and a 40 percent increase in cardiac output. Patients with valvular regurgitation or left-to-right shunts tolerate pregnancy well, so long as pulmonary artery pressures are normal. Patients with cyanosis have difficulty with pregnancy and a high rate of spontaneous abortion. An elevated pulmonary vascular resistance is a contraindication to pregnancy. Patients with Marfan's syndrome and aortic root dilatation are at increased risk as are mothers with significant valvular stenosis.

471. The answer is B. *(pp 1845–1849)*   Patients with coarctation of the aorta have a high recoarctation rate if it is repaired before age 18 months but a higher incidence of persistent hypertension if it is repaired after age 10. Patients with transposition of the great arteries who undergo atrial redirection of blood via the Senning or Mustard techniques still have the right ventricle pumping against systemic pressures and are at risk of congestive failure. Patients with congenitally corrected transposition frequently have ventricular septal defects and pulmonic stenosis. There is a tendency to develop AV conduction problems including complete heart block. Patients with isolated ventricular inversion are at risk for systemic AV valve incompetence and congestive failure. Ebstein's anomaly may be present on the systemic tricuspid AV valve. Patients with Ebstein's anomaly frequently develop cyanosis with right-to-left shunting at the atrial level. There is a high frequency of ventricular preexcitation with symptomatic arrhythmias in 25 to 30 percent of adults, sometimes resulting in sudden death. Patients with tetralogy of Fallot can develop stroke and cerebral abscess as a result of persistent cyanosis and polycythemia. Myocardial fibrosis can result in congestive heart failure and arrhythmic death.

472. The answer is B. *(pp 1834–1835)*   Patients with volume overload, valvular regurgitation, and left-to-right shunts have good exercise tolerance. Patients with pressure overload, valve stenosis, and right-to-left shunts do not tolerate exercise well. Exercise can be fatal in patients with minimal pulmonary vascular resistance of any etiology. All moderate and strenuous exercise is restricted in patients with moderate-to-severe hypertrophic myopathy and patients with Marfan's syndrome and an aortic root larger than 5 cm in diameter.

473. The answer is B (1, 3). *(pp 1715–1716)*   Of the seven septa that allow for partitioning of the normal heart, three form passively: the septum secundum of the atrial septum, the muscular portion of the ventricular septum, and the aorticopulmonary septum. Passive formation occurs when an area of tissue forms a septum because of the rapid, active growth of contiguous tissue. The septum of the atrioventricular (AV) canal, the conal septum, and the truncal septum form actively. The atrial septum begins as a passively formed septum; however, active growth from the endocardial cushions completes the septum.

474. The answer is E (all). *(pp 1715–1719)* All ventricular septal defects are related to an abnormality in completion or misalignment of a septum. Tetralogy of Fallot arises from the anterior displacement of the conal septum, leading to unequal partitioning of the conus at the expense of the right ventricular infundibulum, resulting in right ventricular outflow tract obstruction and failure to close the interventricular foramen. Aorticopulmonary septal defect arises from a failure of fusion between the truncal septum and the aorticopulmonary septum. Double-outlet right ventricle arises from a rightward shift of the atrioventricular (AV) canal, resulting in both AV valves communicating directly with a large right ventricle, which communicates via a basilar ventricular septal defect with the small left ventricle. Persistent AV canal arises from a failure of fusion of superior and inferior endocardial cushions.

475. The answer is C (2, 4). *(pp 1721–1723, Table 95-1)* The aorta and pulmonary roots arise from the truncus arteriosus. The aortic sac gives rise to the ascending aorta, innominate artery, and aortic arch up to the left common carotid. The first and second arches become, respectively, the maxillary and stapedial arteries. The third arches become the common carotids and the proximal segment of the internal carotid arteries. The fourth right arch becomes the proximal segment of the right subclavian, whereas the aortic arch segment between the left common carotid and left subclavian are derived from the fourth left aortic arch. The fifth arotic arch is poorly developed and has no known derivatives.

476. The answer is D (4). *(pp 1742–1743)* Only the congenital heart disease associated with the Ellis-van Creveld syndrome is transmitted by autosomal recessive transmission. Familial atrial septal defect, the Holt-Oram syndrome and supravalvular aortic stenosis are associated with an autosomal dominant mode of inheritance.

477. The answer is B (1, 3). *(pp 1743–1746)* Marfan's syndrome has been mapped to the long arm of chromosome 15 and is transmitted by autosomal dominant transmission. Common cardiac abnormalities include aortic dilatation, leading to aortic dissection or aortic insufficiency, and mitral valve prolapse, leading to mitral regurgitation. Pseudoxanthoma elasticum is a genetic disorder of elastic tissue that involves the skin, eyes, and cardiovascular system. Although endocardial fibroelastosis and mitral valve prolapse may occur, myocardial infarction and ischemia are the major causes of morbidity and mortality. Ehlers-Danlos syndrome is an autosomal dominant disease characterized by looseness of the joints. The abnormality of the heart involves type III collagen and results in aortic rupture and sudden death. Two varieties of autosomal recessive cutis laxa exist. Although pulmonary artery stenosis occurs, most patients die from right-sided heart failure due to pulmonary complications.

478. The answer is E (all). *(pp 1738–1740)* Cardiomyopathy is a feature of virtually all peripheral muscular dystrophies although the age and extent of abnormalities is quite variable. Duchenne muscular dystrophy is the most common type of X-linked muscular dystrophy and is characterized by pseudohypertrophy of the calves, elevated serum creatine kinase, and the late onset of heart failure. The short arm of the X chromosome is the site of the Duchenne muscular dystrophy gene. Patients with Emery-Dreifuss muscular dystrophy develop dilated cardiomyopathy, atrial paralysis, and slow ventricular response rates with atrioventricular (AV) block. Patients with myotonic dystrophy may die of heart failure but are more likely to have AV and bundle branch conduction delays. The gene for myotonic dystrophy is located on chromosome 19. Friedreich's ataxia is the most common of the hereditary ataxias and has been localized to chromosome 9. Hypertrophic cardiomyopathy has been associated with Friedreich's ataxia.

479. The answer is E (all). *(pp 1750–1753)* Hurler's syndrome is a severe form of mucopolysaccharide deposition disease characterized by mental retardation and multiple muscular skeletal deformities. Cardiac manifestations include extensive cardiac involvement culminating in a brief lifespan with congestive heart failure (CHF) and valvular abnormalities. Scheie's syndrome is a milder form of this disorder in which intelligence is normal and though aortic insufficiency is common, the lifespan is preserved. Fabry's disease is a sex-linked recessive disorder in which α-galactosidase deficiency leads to glycolipid deposition in the blood vessels, heart muscle, and viscera. Cardiac manifestations include hypertrophic cardiomyopathy, mitral valve disease, and myocardial infarction. Osteogenesis imperfecta is one of many hereditable connective tissue disorders associated with aortic dilatation and the billowing mitral valve syndrome. Constrictive pericarditis and severe pulmonary hypertension are associated with the glucocerebrosidase deficiency of Gaucher's disease.

480. The answer is E (all). *(pp 1727–1729)* Down's syndrome is due to either an extra chromosome 21 or the presence of only the distal one-half of chromosome 21, band q 22. Approximately 40 to 50 percent of Down's syndrome patients have congenital heart disease, most commonly the endocardial cushion defect or atrioventricular (AV) canal defect. Edward's syndrome is the second most common trisomy. Ninety percent of patients with trisomy 18 have congenital heart disease. Potential combinations of cardiac defects include ventricular septal defect, atrial septal defect, patent ductus arteriosus, pulmonic stenosis, tetralogy of Fallot, bicuspid aortic valve, transposition of the great arteries, and coarctation of the aorta. Turner's syndrome is due to meiotic disjunction, resulting in a single X chromosome. Congenital heart disease occurs in 20 to 50 percent of patients, most commonly coarctation of the aorta, bicuspid aortic valve, aortic stenosis, dilated aorta, and hypoplastic left heart syndrome. The DiGeorge syndrome can be associated with monosomy for the proximal portion of the long arm of chromosome 22 in 5 to 10 percent of cases. In addition to thymic aplasia, mental retardation, and lung abnormalities, there is a frequent association with truncus arteriosus, interrupted aortic arch, and tetralogy of Fallot.

481. The answer is C (2, 4). *(pp 1736–1741)* Familial hypertrophic cardiomyopathy is associated with autosomal dominant inheritance; the putative gene is the beta-myocin heavy chain (β-MHC) gene on chromosome 14. The expression is variable with some members having typical obstructive findings and others only echocardiographic findings. Cardiac involvement is usual in many families with systemic amyloidosis, which is characterized by an autosomal dominant transmission. Patients may present with congestive heart failure (CHF), chest pain, or arrhythmias. The myopathies, such as phytanic acid storage disease (Refsum's disease) and type II glycogen storage disease (Pompe's disease), are transmitted as autosomal recessive traits.

482. The answer is C (2, 4). *(pp 1802–1803)* In Ebstein's anomaly, the anterior leaflet of the tricuspid valve is normally positioned, whereas the posterior and septal leaflets are displaced downward. Thus, the right ventricle is actually smaller than normal, comprised of the apical and outflow tract portions. The proximal part of the right ventricle is contiguous with the right atrium. There is also functional obstruction to the right ventricle as the tricuspid valve is usually regurgitant. An intra-atrial communication (usually a patent foramen ovale) is almost universally present. Although pulmonary pressures are normal, the dominant shunt is right-to-left due to resistance to antegrade flow to the right ventricle; thus, patients are often cyanotic. The electrocardiogram (ECG) reveals giant peaked P waves and a right ventricular conduction delay or right bundle branch block (RBBB). Approximately 10 percent of patients have the Wolff-Parkinson-White syndrome. Left ventricular hypertrophy is not part of the syndrome. The echocardiogram reveals a large tricuspid valve with delayed closure compared to the mitral valve. Cardiac catheterization reveals right-to-left shunting at the atrial level, a prominent V or R wave due to tricuspid regurgitation, and an "atrialized" area of the right ventricle.

483. The answer is A (1, 2, 3). *(pp 1813–1815)* In corrected transposition, the great vessels are transposed to the L position such that the pulmonary arteries arise from the left-sided morphologic right ventricle. In addition to ventricular inversion, there is atrioventricular (AV) valve inversion. In most cases (80 percent) of corrected transposition, a ventricular septal defect is present. In 70 percent of cases, pulmonary atresia or stenosis with or without an intact ventricular septum is present. In 50 percent of cases, the inverted left-sided tricuspid valve shows an Ebstein-like abnormality. An abnormality of the right-sided mitral valve has not been reported.

484. The answer is E (all). *(pp 1800–1802)* Endocarditis prophylaxis is of obvious importance in children with a right-to-left shunt. Fever should be treated aggressively to prevent dehydration, which could lead to thrombotic complications. Hypoxic spells are treated by placing the child in the knee-chest position and administering oxygen, morphine sulfate, and, if the spell is severe, intravenous propranolol. Oral propranolol may prevent episodes. Erythropheresis is indicated if the hematocrit exceeds 70 to 75 percent to prevent thromboses. Prostaglandin infusion may be necessary in the infant with severe tetralogy of Fallot to maintain ductal patency and provide some pulmonary flow until an operation can be performed.

485. The answer is E (all). *(pp 1813–1815)* A ventricular septal defect is present in about 80 percent of cases of corrected transposition of the great arteries. In 70 percent of cases, pulmonary atresia or stenosis is seen. Atrioventricular (AV) block develops in 20 percent of cases if patients are followed over a long time period (20 years). About 10 percent of cases of congenital complete heart block have corrected transposition. The tricuspid valve is left-sided with ventricular inversion. An Ebstein-like malformation can lead to valvular regurgitation and, less likely, stenosis.

486. The answer is E (all). *(pp 1765–1766)* Cyanosis may occur in infancy as a result of pulmonary, central nervous system (CNS), or metabolic disease or methemoglobinemia. Children with respiratory distress syndrome appear dyspneic with grunting respirations and tachypnea. The chest roentgenogram reveals reticulonodular infiltrates and air bronchograms. Children with cyanosis due to CNS disease often exhibit periodic breathing and vasomotor instability. The blood of children with methemoglobinemia when exposed to air turns brown rather than bright red. In cyanotic heart disease, hypoxia leads to secondary polycythemia. Most complications of cyanosis result from polycythemia or paradoxical embolism. With polycythemia, hyperuricemia with secondary gout can occur. With dehydration or febrile states, cerebrovascular accidents are more frequent. Thrombosis, embolism, and hemorrhage can all cause cerebrovascular accidents. Brain abscesses that result from paradoxical embolism are rare before age 2.

487. The answer is E (all). *(pp 1767–1768)* Despite excellent surgical results, some sequelae are unavoidable following repair of congenital heart disease. Pulmonary valve regurgitation and late complete heart block are not unexpected sequelae of repair of tetralogy of Fallot. Serious ventricular dysrhythmias resulting in sudden death can also occur as a late sequela of tetralogy repair. Mild valvular regurgitation can follow repair of atrioventricular (AV) or aortic valves. Small (hemodynamically insignificant) left-to-right shunts may be present following repair of atrial, ventricular, or AV canal defects. Repair of coarctation of the aorta may be followed by hypertension either idiopathically or as the conduit narrows once again.

488. The answer is B (1, 3). *(pp 1795–1796)* Abnormalities of the aortic arch range from asymptomatic variants, such as a common origin of the innominate and left common carotid, to complex vascular rings compromising cardiac and respiratory status. A right aortic arch occurs in 0.1 to 0.14 percent of the population. When mirror-image branching occurs, there is a 98 percent incidence of congenital heart disease, mostly tetralogy of Fallot. Most patients with double aortic arch (persistence of two aortic arches) have respiratory symptoms, whereas only 20 percent have congenital heart disease, especially ventricular septal defect and tetralogy of Fallot. Pulmonary artery sling is characterized by a left pulmonary artery arising from the distal right pulmonary artery arching over the right main stem branches and behind the trachea. There is a 60 to 80 percent incidence of cardiovascular abnormalities, including tetralogy of Fallot, and a 50 percent incidence of tracheobronchial abnormalities, including tracheomalacia, tracheal stenosis, and respiratory obstruction. Patients with a cervical aortic arch have an aortic arch that lies at a more cephalad level than normal. A pulsating mass in the supraclavicular area is noted; however, no other significant pathological conditions occur.

489. The answer is B (1, 3). *(pp 1775–1776)* Surgical closure of secundum atrial septal defect is recommended for patients with a pulmonary/systemic blood flow ratio $(\dot{Q}_p/\dot{Q}_s)$ of 1.5 to 1 in the absence of significant left-sided heart disease. Surgery would be recommended for a $(\dot{Q}_p/\dot{Q}_s)$ of greater than 1.5 to 1 in the presence of pulmonary hypertension as long as the systemic arterial oxygen saturation is greater than 92 percent and the total pulmonary resistance is less than 15 Wood units/m². Closure is advised prior to pregnancy or use of contraceptives since pulmonary vascular resistance may accelerate in these settings. Genetic counseling is warranted since the risk of the patient described in the question of having an affected child is about 10 percent. The risk of two unaffected parents having a second child with secundum atrial septal defect is also increased (2.5 percent).

490. The answer is B (1, 3). *(pp 1782–1784)* There is a higher incidence of patent ductus arteriosus in girls, in children with birth asphyxia or respiratory distress syndrome, and in children with maternal exposure to rubella in the first trimester. Commonly associated defects include coarctation of the aorta and ventricular septal defect. The magnitude of the shunt is determined both by the cross-sectional area and the length of the ductus. If the shunt is large, pulmonary vascular resistance can increase dramatically. With reversal of blood flow through the patent ductus, deoxygenated blood is preferentially distributed to the legs. Arterial oxygen saturation is higher in the arms, especially the right arm.

491. The answer is A (1, 2, 3). *(pp 1783–1784)* Current indications for closure of a patent ductus arteriosus include uncontrollable congestive heart failure (CHF) in a neonate, growth retardation, and signs of a significant ductus in an infant. Persistence of a patent ductus after the age of 6 months is an indication for surgery due to the threat of infection of the ductus. Complications of infections can include septic pulmonary emboli, compression of the laryngeal nerve, and rupture of the ductus. The risk of endocarditis increases with age, whereas the operative mortality in skilled hands approaches zero. The high resistance in a pulmonary artery indicates irreversible pulmonary hypertension, and thus, the patient is inoperable.

492. The answer is B (1, 3). *(pp 1790–1792)* A measured pulse pressure of less than 20 mmHg suggests severe aortic stenosis. A systolic thrill along the right upper sternal border is usually present, in very young patients with significant aortic stenosis, whereas the absence of a thrill suggests a systolic gradient of less than 30 mmHg. Paradoxical splitting (a rare finding) is due to delayed aortic closure associated with severe valvular obstruction or left ventricular dysfunction. Left ventricular hypertrophy by voltage alone does not separate mild-to-moderate from severe obstruction. Absence of R waves in V_1 and V_2, loss of Q waves in V_6, and abnormal ST-segment and T-wave changes anterolaterally are more frequently seen in patients with severe valvular aortic stenosis as compared to those with mild aortic stenosis. However, severe stenosis can be present in the absence of any or all of these electrocardiographic (ECG) findings.

493. The answer is D (4). *(pp 1793–1794)* Evidence of outflow obstruction is common to valvular, subvalvular, and supravalvular stenoses. An ejection click at the apex is the hallmark of valvular aortic stenosis and is not heard in patients with subvalvular aortic stenosis. Half of all patients with discrete subvalvular aortic stenosis have an early diastolic murmur associated with aortic regurgitation due to nonsupport of the aortic leaflets. Supravalvular aortic stenosis is associated with the characteristic facies and mental retardation in the Williams syndrome. Hypercalcemia is not usually a part of this syndrome if recognized beyond infancy. Poststenotic dilatation of the aorta is characteristic of valvular aortic stenosis. Left ventricular hypertrophy is common to all forms of outflow obstruction.

494. The answer is A (1, 2, 3). *(pp 1773–1774)* In an atrial septal defect, the mean left atrial pressure is usually less than 3 mmHg higher than the right atrial pressure. The larger the interatrial defect, the less the resistance to flow, and, thus, the smaller the pressure difference between the atrium. Thus, resistance to flow determines the direction and magnitude of shunt flow. Atrial distensibility, atrial ventricular valve distensibility, and ventricular compliance all contribute to the determination of shunt flow.

495. The answer is E (all). *(pp 1771–1772)* Criteria for closure of ventricular septal defect include: (1) schoolchildren with a $\dot{Q}_p/\dot{Q}_s$ greater than 1.8 to 1 or a $\dot{Q}_p/\dot{Q}_s$ greater than 1.4 to 1 if cardiomegaly or other symptoms are present and (2) adults with a $\dot{Q}_p/\dot{Q}_s$ greater than 1.4 to 1 in the absence of severe pulmonary hypertension. Criteria for closure in the presence of pulmonary hypertension include children older than age two with pulmonary artery pressure greater than half systolic, a mean pulmonary artery pressure above 20 mmHg, or a pulmonary/systemic vascular resistance of greater than 0.2 to 1 but less than 0.7 to 1 with a $\dot{Q}_p/\dot{Q}_s$ ratio of more than 1.5 to 1. Surgery becomes too great a risk in children if their pulmonary vascular resistance is greater than 11 Wood units/m^2 or in an adult with a pulmonary vascular resistance greater than 800 dynes·sec·cm^{-5}.

496. The answer is A (1, 2, 3). *(pp 1768–1773)* Patients with small ventricular septal defects (less than 0.5 cm^2/m^2) have small left-to-right shunts often undetectable by pressure or oximetric measurements. Since they are not hemodynamically impaired, only infective endocarditis is a concern. Patients with moderate defects (0.5 to 1.0 cm^2/m^2) have significant left-to-right shunts but are unlikely to develop pulmonary vascular disease since the defect is restricted. The right ventricular pressure is generally less than 80 percent of the left ventricular pressure. Patients with large defects (greater than 1.0 cm^2/m^2) have equal systolic pressures in both ventricles and in both great vessels if no other outflow obstruction is present. The development of pulmonary vascular disease is of greatest risk in this group.

497. The answer is A (1, 2, 3). *(pp 1767–1768)* Despite surgical intervention for palliation or correction of congenital heart disease, long-term sequelae may still occur, such as patients with persistent hypertension or restenosis after coarctation repair or patients with valvular regurgitation after repair of aortic or pulmonary stenosis. Patients with complex cyanotic heart disease may have long-term sequelae of persistent cyanosis, dysrhythmias, and postoperative atrioventricular (AV) block. Interatrial repair for transposition (Mustard) and congenitally corrected transposition both result in an anatomic right ventricle that pumps against systemic pressures, leaving it vulnerable to serious ventricular dysfunction and venous obstruction. The left ventricle in corrected tricuspid atresia is overburdened as well. Patients with corrected tetralogy of Fallot are at risk for late complete heart block and arrhythmias.

498. The answer is B (1, 3). *(p 1766)* Pulmonary arterial hypertension can result from either severe obstruction to blood flow through the left side of the heart or as a result of direct transmission of systemic arterial pressure to the right ventricle or pulmonary arteries via a large left-to-right shunt. Increased pulmonary artery pressure stimulates persistence of the thick medial layer present in the smaller arteries of the newborn infant. The smooth muscle then extends into the small and more peripheral arteries. Patients with large intracardiac or extracardiac shunts have increased pulmonary flow unless there is concomitant outflow tract obstruction to the pulmonary arteries. Patients with tetralogy of Fallot or Ebstein's anomaly have normal pulmonary artery pressures and diminished pulmonary blood flow.

499. The answers are: A-N, B-N, C-N, D-Y, E-Y. *(pp 1746–1750)* Lipoproteins are composed of a central core of cholesterol or triglycerides surrounded by a layer of phospholipid and cholesterol in which apolipoproteins are imbedded. Both chylomicrons and very low-density lipoprotein (VLDL) contain apolipoprotein B (apo B), which is needed to form a hydrophobic core. High-density lipoprotein (HDL) is synthesized predominantly in the liver and small intestine. Hepatic HDL contains apolipoprotein E (apo E), and small intestine HDL contains apolipoprotein A (apo A). Apolipoproteins were originally thought to serve a structural role in the formation and stabilization of lipoprotein particles, but they are now felt to have a functional role in the regulation of enzymes or receptor interaction in peripheral tissues designed to catabolize lipoproteins. Lipoprotein[a] (Lp[a]) is a variant of low-density lipoprotein (LDL) which contains apo (a) bound to apolipoprotein B-100 (apo B-100). High levels of Lp(a) are associated with an increased incidence of atherosclerosis, especially if the LDL level is elevated. Apo (a) is related to plasminogen, but how exactly the lipoproteins relate to the clotting mechanism is uncertain.

500. The answers are: A-Y, B-Y, C-N, D-Y, E-N.   *(pp 1799–1802)*   The 8-year-old boy who presented with cyanotic heart disease has physical findings compatible with tetralogy of Fallot. The electrocardiogram (ECG) reveals right ventricular hypertrophy, and the chest roentgenogram reveals the configuration of a *couer en sabot* with diminished pulmonary blood flow. Congestive heart failure (CHF) is unusual unless either anemia or endocarditis is present. The outflow tract is dynamic, and drugs that increase contractility or decrease the volume cause an increase in right ventricular outflow obstruction. Overriding of the aorta is characterized echocardiographically by anterior displacement of the anterior aortic wall with loss of continuity with the interventricular septum. However, the anterior mitral valve leaflet and the posterior aortic wall remain continuous even if only a band of fibrous tissue is present. The ventricular septal defect is large; therefore, the right and left ventricular systolic pressures are equal. Outflow obstruction is always present by definition to such a degree that pulmonary hypertension is not present. Cardiac catheterization may be useful in corroborating the diagnosis and excluding other intracardiac defects. Aortography is essential prior to surgical repair to identify the coronary anatomy because of the associated high incidence of coronary anomalies.

XII. Pulmonary Hypertension and Pulmonary Heart Disease

DIRECTIONS: Each question below contains five suggested responses. Select the **one best** response to each question.

501. All the following statements about the causes of pulmonary hypertension are true EXCEPT

(A) left ventricular failure is the most common cause of pulmonary hypertension

(B) right ventricular failure occurring secondary to left ventricular failure is usually secondary to very high pulmonary artery pressures

(C) the major cause of pulmonary hypertension in congenital heart disease is an increase in blood flow combined with an increase in resistance to blood flow

(D) pregnant patients with congenital heart disease and pulmonary hypertension are at increased risk of sudden death during delivery and in the postpartum period

(E) vasodilators have no role in the treatment of pulmonary hypertension associated with interstitial pulmonary fibrosis

502. The most common syndrome associated with thromboembolic pulmonary hypertension in the United States is

(A) schistosomiasis

(B) occlusion of intermediate pulmonary arteries by emboli

(C) tumor emboli from extrapulmonary sites

(D) occlusion of small muscular arteries and arterioles by organized thrombi

(E) acute massive proximal pulmonary thromboembolism

503. The clinical picture of patients with primary pulmonary hypertension includes all the following physical findings EXCEPT

(A) prominent A wave in the jugular venous pulse

(B) parasternal heave

(C) soft widely split second heart sound (S_2)

(D) fourth heart sound (S_4) emanating from the right ventricle

(E) jugular venous distention and third heart sound (S_3) gallop, which increases with inspiration

504. All the following statements about pulmonary embolism are correct EXCEPT

(A) hemoptysis occurs in very few patients with pulmonary infarction

(B) massive pulmonary embolism will usually cause right ventricular systolic pressures of greater than 65 mmHg

(C) a normal P_{O_2} does not preclude the diagnosis of pulmonary embolism

(D) both the ECG and chest x-ray may be normal in pulmonary embolism

(E) acute cor pulmonale may occur with pulmonary embolism when over 60 percent of the pulmonary circulation is obstructed

505. Which of the following statements regarding therapy of pulmonary embolism is true?

(A) Heparin-associated thrombocytopenia usually occurs within 24 h of onset of heparin therapy

(B) A 62-year-old man being treated for a pulmonary embolus has a recurrent pulmonary embolus 2 weeks after the initial event. His prothrombin time is 14 s with a control of 11.9 s and he has been taking Coumadin. Appropriate therapy is venous interruption

(C) Embolic obstruction of a pulmonary artery resolves by 10 to 20 percent during the first 24 h after acute pulmonary embolism

(D) Thrombolytic therapy reduces the mortality of patients with pulmonary embolism when compared with heparin therapy alone

(E) The preferred therapy of fat embolism is heparin infusion

506. All the following statements regarding signs and symptoms of cor pulmonale are true EXCEPT

(A) the most sensitive sign of pulmonary hypertension associated with cor pulmonale is an accentuated pulmonic component of the second heart sound (S_2)

(B) patients with cor pulmonale may demonstrate S waves deeper than R waves in V_5 and V_6 rather than classic findings of right ventricular hypertrophy

(C) the most sensitive indicator of pulmonary hypertension on the chest roentgenogram is right ventricular enlargement

(D) morning headaches, loud snoring, daytime somnolence, personality disturbances, and sleep deprivation may indicate a disorder associated with the development of cor pulmonale

(E) cor pulmonale may be associated with chest pain in the absence of coronary disease

DIRECTIONS: Each question below contains five suggested responses. For **each** of the **five** responses listed with every question you are to respond either YES (Y) or NO (N). In a given item **all, some, or none of the alternatives may be correct.**

507. True statements regarding primary pulmonary hypertension include which of the following?

(A) Pulmonary hypertension is more common in young men than women

(B) Survival of patients can be predicted on the basis of the New York Heart Association functional classification

(C) High cardiac output is typically found

(D) Sudden death is uncommon in patients with primary pulmonary hypertension

(E) Chest pain, breathlessness, and syncope on effort are common symptoms of primary pulmonary hypertension

508. True statements regarding pulmonary vascular hemodynamics include which of the following?

(A) Pulmonary artery pressure and resistance depend on atmospheric pressure

(B) The pulmonary vascular bed provides significant resistance to flow and a significant drop in pressure from the right ventricle to the left atrium

(C) In the absence of intrinsic lung disease, the pulmonary capillary wedge pressure can be substituted for the left atrial pressure

(D) Any condition that causes a considerable increase in cardiac output causes a considerable increase in pulmonary artery pressure in the normal person

(E) Hypoxia and acidosis can lead to vasoconstriction of the pulmonary vascular tree and elevated pulmonary artery pressures

509. Correct statements regarding the therapy of primary pulmonary hypertension include which of the following?

(A) Oral anticoagulants have been shown in a nonrandomized clinical trial to improve long-term survival

(B) Single-lung transplantation has evolved as the operation of choice for end-stage primary pulmonary hypertension

(C) Mild decreases in pulmonary vascular resistance associated with vasodilator agents have been shown to improve survival in patients with pulmonary hypertension

(D) Most patients with primary pulmonary hypertension respond to pulmonary vasodilator therapy

(E) Prostacyclin (PGI_2), a potent pulmonary vasodilator, can be used in responsive patients until lung or heart-lung transplantation

510. True statements regarding thromboembolic disease include which of the following?

(A) If a ventilation-perfusion lung scan is nonspecific and impedance pletnysmography is positive, pulmonary angiography should be performed

(B) In patients with acute cor pulmonale due to massive pulmonary embolism, selective or subselective injections should be into areas shown to have perfusion defects by lung scan

(C) Thrombophlebitis migrans is frequently associated with occult cancer

(D) The most common intracardial defect associated with paradoxical embolism is an atrial septal defect

(E) Paradoxical pulmonary embolism is usually associated with massive pulmonary embolism

511. True statements regarding deep venous thrombosis and pulmonary embolism include

- (A) the mortality of untreated pulmonary embolism is about 20 to 30 percent
- (B) in men undergoing urologic procedures, 5000 units subcutaneous heparin every 12 h offers adequate protection from deep venous thrombosis
- (C) impedence plethysmography is a relatively insensitive method of detecting deep venous thrombosis
- (D) pulmonary embolism occurs in about 50 percent of patients with proximal deep venous thrombosis (above the knee)
- (E) pregnancy, oral contraceptives, and obesity all predispose patients to deep venous thrombosis

512. True statements regarding cor pulmonale include which of the following?

- (A) In chronic obstructive pulmonary disease (COPD), pulmonary artery pressure is related to the level of hypoxemia
- (B) Home oxygen therapy has been shown to be effective in reducing elevated pulmonary pressures in patients with cor pulmonale
- (C) Digoxin has been demonstrated to improve left ventricular function in cor pulmonale
- (D) In patients with cor pulmonale, heart rate can be used as a measure of the level of digitalization
- (E) Right ventricular systolic function has been shown to improve following successful lung transplantation

XII. Pulmonary Hypertension and Pulmonary Heart Disease

Answers

501. The answer is B. *(pp 1860–1866)* The most common cause of pulmonary hypertension is left ventricular failure, either secondary to myocardial disorders or lesions of the aortic and mitral valves. These lesions lead to an increase in pulmonary venous pressure that evokes an increase in pulmonary artery pressure. Although left ventricular failure is the most common cause of right ventricular failure, the etiology is usually attributed to failure of the muscle in the shared ventricular septum and not to the elevated pulmonary artery pressures that accommodate left ventricular failure. Congenital defects of the heart are commonly associated with pulmonary hypertension, the underlying causes of which are an increase in blood flow, an increase in resistance to blood flow, or both. Pregnant women with pulmonary hypertension are at high risk for sudden death during delivery and in the postpartum period. Interstitial fibrosis from any number of diseases, including radiation, asbestosis, or sarcoidosis, generally develops at the end of the illness when hypoxia is present and the patient develops hypercapnia. Right ventricular enlargement and failure are common sequelae. Oxygen can decrease the hypoxic pulmonary pressure response; however, vasodilators such as calcium blockers and hydralazine do not improve the pulmonary hypertension associated with interstitial fibrosis. The advent of single-lung transplantation has improved the overall therapeutic outlook for patients with widespread interstitial fibrosis.

502. The answer is B. *(pp 1862–1863)* In the United States, pulmonary thromboembolic disease is the third most common cause of occlusive pulmonary vascular disease. Infectious etiologies, such as schistosomiasis and filariasis, are common in other parts of the world but not in the United States. The most common syndrome associated with thromboembolic pulmonary hypertension is due to repeated blood clots that progressively amputate more and more of the pulmonary arterial tree. These clots almost invariably arise from the vessels in the upper legs and thighs. Ventilation perfusion scans and pulmonary arteriography demonstrate the extent of pulmonary vascular occlusion. Treatment with oral anticoagulants is usually indicated. Massive acute pulmonary embolism can cause severe hemodynamic abnormalities. In survivors, the large clots can become incorporated into the walls of the major pulmonary arteries, leading to pulmonary hypertension. It is important to recognize proximal major pulmonary thromboembolism as a cause of pulmonary hypertension, because relieving the pulmonary hypertension by surgical intervention usually leads to hemodynamic improvement. Organized thrombi in the minute vessels of the lungs can lead to occlusion of small muscular arteries and arterioles. Thrombi in these small arteries are common postmortem findings in pulmonary hypertensive patients who develop right-sided heart failure. This syndrome is somewhat rare and generally misdiagnosed as "primary pulmonary hypertension."

503. The answer is C. *(pp 1868–1869)* Physical examination of patients with primary pulmonary hypertension reveal all of the findings of increased pressure in the right ventricle. The right ventricular hypertrophy causes a heave along the left sternal border. Occasionally a distinct systolic impulse is palpable over the region of the main pulmonary artery. A prominent A wave in the venous pulsation is usually present. The second heart sound (S_2) is usually quite loud and narrowly split. An ejection click is frequently heard in the pulmonic area. As the right ventricle hypertrophies, a fourth heart sound (S_4) can be heard along the left sternal border. Once the right ventricle begins to fail, marked jugular venous distention and a third heart sound (S_3) can be heard. Inspiration intensifies this gallop, distinguishing it from an S_3 arising from the left ventricle.

504. The answer is B. *(pp 1878–1881)* Pulmonary infarction occurs in more than 50 percent of patients in whom pulmonary embolism is diagnosed. Pulmonary hemorrhage in this situation is caused by bronchial arterial collateral flow into ischemic lung parenchyma. This may cause a pulmonary infiltrate with a small pleural effusion visible on chest x-ray, but only a small number of these patients in fact experience hemoptysis. The pleural effusion may or may not be bloody. Acute cor pulmonale may be the presenting feature of pulmonary embolism when more than 60 percent of the pulmonary arterial tree is occluded. In this setting, physical examination will reveal distended neck veins, a parasternal heave, and a right-sided S_3 gallop. The right ventricle responds to this massive obstruction by attempting to maintain cardiac output through elevation of right ventricular systolic pressure. However, the right ventricle can acutely elevate its systolic pressure to only 50 to 60 mmHg. Increases in pressure beyond this lead to right ventricular dilatation and increasing right ventricular filling pressures, thereby decreasing right ventricular stroke volume and cardiac output. Patients presenting with dyspnea due to acute pulmonary embolism are generally hypoxic. However, if submassive pulmonary embolism has occurred in a patient without underlying pulmonary disease, the P_{O_2} may be normal. Since tachypnea is nearly always present with pulmonary embolism, the ECG may demonstrate any of the following: sinus tachycardia, $S_1Q_3T_3$ pattern, incomplete right bundle branch block, or nonspecific ST and T wave changes. It may, however, remain normal. Likewise, while the chest x-ray may demonstrate a pulmonary infiltrate, pleural effusion, or an elevated hemidiaphragm, it may also be perfectly normal.

505. The answer is C. *(pp 1878–1888)* Heparin can cause an immunologically mediated thrombocytopenia in about 5 to 22 percent of patients receiving intravenous heparin. Onset of this usually occurs 6 to 12 days after initiation of therapy. This heparin-associated thrombocytopenia may be associated with life-threatening arterial thrombosis. The patient presented in choice B is not adequately anticoagulated and should not be considered for vena caval interruption but should have his anticoagulation adjusted. The indications for venous interruption are (1) recurrent emboli on adequate anticoagulation, (2) contraindication of anticoagulants, (3) persistent disease state predisposing to emboli, (4) septic embolization from below the heart, and (5) certain patients with massive emboli in whom a further embolus would be fatal. Resolution of pulmonary embolus occurs by fibrinolysis and mechanical changes in the location of clots within the vascular bed. Embolic obstruction resolves by about 10 to 20 percent in the first 24 h and can be completely resolved as soon as 14 days after the acute event. Thrombolytic therapy is potentially most useful in a small group of patients with documented massive pulmonary embolism with severe hemodynamic compromise. Except for this situation, thrombolytic therapy has not reduced the mortality in pulmonary embolism when compared with heparin therapy alone. Fat embolization occurs usually after fractures of long bones and consists of the development of acute respiratory distress syndrome with altered levels of consciousness, delirium, seizures, coma, and development of petechiae. The most important therapy is maintenance of oxygenation. Heparin is not beneficial and may even be detrimental in that the lipase activity might increase the toxic fatty acids in the lungs.

506. The answer is C. *(pp 1895–1904)* The early signs of cor pulmonale are those associated with long-standing pulmonary hypertension. The most sensitive sign for pulmonary hypertension is an accentuated pulmonary component of the second heart sound (S_2). The pulmonic component of S_2 may be palpable in some patients, and a parasternal lift of the right ventricle may be noted. Classical changes of right ventricle hypertrophy may be absent on the electrocardiogram (ECG), but S waves larger than R waves in V_5 and V_6 may be noted with right axis deviation, qR in aVR, and P pulmonale. On chest roentgenogram, the most sensitive indicator of pulmonary hypertension is enlargement of the dimensions of the right pulmonary artery. Right ventricular enlargement may be difficult to detect on the chest roentgenogram, particularly when the cardiac silhouette is vertical from hyperexpanded lung fields. Patients with sleep apnea, or pick-wickian syndrome, develop alveolar hypoventilation and hypoxia that may lead to pulmonary hypertension and cor pulmonale. Leg edema, atypical chest pain, dyspnea on exertion, morning headaches, daytime somnolence, loud snoring, periodic apnea during sleep, and personality disturbances are characteristic symptoms of this disorder.

507. The answers are: A-N, B-Y, C-N, D-N, E-Y. *(pp 1866–1872; D'Alonzo, Ann Intern Med 115:343–349, 1991)* Primary pulmonary hypertension is generally more common in women between the ages of 10 and 40. Prior to puberty, no sex difference is discernible. In general, the median survival of patients with primary pulmonary hypertension can be predicted on the New York Heart Association functional classification. Patients with class IV heart failure have a median survival of about 6 months. The hemodynamic hallmarks of primary pulmonary hypertension include an elevated pulmonary artery pressure, a normal or low cardiac output, and a normal left atrial or pulmonary wedge pressure. Therefore, the calculated pulmonary vascular resistance is high. During exercise as cardiac output increases, pulmonary artery pressures increase further, and the incremental increase in pulmonary artery pressure is much more striking than in the normal population. Sudden cardiac death is not uncommon in patients with severe pulmonary hypertension. Death has occurred unexpectedly during normal activities, cardiac catheterization, and after the administration of different anesthetic agents. Initial complaints of easy fatigability and chest discomfort in young patients presenting with this disease are often disregarded. When the disease is advanced, incapacitating dyspnea, a nondescript type of chest pain, breathlessness, syncope, weakness, and fatigue are common.

508. The answers are: A-Y, B-N, C-Y, D-N, E-Y. *(pp 1857–1859)* The normal pulmonary hemodynamics of adults depends in part on the atmospheric pressure. At sea level, a cardiac output of 5 to 6 liters/min in a normal person is associated with mean pulmonary artery pressures of about 15 mmHg. However, at 15,000 feet of altitude, the same level of blood flow is associated with an elevated mean pulmonary arterial pressure of about 25 mmHg. This occurs because of an increase in pulmonary vascular resistance. Although a large volume of blood crosses through the right ventricle and into the pulmonary bed, only a modest drop in pressure between the pulmonary artery and the left atrium occurs. This is because in a healthy person, the pulmonary vascular tree is a low-resistance organ. The pulmonary vascular resistance is calculated as the ratio between the difference in mean pressures between the pulmonary artery and the left atrium. Specifically, the pulmonary artery pressure minus left atrial pressure divided by the cardiac output equals the pulmonary vascular resistance. In the absence of intrinsic lung disease, the pulmonary capillary wedge pressure directly reflects the left atrial pressure and is generally substituted for left atrial pressure in calculations used to determine pulmonary vascular resistance. In the normal lung, increases in cardiac output up to three times resting cardiac output are associated with minimal increases in pulmonary artery pressure. However, in patients with pulmonary hypertension, the diseased pulmonary vascular bed cannot accommodate this increased flow and lesser increments in pulmonary blood flow elicit more striking increases in pulmonary artery pressure. The pulmonary vascular bed is a reactive organ with multiple factors playing a role in determining the degree of vasoconstriction or vasodilation. Autonomic nerves play a much less important role in mediating a vascular tone than hypoxia and acidosis do. Furthermore, acidosis tends to reinforce the hypoxic pressor effect. Treatment of patients with pulmonary hypertension with oxygen can often lead to decreased pulmonary pressures and improved right-sided cardiac function.

509. The answers are: A-Y, B-Y, C-N, D-N, E-Y. *(pp 1870–1872)* There is a high incidence of clots found in the small pulmonary arteries and arterioles of patients with primary pulmonary hypertension. This supports some of the clinical studies that recommend anticoagulation in patients with pulmonary hypertension, especially when right ventricular failure is present. One nonrandomized clinical trial showed enhanced long-term survival in patients receiving anticoagulant therapy. Single-lung transplantation can drop pulmonary artery pressures to near normal levels and can improve right ventricular function rapidly and dramatically. Transplantation, although effective, can be associated with serious postoperative complications, chronic rejection, and limited organ availability. The primary vasodilator therapy that continues to hold promise for oral therapy is calcium channel blocking agents. However, prospects for survival do not seem to be related to the test response to calcium blockers unless a dramatic fall in pulmonary vascular resistance is achieved. Verapamil has fallen into disuse largely because of its undesirable negative inotropic effects, and recent studies have concentrated on the use of nifedipine and diltiazem. Only one-third of patients with primary pulmonary hypertension are responsive to pulmonary vasodilator therapy. Epoprostenol [prostacyclin (PGI$_2$)] is an arachidonic acid metabolite. PGI$_2$ has a very short half-life and needs to be administered by continuous intravenous infusion; however, it is a potent pulmonary dilator, and it inhibits proliferation of vascular smooth muscle. Currently its most effective use is as a bridge to lung or heart-lung transplantation in patients who respond to its pulmonary vasodilator effects.

510. **The answers are: A-Y, B-N, C-Y, D-N, E-Y.** *(pp 1880–1882)*   Impedance plethysmography is particularly helpful when the lung scan is nonspecific. When impedance plethysmography is negative, it is usually appropriate to conclude that the patient does not have pulmonary embolism. If impedance plethysmography is unilaterally positive, the diagnosis of pulmonary embolism should be pursued by performance of pulmonary angiography. In patients with submassive pulmonary emboli, selective or subselective injections should be made at pulmonary angiography in areas shown to have perfusion defects by lung scan. In patients with acute cor pulmonale due to massive pulmonary embolism in whom pulmonary embolectomy may be indicated, mainstream injection into the main pulmonary artery performed at angiography to visualize the total pulmonary circulation is safer than selective injections. Thrombophlebitis migrans is an unusual form of venous thrombosis and may be associated with an occult malignancy. This involves the superficial veins often at atypical sites such as the arms, is migratory, and may be resistant to anticoagulant therapy. Paradoxical embolism of the systemic circulation is a rare complication of deep venous thrombosis that may occur in patients with an intracardiac defect such as an atrial septal defect, ventricular septal defect, or most commonly a patent foramen ovale, which occurs in about 27 percent of the adult population. In order for a venous thrombus to cross a patent foramen ovale into the systemic circulation, pressure in the right atrium must exceed pressure in the left atrium. The usual clinical profile is of a patient experiencing a massive pulmonary embolism that causes acute cor pulmonale.

511. **The answers are: A-Y, B-N, C-N, D-Y, E-Y.** *(pp 1875–1876)*   About 200,000 deaths per year in the United States are caused by pulmonary embolism. In nearly all of these cases, the embolus arises from deep venous thrombosis in the proximal venous system of the leg. Prevention of deep venous thrombosis is the cornerstone of prevention of pulmonary embolism. Bed rest, surgical procedures, congestive heart failure, pregnancy, advanced age, oral contraceptive agents, obesity, and a prior history of venous thrombosis are all predisposing factors for the development of venous thrombosis. While 5000 units of subcutaneous heparin every 12 h is adequate protection from deep venous thrombosis in general medical patients, it is not adequate protection in patients with hip fractures and those undergoing hip replacement or men undergoing urologic procedures. In these high-risk groups, intravenous dextran or the combination of dihydroergotamine and low-dose heparin is the appropriate prophylactic measure. Venography, while the most sensitive and specific test for deep venous thrombosis, is very painful. Impedance plethysmography is also very sensitive. A positive test is over 90 percent specific for deep venous thrombosis. This test is based on the principle that electrical impedance in the lower extremities is related to venous volume. When a cuff occluding venous return is released, electrical impedance in the lower extremity returns to baseline more slowly than normal if the deep venous system is occluded. Approximately 50 percent of patients with proximal deep venous thrombosis will suffer a pulmonary embolism. The mortality of untreated pulmonary embolism is about 20 to 30 percent. If intravenous heparin therapy is instituted, the mortality diminishes to less than 10 percent.

512. **The answers are: A-Y, B-Y, C-Y, D-N, E-Y.** *(pp 1895–1904)*   In chronic obstructive pulmonary disease (COPD), the pulmonary artery pressure is related to a high level of hypoxemia and is usually de-

creased by oxygen administration. Adequate oxygenation in patients with COPD may prevent the onset of right ventricular failure. All patients with cor pulmonale should be given home oxygen therapy in order to restore P_{O_2} to levels greater than 60 torr. Studies show that continuous nocturnal home oxygen therapy is beneficial in keeping patients with severe COPD functional for longer periods. Although susceptibility to digoxin therapy appears to be increased in COPD, some studies have demonstrated that digoxin improves left ventricular function in cor pulmonale. Tachycardia in patients with COPD may be secondary to hypoxia and will not respond to digitalis. Likewise, the multifocal atrial tachycardia seen in some COPD patients does not respond to digitalis or other antiarrhythmics. The success rate for single and double lung transplantation is over 60 percent in most large centers. Lung transplantation is most often performed for the following preoperative diagnoses: primary pulmonary hypertension, idiopathic pulmonary fibrosis, and cystic fibrosis. Interestingly, right ventricular systolic function following lung transplantation has been shown to improve even when the preoperative right ventricular function was severely impaired.

XIII. The Heart and Systemic Disease or Conditions

DIRECTIONS: Each question below contains five suggested responses. Select the **one best** response to each question.

513. The systemic arterial hypertension found in patients with primary hyperparathyroidism

    (A) is a distinctive entity associated with the disease state
    (B) responds dramatically to surgical removal of the parathyroid gland
    (C) should be treated with thiazides as the diuretic of choice
    (D) is usually associated with concomitant Hashimoto's thyroiditis
    (E) should be treated with loop diuretics as the diuretic of choice

514. Compared to an ethnic, age-, and sex-matched population, a predominant cardiovascular manifestation in patients with acromegaly is

    (A) hypertriglyceridemia
    (B) accelerated coronary atherosclerosis
    (C) dilated cardiomyopathy
    (D) systemic arterial hypertension
    (E) mitral valve prolapse

515. In postmenopausal women, replacement therapy with a combination of estrogen and progestin, compared to estrogen therapy alone

    (A) reduces the potential incidence of endometrial carcinoma
    (B) increases the protective effect against the development of coronary atherosclerotic heart disease
    (C) reduces the potential incidence of breast cancer
    (D) increases the incidence of deep vein thrombophlebitis and thromboembolism
    (E) increases the incidence of thrombotic coronary artery events

516. In a patient receiving amiodarone therapy, the most helpful test to detect the possibility of primary hypothyroidism would be

    (A) triiodothyronine (T_3) levels
    (B) biologically inactive triiodothyronine (rT_3) levels
    (C) thyroxine (T_4) levels
    (D) biologically inactive thyroxine (rT_4) levels
    (E) thyroid-stimulating hormone (TSH) levels

517. Each of the following statements regarding cardiac involvement in polyarteritis nodosa is true EXCEPT

(A) coronary artery involvement in polyarteritis nodosa may lead to myocardial infarction

(B) conduction tissue is spared in polyarteritis nodosa with only rare instances of conduction disturbances

(C) congestive heart failure is often seen in patients with polyarteritis nodosa

(D) pericarditis is an unusual primary manifestation of polyarteritis nodosa

(E) systemic arteriolar hypertension occurs in about 90 percent of patients with polyarteritis nodosa

518. All the following statements regarding cardiac involvement with progressive systemic sclerosis are true EXCEPT

(A) patchy fibrosis noted in the hearts of patients with scleroderma is secondary to occlusion of small coronary vessels caused by vascular intimal proliferation

(B) cold-induced myocardial perfusion defects as well as cold-induced left ventricular dysfunction have been noted in patients with scleroderma

(C) pericarditis occurs in up to 20 percent of patients with scleroderma

(D) cardiac involvement with scleroderma may present as a dilated, congestive cardiomyopathy

(E) left ventricular hypertrophy is a common finding in patients with scleroderma

519. When extremely obese patients lose weight, they are least likely to

(A) improve glucose tolerance
(B) lessen insulin resistance
(C) reduce circulating blood volume and cardiac output
(D) regress myocardial hypertrophy
(E) lessen blood pressure

520. Which of the following statements regarding cardiac involvement in systemic lupus erythematosus is most accurate?

(A) Pericardial involvement in systemic lupus erythematosus generally causes bothersome symptoms for the patient

(B) Libman-Sachs lesions of systemic lupus erythematosus are generally associated with valvular dysfunction

(C) Unlike other connective tissue disorders, the serum complement level is usually elevated in systemic lupus erythematosus

(D) The major cause of cardiac enlargement and heart failure in systemic lupus erythematosus is the myocarditis associated with this disease

(E) Rhythm and conduction disturbances have been associated with systemic lupus erythematosus

521. Regarding alcohol-induced cardiomyopathy, which of the following is true?

(A) In the early, presymptomatic stages of alcoholic cardiomyopathy, global systolic dysfunction is the predominant physiologic abnormality

(B) Chest pain is rare and angina indicates the presence of atherosclerotic coronary artery disease

(C) Patients who drink mixed drinks are more likely to develop alcoholic cardiomyopathy than those patients who consume beer and wine

(D) Patients with alcohol-induced cirrhosis and peripheral neuropathy rarely develop alcohol-related cardiomyopathy

(E) By the time symptoms of alcohol-induced cardiomyopathy ensue, the left ventricular walls are usually hypertrophied

522. The effects of alcohol on the heart are correctly characterized by which of the following?

(A) Ventricular arrhythmias are more common than atrial arrhythmias

(B) Mechanisms of cardiac arrhythmias in alcoholics include high levels of circulating cathecholamines, electrolyte abnormalities, and abnormal delays in normal conduction

(C) Alcohol does not have a direct toxic effect on cardiac myocytes, but indirectly causes cardiac pathology by neurohormonal influences on the heart

(D) In female alcoholics, it is more common to have alcohol-induced cardiomyopathy in premenopausal women and cirrhosis in postmenopausal women

(E) In experimental animals, alcohol impairs protein synthesis in myocytes

523. All the following statements concerning systemic arterial hypertension and renal disease are correct EXCEPT

(A) 80 to 90 percent of patients with end-stage renal disease develop hypertension prior to beginning dialysis

(B) hypertension associated with end-stage renal disease is characterized by normal cardiac output and high peripheral resistance

(C) hypertension is generally responsive to vigorous dialysis in most patients with end-stage renal disease

(D) dialysis-resistant hypertension is characterized by high plasma renin activity

(E) blood pressure in dialysis-resistant hypertension may become volume-sensitive after bilateral nephrectomy

524. Correct statements concerning cardiac risk factors in patients with chronic renal insufficiency include all the following EXCEPT

(A) diabetic patients with chronic renal failure have a higher mortality on dialysis than nondiabetics

(B) lipid levels should be drawn after a 12-h fast but prior to heparin injection for dialysis

(C) triglyceride levels are not affected by peritoneal dialysis as they are by hemodialysis

(D) elevated triglyceride levels are due to impaired degradation of very low-density lipoproteins by lipoprotein lipase

(E) diuretics and beta blockers used to control blood pressure may also elevate serum lipids

525. Causes of hypotension during dialysis include all the following EXCEPT

(A) pericardial tamponade

(B) aortic stenosis

(C) autonomic neuropathy

(D) use of bicarbonate-based dialysis solutions

(E) hypersensitivity to ethylene oxide

526. The phase of syphilitic infection in which luetic cardiovascular disease becomes clinically manifest is the

(A) primary stage

(B) secondary stage

(C) tertiary stage

(D) quaternary stage

(E) primary stage and secondary stage

DIRECTIONS: Each question below contains four suggested responses of which **one or more** is correct. Select

A	if	**1, 2, and 3**	are correct
B	if	**1 and 3**	are correct
C	if	**2 and 4**	are correct
D	if	**4**	is correct
E	if	**1, 2, 3, and 4**	are correct

527. Cardiovascular manifestations of a significant hyperthyroid state include

(1) increased total peripheral resistance
(2) increased sensitivity to digitalis glycosides
(3) accelerated coronary atherosclerosis
(4) increased sensitivity to β-adrenergic agonists

528. In most patients with significant hypothyroidism, the serum lipid profile will reflect an elevation of

(1) low-density lipoproteins (LDL)
(2) very low-density lipoproteins (VLDL)
(3) triglycerides
(4) high-density lipoproteins (HDL)

529. The cardiovascular complications of Addison's disease (adrenocortical insufficiency) include

(1) systemic arterial hypertension
(2) hyperkalemic depression of the myocardium
(3) increased cardiac output
(4) vascular collapse when stressed

530. Severe autonomic neuropathy in diabetic individuals may be suggested by

(1) a resting bradycardia
(2) a decreased variation in heart rate with respiration
(3) QT shortening on the electrocardiogram (ECG)
(4) postural hypotension

531. True statements regarding the cardiovascular manifestations of scleroderma include which of the following?

(1) Pulmonary vasodilators such as tolazoline are frequently effective in lowering pulmonary hypertension associated with scleroderma
(2) The chest x-ray normally demonstrates bilateral pulmonary infiltrates when patients with scleroderma develop rapidly progressive dyspnea and right-sided congestive heart failure
(3) The CREST syndrome is a variant of scleroderma that is not associated with pulmonary involvement
(4) Histologically the pulmonary vascular lesions of scleroderma resemble those of idiopathic primary pulmonary hypertension

532. Pathophysiological and echocardiographic features of the cardiomyopathy of obesity may include

(1) diffuse left ventricular hypertrophy
(2) right ventricular hypertrophy
(3) diastolic dysfunction
(4) reactive pulmonary hypertension

533. The clinical manifestations of cardiovascular syphilis may involve the pathophysiological consequences of

(1) coronary artery aneurysm
(2) aortic regurgitation
(3) mitral regurgitation
(4) coronary ostial disease

SUMMARY OF DIRECTIONS

A	B	C	D	E
1, 2, 3 only	1, 3 only	2, 4 only	4 only	All are correct

534. Correct statements regarding nutritional heart disease include

(1) left ventricular mass in patients with anorexia nervosa is diminished by one-half to two-thirds that of age- and sex-matched controls

(2) systolic function of the left ventricle is not compromised in patients with anorexia nervosa

(3) thiamine deficiency can result in significant elevation of left ventricular and diastolic and pulmonary capillary wedge pressures

(4) adults with chronic undernutrition without underlying heart disease may develop heart failure during hyperalimentation

535. Regarding vitamin deficiencies and heart disease, true statements include

(1) the cardiomyopathy caused by selenium deficiency, Keshan's disease, is a rare disease that is most often seen in Chinese children and young adults

(2) in most patients suffering with anorexia nervosa, the QT interval is markedly prolonged

(3) scurvy, or vitamin C deficiency, does not affect the heart

(4) patients who develop severe malnutrition and are then abruptly refed can develop congestive heart failure

536. Syphilitic aortic aneurysms have which of the following characteristics?

(1) They occur predominantly in the thoracic aorta

(2) They are in danger of erosion or rupture

(3) They tend to be saccular or fusiform

(4) They have a high incidence of dissection

537. In the absence of atherosclerosis, angina may occur in syphilitic cardiovascular disease as a result of

(1) diffuse coronary arteritis

(2) rupture of the sinus of Valsalva

(3) coronary artery dissection

(4) coronary ostial stenosis

538. Treatment of a hypotensive patient on dialysis who is experiencing angina pectoris should include

(1) stopping ultrafiltration

(2) reducing blood flow through the dialyzer

(3) nasal oxygen therapy

(4) nitroglycerin sublingually

539. Cimetidine increases the blood levels of which of the following beta blockers?

(1) Sotalol

(2) Metoprolol

(3) Nadolol

(4) Propranolol

540. Which of the following drugs increase blood levels of verapamil?

(1) Beta blockers

(2) Quinidine

(3) Digoxin

(4) Cimetidine

541. Amiodarone predisposes patients to a proarrhythmic condition that leads to torsades de pointes when it is coadministered with which of the following drugs?

(1) Quinidine

(2) Thiazide diuretics

(3) Tricyclic antidepressants

(4) Digitalis

DIRECTIONS: Each question below contains five suggested responses. For **each** of the **five** responses listed with every question you are to respond either YES (Y) or NO (N). In a given item **all, some, or none of the alternatives may be correct.**

542. Each of the following statements concerns cardiac involvement in rheumatoid arthritis and ankylosing spondylitis. True statements include

(A) pericarditis may occur in up to 30 percent of cases of rheumatoid arthritis

(B) aortic regurgitation may occur in rheumatoid arthritis as a result of rheumatoid involvement of the aortic valve annulus

(C) aortic insufficiency associated with ankylosing spondylitis results from inflammatory lesions of the aortic valve leaflet

(D) ankylosing spondylitis may result in mitral valve insufficiency

(E) corticosteroid therapy may limit the inflammatory process and progression of aortic insufficiency in ankylosing spondylitis

543. Correct statements concerning obesity and heart disease include which of the following?

(A) In extremely obese patients, adipose flow may constitute one-half of resting cardiac output

(B) Weight loss in obese patients reduces both number and size of adipocytes

(C) Correlation between obesity and hypertension is highest in young men and black women

(D) A predominantly abdominal distribution of body fat correlates better with hypertension than relative weight or body mass

(E) Most extremely obese patients have concomitant hypertension as a risk for coronary disease

544. Correct statements regarding the commonly recognized cardiovascular abnormalities associated with the acquired immunodeficiency syndrome (AIDS) include

(A) pericardial effusion is the most commonly recognized abnormality

(B) myocardial involvement with lymphocytic infiltration may result in the development of a dilated cardiomyopathy

(C) development of nonbacterial thrombotic endocarditis is commonly recognized

(D) metastatic Kaposi's sarcoma may be seen at autopsy findings on the pericardium

(E) cardiac involvement is the most common cause of death

XIII. The Heart and Systemic Disease or Conditions

Answers

513. The answer is E. *(p 1913)* The incidence of systemic arterial hypertension appears to be higher in hypercalcemic patients compared to the normal population. However, estimates of the prevalence of hypertension in patients with primary hyperparathyroidism vary, and in general, it remains uncertain whether there is a true association between hypertension and hyperparathyroidism. Surgical removal of the hyperactive parathyroid gland does not have a distinctive beneficial effect on hypertension but may improve the management of hypertension with medical therapy. When diuretics are necessary for the treatment of hypertension associated with hyperparathyroidism, thiazide diuretics should be avoided since they may further increase serum calcium (Ca^{2+}) levels. Loop diuretics should be the agents of choice since they are calciuric agents.

514. The answer is D. *(pp 1907–1908)* Autopsy studies in acromegalic patients have been unable to show a characteristic form of cardiac pathology. Although visceral enlargement is characteristic, this is usually reflected in left ventricular hypertrophy or congestive heart failure (CHF) rather than a dilated cardiomyopathy. Hypertension occurs in acromegaly three times more frequently than in the general population. It tends to be mild, responsive to conventional therapy, and regression may occur after successful treatment of growth hormone excess. The etiology of the hypertension in acromegaly is thought to be secondary to growth hormone–mediated sodium (Na^+) retention associated with low plasma renin. However, the possibility of a pheochromocytoma or hyperaldosteronism should also be kept in mind since acromegaly could be a variant of a multiple endocrine neoplasia syndrome. Ironically, in spite of the high incidence of glucose intolerance and hypertension, the occurrence of coronary artery disease or peripheral vascular disease is not higher than that of a comparable matched population.

515. The answer is A. *(p 1915)* The benefits of estrogen replacement therapy in postmenopausal women to relieve menopausal symptoms and reduce bone loss have been clearly established. In addition, estrogen therapy has been documented both by population studies and angiographic studies to reduce the incidence of coronary atherosclerotic heart disease by as high as 40 to 50 percent. However, estrogen replacement therapy is associated with a 6-fold increase in endometrial cancer and a 1.3-fold increase in breast cancer. The addition of progestin to estrogen replacement therapy reduces the increased risk of endometrial cancer but does not appear to prevent the potential increased incidence of breast cancer. Unfortunately, the combination of estrogen and progestins decrease the protective effect against coronary atherosclerotic heart disease since progestins have an adverse effect on serum lipoproteins. There is a high incidence of thrombotic vascular disease in premenopausal women who take oral contraceptives. However, this thromboembolic risk is not seen in postmenopausal women who receive estrogen replacement therapy.

516. The answer is B. *(pp 1912–1913)*   Amiodarone is an important source of exogenous iodine as it contains 37 percent iodine and provides 75 mg of iodine per 200-mg tablet. Iodine administration in these high doses may alter thyroid hormone production in patients with underlying thyroid disease. Administration of milligram quantities of iodide results in a transient reduction of thyroid hormone secretion and a concomitant increase in thyroid-stimulating hormone (TSH). In a euthyroid patient receiving amiodarone, a new equilibrium may be reached in which thyroxine (T_4) levels are high, triiodothyronine (T_3) levels remain normal, and TSH is increased. At times, this may be difficult to differentiate from true hyperthyroidism. Since TSH is generally elevated in patients receiving amiodarone, the most helpful test for detecting primary hypothyroidism is the measurement of biologically inactive triiodothyronine (rT_3) concentrations. This is generally elevated in patients receiving amiodarone. Failure to show high serum levels of rT_3 in a patient receiving amiodarone may indicate hypothyroidism.

517. The answer is B. *(pp 1925–1926)*   Polyarteritis nodosa causes segmental necrotizing inflammation of medium-to-small arteries throughout various organs of the body including the heart. This vasculitis involves the coronary arteries primarily at the distal extramural and subepicardial coronary arteries just as they penetrate the myocardium. The media and adventitia are involved with an inflammatory infiltrate that eventually causes necrosis and inflammation of the full thickness of the artery and surrounding connective tissue. Thrombosis and aneurysmal dilatation of the coronary arteries result and myocardial infarcts may occur as a result of these changes. Additionally, the coronary lumen is narrowed by internal proliferation during the healing phase of the inflammatory reaction. The sinoatrial node and atrioventricular node arteries are frequently involved in polyarteritis and both the atrioventricular and sinoatrial nodes may be involved in the inflammatory process since the nodal tissue surrounds these arteries. Both atrial and ventricular conduction abnormalities result. Because of the renal involvement that occurs with polyarteritis nodosa, systemic arteriolar hypertension is present in about 90 percent of these patients. Hypertension is the primary cause of congestive heart failure that is frequently seen in these patients and may lead to other manifestations of renal failure such as uremic pericarditis. Pericarditis, as a manifestation solely of polyarteritis, is unusual. As mentioned above, myocardial infarction may occur as a result of thrombosis of the coronary arteries. However, coronary atherosclerotic vascular disease may also be the cause of infarction in this population of typically middle-aged males who are often treated with steroids.

518. The answer is A. *(pp 1929–1931)*   When the heart is involved in scleroderma a patchy myocardial fibrosis is found that bears no relationship to large- or small-vessel occlusion or other anatomic abnormalities. All levels of myocardium are involved and the right ventricle is involved as often as the left. The type of necrosis seen is myofibrillar degeneration or contraction band necrosis. These lesions develop when the myocardium is subjected to transient occlusion with reperfusion. It is presently thought that the most likely etiology of the cardiac sclerosis noted in patients with scleroderma is a consequence of focal intermittent and progressive ischemic injury resulting from recurrent vasospasm (a Raynaud's phenomenon) of the coronary arteries. This phenomenon has also been noted in renal arterioles of the coronary vasculature. In keeping with this, transient perfusion defects on thallium studies have been noted in patients with scleroderma and patent coronary arteries with symptomatic cardiac disease. Reversible cold-induced myocardial perfusion defects and reversible left ventricular dysfunction have been noted in these patients with scleroderma. In two-thirds of these patients, the pericarditis is secondary to renal failure. Occasionally, very large pericardial effusions occur with scleroderma. When myocardial injury due to scleroderma is extensive, dilated hypodynamic ventricles result, simulating the picture of a congestive cardiomyopathy. Atrial and ventricular arrhythmias, angina pectoris, myocardial infarction, and sudden death may all be associated clinical features of myocardial sclerosis. One of the most frequent results of scleroderma is systemic arteriolar hypertension due to renal parenchymal involvement. Therefore, left ventricular hypertrophy is often associated with scleroderma. Myocardial infarction and angina may be the result of microvascular spasm or coronary atherosclerotic disease. Sudden death may be the result of pulmonary hypertension or myocardial infarction.

519. The answer is E. *(p 1938)*   Weight loss in patients with obesity hypertension correlates poorly with the decrease in pressure. The blood pressure may drop early and then plateau as further weight is lost. Other potentially desirable effects include improved glucose tolerance, lessened insulin resistance, reduction of blood volume and cardiac output, and regression of ventricular hypertrophy.

520. The answer is E. *(pp 1921–1925)*   Systemic lupus erythematosus may cause a pancarditis with involvement of the pericardium, endocardium, myocardium, and coronary arteries. The pericardium is most frequently involved and pericardial effusion occurs during the course of the illness in over 50 percent of these patients. Pericarditis is the presenting feature of the illness in about 4 percent of the patients with systemic lupus erythematosus, but generally pericardial involvement causes no symptoms. Rarely constriction and tamponade have occurred in these patients. Purulent pericarditis is a serious complication associated with systemic lupus, and this occurs most frequently in patients with renal failure and immunocompromised patients being treated with steroids or cytotoxic agents. Fibrofibrinous sterile vegetations known as Libman-Sachs vegetations are observed at autopsy in up to 40 percent of patients with systemic lupus erythematosus. They occur most commonly on the aortic and mitral valves and favor the ventricular surface of the mitral valve. They differ from marantic endocarditis in that they may lead to focal necrosis of valve leaflets with scarring. Generally, there is no valvular dysfunction associated with Libman-Sachs endocarditis, but the risk of bacterial endocarditis is increased with the presence of these vegetations. The serum complement level is decreased in most patients with systemic lupus erythematosus, and this may serve as a useful diagnostic test since complement level is usually increased in other connective tissue disorders. Myocarditis is an uncommon manifestation of systemic lupus erythematosus, and the most common cause of heart failure is systemic arteriolar hypertension frequently associated with renal involvement. Rhythm and conduction disturbances may occur in systemic lupus due to arteritis involving the sinus node artery with scarring of the sinus and atrioventricular nodes. Generally, coronary artery arteritis is uncommon but small intramural vessels may demonstrate fibrinoid necrosis and thromboembolic occlusion. Coronary atherosclerosis may occur in the young patient with systemic lupus erythematosus who has had long-standing hypertension, renal failure, or steroid treatment.

521. The answer is D. *(pp 1943–1948)*   Chronic alcohol abuse can cause significant myocardial dysfunction prior to the onset of clinical symptoms. In the early, preclinical phases of the disease, myocardial hypertrophy and diastolic dysfunction predominate. Only late in the disease process, when symptoms finally appear, does the ventricle dilate and the ventricular walls thin and systolic function decline. Symptoms of left-sided heart failure are often the presenting symptoms, but it is not uncommon for the first symptoms to be chest pain (occasionally anginal in nature). The etiology of the chest pain is not clear since most patients do not have occlusive coronary disease seen on angiography. The pattern of alcohol intake (i.e., binge versus regular, constant imbibing) and the type of alcohol consumed (i.e., beer versus wine versus mixed drinks) do not predict who will develop the dilated cardiomyopathy of alcoholism. However, it has been observed that patients who develop neuropathy and cirrhosis rarely acquire alcoholic cardiomyopathy.

522. The answer is B. *(pp 1943–1948)*   Arrhythmias are common in patients who abuse alcohol. Indeed arrhythmias may often be the first presenting symptom in patients with alcohol-induced cardiac dysfunction. In general, atrial arrhythmias predominate, although ventricular premature contractions and sudden cardiac death have been reported. The mechanisms of cardiac dysrhythmias in the alcoholic are not known with certainty. However, elevated levels of catecholamines, delays in native conduction, and electrolyte abnormalities (hypokalemia and hypomagnesemia) have been implicated. There is a direct toxic effect of alcohol on myocytes, but in animals, alcohol does not impair protein synthesis of cardiac myocytes. Female alcoholics are more likely to develop cardiomyopathy after the menopause.

523. The answer is B. *(p 1961)*   The majority (80 to 90 percent) of patients with end-stage renal disease have systemic hypertension prior to beginning dialysis. The hypertension is due to sodium retention and extracellular volume expansion. These patients have an increased cardiac output and a low vascular resistance, unlike patients with hypertension and normal renal function who have a normal cardiac output and high peripheral resistance.

The hypertension in these patients rapidly resolves after commencement of vigorous dialysis, showing the effect of increased volume. Ten to twenty percent of cases remain dialysis-resistant but do respond to drugs that inhibit plasma renin activity. Bilateral nephrectomy may be necessary to decrease renin levels and control blood pressure. After nephrectomy, volume sensitivity may return in this subset of patients.

524. The answer is C. *(p 1962)* Coronary artery disease is the likely cause of the significantly higher mortality of diabetics on dialysis compared with age-matched nondiabetics on dialysis. Analysis of lipid levels demands a 12-h fast prior to analysis. Heparin given to prevent clot formation in the dialyzer increases lipoprotein lipase and thus decreases plasma triglycerides. The high concentration of glucose in the peritoneal dialysate complicates analysis of triglycerides because glucose is converted to triglycerides. Impaired degradation of very low-density lipoproteins by lipoprotein lipase appear to be the major cause of hypertriglyceridemia. Patients who are taking diuretics or beta blockers or patients with end-stage renal disease have exaggerated levels of lipids partially due to side effects of the drugs.

525. The answer is D. *(p 1962)* Dialysis-induced hypotension may be due to antihypertensive medications, overdiuresis, and too vigorous dialysis. Anaphylaxis due to hypersensitivity to ethylene oxide (used to sterilize dialyzers) is another cause. Until recently, acetate buffers in dialysis solutions predisposed to hypotension (a vasodilator effect), hypoventilation, and hypoxemia. Other factors include (1) decreased cardiac output (due to left ventricular dysfunction, valvular stenosis, or pericardial tamponade); (2) decreased myocardial contractility due to potassium or calcium imbalance; (3) autonomic neuropathy (especially in diabetics); (4) sepsis; and (5) occult hemorrhage (GI or retroperitoneal bleeding).

526. The answer is C. *(p 1949)* The primary stage of syphilitic infection is characterized by a chancre (primary lesion). Four to eight weeks later, widespread vascular dissemination of the spirochete occurs in the secondary stage, which is characterized by skin rash, malaise, fever, mucocutaneous ulcers, and other systemic signs. As a result of this process, arteritis develops but lays dormant until the tertiary stage of infection. In the tertiary stage, which may occur a few years to decades after the primary stage, the clinical manifestations of luetic cardiovascular disease become apparent. Classically, there has not been a designated quarternary stage.

527. The answer is D (4). *(pp 1908–1910)* There is evidence that thyroid hormone increases total body oxygen consumption, increases sensitivity of the heart to β-adrenergic stimuli, and has a direct inotropic and chronotropic effect on cardiac muscle. As a result of this, the clinical manifestations of a hyperthyroid state include an increase in cardiac output, an increase in stroke volume, an increase in heart rate, an increase in systolic ejection rate, a decrease in peripheral vascular resistance, and a widened pulse pressure. Myocardial sensitivity to digitalis glycosides is decreased, and as a result large doses of digitalis are usually required to control atrial arrhythmias. It is thought that an increased number of as well as an increased affinity for β-adrenergic receptors is responsible for the increased sensitivity to β-adrenergic agonists on the heart in hyperthyroid patients.

528. The answer is E (all). *(p 1911)* Approximately 95 percent of patients with significant hypothyroidism have significant hypercholesterolemia and hypertriglyceridemia. When hypercholesterolemia in hypothyroidism is present, all cholesterol subfractions are increased including low-density lipoproteins (LDL), very low-density lipoproteins (VLDL), and even the protective high-density lipoproteins (HDL). The elevation of LDL cholesterol is thought to be secondary to a decreased concentration of LDL receptors, resulting in decreased clearance of LDL cholesterol. Accumulation of VLDL is thought to be secondary to decreased activity of lipoprotein lipase without being sufficiently reduced as to cause fasting chylomicronemia. An elevated HDL cholesterol is explained by reduced hepatic triglyceride lipase. Overall, since the increased LDL cholesterol is not accompanied by a proportional increment in total HDL cholesterol, an unfavorable HDL-LDL cholesterol ratio results.

529. The answer is C (2, 4).   *(pp 1913–1914)*   A deficiency of both cortisol and aldosterone is the primary effect of adrenocortical insufficiency (Addison's disease). Sodium (Na⁺) resorption and potassium (K⁺) secretion are impaired as a result of the aldosterone deficiency. There is an inherent inability to conserve Na⁺ with a resultant tendency to be prone to volume depletion. The effect of both glucocorticoid and aldosterone deficiency causes a decrease in cardiac output with a tendency to develop hypotension and complete vascular collapse when stressed. The tendency to develop hyperkalemia has a depressive effect on the myocardium.

530. The answer is C (2, 4).   *(p 1916)*   An increase in resting heart rate and a decrease in the variation of heart rate with respiration are reflections of defective parasympathetic innervation in patients with significant diabetic cardiac autonomic neuropathy. It has recently been shown that there is a high incidence of QT prolongation in this entity. This is probably a result of autonomic imbalance and may be the etiology of an increased tendency to ventricular arrhythmias and sudden death in these individuals. Postural hypotension is another manifestation of significant autonomic neuropathy in diabetic patients.

531. The answer is D (4).   *(pp 1929–1931)*   Both pulmonary fibrosis secondary to parenchymal disease and a "primary" pulmonary vascular disease occur in patients with scleroderma and contribute to arterial vasospasm in these patients. Pulmonary arterial vasospasm is felt to be a major component of primary pulmonary hypertension. Patients with this vascular lesion often develop rapidly progressive dyspnea and right-sided congestive heart failure in the setting of clear lungs. Because the etiology of this "primary" pulmonary hypertension is vasospasm rather than parenchymal fibrosis, the lungs are clear. Occasionally, vasodilators such as tolazoline may induce partial lowering of pulmonary pressures, but the fixed pulmonary lesions and focal thrombotic occlusions that always accompany the advanced stages of pulmonary hypertension with scleroderma make restoration of lower pulmonary pressures unlikely. Histologically, the pulmonary arterial lesions show medial and intimal hyperplasia, plexiform lesions, and necrotizing arteritis seen in Eisenmenger syndrome and idiopathic primary pulmonary hypertension. A variant of scleroderma, the CREST syndrome (calcinosis, Raynaud's phenomenon, esophageal abnormalities, sclerodactyly, telangiectasia), manifests relatively mild skin changes limited to face and fingers but may result in severe pulmonary hypertension due to "primary" pulmonary hypertension.

532. The answer is E (all).   *(pp 1938–1939)*   Patients with the cardiomyopathy of obesity have left ventricular hypertrophy, diastolic dysfunction, and sometimes systolic dysfunction. If an increased left atrial pressure is transmitted back to the right heart, right ventricular hypertrophy and pulmonary hypertension may occur. On occasion, a disproportionate increase in pulmonary hypotension may occur such that an increased transpulmonary gradient (mean pulmonary artery pressure − pulmonary capillary wedge pressure) exists.

533. The answer is C (2, 4).   *(pp 1949–1950)*   The three major manifestations of cardiovascular syphilis are aortic regurgitation, aortic aneurysm formation, and coronary ostial disease. These are a reflection of an arteritis that predominantly invades the vasa vasorum of the proximal aorta. Aortic regurgitation occurs as a result of dilatation of the ascending aorta and inflammation just above the sinus of Valsalva. Distal aortic involvement, myocarditis, pulmonary arteritis, and myocardial gummata are less common manifestations of syphilitic cardiovascular disease. Proximal coronary ostial stenoses and ectasia are present in tertiary lues. Extensive coronary artery aneurysms are not found in syphilitic cardiovascular disease but are more common in widespread atherosclerosis or Kawasaki's disease.

534. The answer is E (all).   *(pp 1946–1947)*   Two-dimensional echocardiography has documented a reduction of left ventricular mass by one-half to two-thirds that of normal in patients with anorexia nervosa. This reduction was even greater when left ventricular mass was considered in relation to total body weight. Left ventricular systolic and diastolic volumes are significantly decreased, although the shape of the left ventricular cavity remains normal. However, indexes of the systolic ejection phase of left ventricular function are normal and respond normally to exercise. Left ventricular afterload is reduced in patients with anorexia nervosa. Thiamine deficiency results in a high cardiac output associated with arteriolar vasodilatation. Several studies have documented significant elevation of left ventricular end-diastolic and pulmonary capillary wedge pressures, which is reversible with thiamine therapy. Chronically malnourished persons undergoing hyperalimentation may develop symptoms of heart failure even with no underlying cardiac disease. This resembles a high-output type of congestive heart failure characterized by hypermetabolism, ventricular gallops, augmented cardiac output, and normal ejection fraction. This situation is treated by slowing the rate of hyperalimentation, diuresis, and sodium restriction.

535. The answer is B (1, 3). *(pp 1943–1948)* Vitamin deficiencies and malnutrition states can adversely affect normal cardiac physiology. Perhaps the most well known of these is thiamine deficiency, or beriberi. This results in high-output right and left heart failure. Vitamin C deficiency, or scurvy, results in PR prolongation, ST-segment abnormalities, and dyspnea and chest pain. In China, children fed grains grown on soil deficient in selenium develop a cardiomyopathy characterized by necrosis, fibrosis, and hypercontraction bands. Supplementation of the diet with selenium prevents this disease. Vitamin A and niacin deficiencies have not been unequivocally related to diseases of the heart in man. Patients who develop severe undernutrition and who are then hyperalimented can develop a syndrome of high-output heart failure characterized by an S_3, but with normal systolic function. The psychiatric condition of anorexia nervosa has been associated with a number of cardiac abnormalities. However, the ECG is usually normal. A prolonged QT interval is seen in a small number of patients with anorexia nervosa.

536. The answer is A (1, 2, 3). *(pp 1949–1950)* Syphilitic aortic aneurysms occur most commonly in the ascending thoracic aorta and tend to be saccular or fusiform in morphology. Since syphilitic aortitis results in dense scarring of the media, true aortic dissection is uncommon. However, syphilitic aortic aneurysms may erode into the sternum or vertebral bodies and may rupture into adjacent structures, leading to rapid collapse and death.

537. The answer is C (2, 4). *(pp 1950–1951)* Angina may be due to coronary artery stenosis, which occurs as a late sequela of syphilitic aortitis. The aortitis does not extend distally along the coronary arteries beyond 1 cm. Coronary artery dissection and widespread active coronary arteritis are uncommon. Severe aortic regurgitation as a result of rupture of the sinus of Valsalva in syphilitic cardiovascular disease may also cause angina.

538. The answer is A (1, 2, 3). *(p 1963)* The management of angina pectoris in uremic patients should be tempered by the volume status since in the setting of hypervolemia, agents such as nitrates, beta blockers, and calcium antagonists may create unwanted hypotension. The hematocrit should be increased to above 30, preferably by erythropoietin and iron supplements. Treatment of angina pectoris that develops during hemodialysis includes (1) stopping the ultrafiltration, (2) reducing blood flow through the dialyzer, and (3) administering supplemental nasal oxygen. The patient should be placed in the Trendelenburg position and given intravenous saline. Sublingual nitroglycerin given in the setting of hypotension will only aggravate the condition.

539. The answer is C (2, 4). *(p 1971)* Cimetidine reduces hepatic flow and thus increases blood levels of propranolol and metoprolol, which are metabolized by the liver. Atenolol, nadolol, and sotalol are not affected by administration of cimetidine since they are not degraded by the liver.

540. The answer is D (4). *(p 1973, Table 109-2)* Combined treatment with verapamil and beta blockers leads to sinoatrial (SA) and atrioventricular (AV) nodal inhibition as well as suppression of left ventricular function by the direct effect of the two drugs. Drug levels are not affected. Cimetidine increases blood verapamil levels by a hepatic metabolic interaction. Verapamil decreases digoxin clearance, leading to digitalis toxicity, and quinidine clearance, leading to increased quinidine levels. Additional alpha-receptor inhibition leads to hypotension.

541. The answer is A (1, 2, 3). *(pp 1975–1978)*   Drugs that prolong the QT interval provide pharmacologically additive effects, which lead to torsades de pointes. These include the antiarrhythmics (i.e., quinidine, procainamide, and disopyramide), tricyclic antidepressants, thiazide diuretics (via hypokalemic effects), and sotalol. Amiodarone also leads to increased quinidine and procainamide levels. Amiodarone increases digoxin levels, thereby potentially suppressing sinoatrial (SA) node function. Digoxin does not facilitate torsades de pointes since it tends to shorten the QT interval.

542. The answers are: A-Y, B-N, C-N, D-Y, E-N. *(pp 1926–1929)*   Pericarditis occurs in about 30 percent of patients with rheumatoid arthritis. Usually the pericarditis is not symptomatic and the patient is more bothered by synovitis or pleuritis. Occasionally, large pericardial effusions may require pericardiocentesis, and constriction requiring pericardiectomy has occurred. Chronic pericarditis may occur and respond to corticosteroid therapy. Rheumatoid nodules may occasionally infiltrate the myocardium and each of the four cardiac valves. A rheumatoid nodule developing in an aortic leaflet may lead to aortic regurgitation, and perforation of the leaflet may occur if the nodule becomes necrotic. Valvular infiltration is felt to occur in about 1 to 2 percent of patients with rheumatoid arthritis. Rheumatoid myocarditis is very rare but may lead to heart failure. Ankylosing spondylitis may lead to a sclerosing inflammatory process that is limited to the aortic root extending immediately above and below the valve. This involvement of the aortic root leads to aortic regurgitation in as many as 10 percent of patients with ankylosing spondylitis. Aortic insufficiency is present in 2 percent of patients with this disease for 10 years and 10 percent of patients at 30 years. The inflammatory process may extend below the aortic valve and infiltrate the basal portion of the mitral valve, causing mitral insufficiency. Reiter's syndrome and psoriatic arthropathy may also be associated with an inflammatory process of the aortic root and lead to aortic regurgitation. The inflammatory lesion of the aortic root is clinically silent until aortic insufficiency occurs, at which point the inflammatory process has resolved. Therefore, while corticosteroids are used in iritis associated with ankylosing spondylitis, they are not useful in the treatment of aortic regurgitation.

543. The answers are: A-Y, B-N, C-Y, D-Y, E-N. *(pp 1937–1938)*   In extremely obese patients, there is both adipocyte hyperplasia and hypertrophy. In these patients, adipose tissue flow can approximate 50 percent of total resting cardiac output. Weight loss results in a decrease in adipocyte size but not number. Obesity is a health risk for hypertension, but the correlation is generally low with the best correlation seen in young men and black women. Those with a predominantly abdominal distribution of body fat have the greatest correlation with the presence of hypertension, better than relative weight or body mass. Even extremely obese patients have only a 15 percent incidence of hypertension. The incidence is much lower in moderately obese patients.

544. The answers are: A-Y, B-Y, C-Y, D-Y, E-N. *(pp 1953–1955)*   Cardiac involvement is common in the acquired immunodeficiency syndrome (AIDS). The most common abnormality is a pericardial effusion, which may be related to metastatic Kaposi's sarcoma on the pericardium. Lymphocytic infiltration in the myocardium is commonly seen and may result in a left ventricular cardiomyopathy. Nonbacterial thrombotic endocarditis is occasionally seen and may result in systemic embolization. The most common cause of death in patients with AIDS is respiratory failure and infection; cardiac involvement causes death in less than 5 percent of patients.

XIV. Miscellaneous Causes of Heart Disease

DIRECTIONS: Each question below contains five suggested responses. Select the **one best** response to each question.

545. All the following statements regarding carcinoid heart disease are true EXCEPT

(A) the primary cardiac manifestations are pulmonic insufficiency and tricuspid stenosis

(B) a holosystolic murmur increasing in intensity with inspiration associated with a diastolic flow rumble are common physical findings

(C) echocardiography often reveals distinctive findings

(D) the carcinoid syndrome is most often associated with ileal carcinoid

(E) a *v* wave with distended neck veins, a parasternal heave, and multinodular irregularity of the liver are clinical features that may be seen

546. Cardiac manifestations of left atrial myxoma include all the following EXCEPT

(A) a low-pitched apical diastolic murmur

(B) an early diastolic low-pitched sound, occurring later than an opening snap

(C) a faint first heart sound (S_1)

(D) a rapid *y* descent in the pulmonary capillary wedge tracing

(E) a large *v* wave in the pulmonary capillary wedge tracing

547. The cardiomyopathy seen with doxorubicin is best characterized by which statement?

(A) Significant increases in QRS voltage often indicate the onset

(B) A total dose of over 550 mg/m² is associated with a high incidence

(C) Preexisting heart disease does not appear to increase the incidence

(D) Prior radiation therapy does not increase the incidence

(E) Most patients improve clinically with discontinuation of doxorubicin

548. The cardiovascular effects of electrical injuries including lightning are best characterized by which of the following statements?

(A) The path of the electrical current (entry to exit sites) is not important in determining the cardiac effects

(B) Evidence of myocardial damage is very unusual

(C) Both significant left ventricular dysfunction and a return to normal ventricular function can be seen following successful recovery of the patient

(D) Despite catecholamine release following the injury, hypertension and tachycardia are not seen

(E) Direct current even of low voltage is of greater hazard than an alternating current because of the "let go" phenomenon

549. All the following statements regarding penetrating cardiac injuries are true EXCEPT

  (A) over 50 percent of patients succumb shortly after injury
  (B) recurrent post-traumatic pericarditis occurs in approximately 20 percent of cases
  (C) the treatment of missiles in the heart is surgical removal irrespective of the clinical situation
  (D) delayed sequelae include the formation of ventricular aneurysm
  (E) traumatic arteriovenous fistulas can be complicated by a bacterial endarteritis

550. Penetrating wounds of the free cardiac wall usually involve the

  (A) right atrium
  (B) right ventricle
  (C) left atrium
  (D) left ventricle
  (E) interventricular septum

DIRECTIONS: Each question below contains four suggested responses of which **one or more** is correct. Select

A	if	**1, 2, and 3**	are correct
B	if	**1 and 3**	are correct
C	if	**2 and 4**	are correct
D	if	**4**	is correct
E	if	**1, 2, 3, and 4**	are correct

551. Cardiac effects of the tricyclic antidepressants include

(1) orthostatic hypotension
(2) prolongation of the QT interval
(3) mild depression of left ventricular function
(4) mild decrease in heart rate

552. The effects of oral contraceptives that may increase the incidence of myocardial infarction include

(1) changes in lipid metabolism
(2) increased incidence of hypertension
(3) hypercoagulability
(4) coronary spasm

553. Cardiac effects of cocaine include

(1) enhancement of the myocardial sodium channel
(2) increase in the release of and blocking of the reuptake of catecholamines
(3) a direct positive inotropic effect on the myocardium
(4) coronary vasoconstriction of both diseased and nondiseased coronary artery segments

554. The cardiac effects of caffeine cause

(1) a sympathomimetic amine effect on the heart
(2) an increase in heart rate
(3) an increase in blood pressure
(4) an antiarrhythmic effect on the heart

555. Correct statements regarding cardiac contusion from nonpenetrating injuries include which of the following?

(1) Hemopericardium invariably causes cardiac tamponade
(2) Patients are frequently asymptomatic
(3) Coronary thrombosis is a common complicating factor
(4) Patients may have all the clinical features of a well-developed myocardial infarction

556. Correct statements regarding traumatic rupture of the aorta include which of the following?

(1) The most common sites of rupture are the aortic isthmus and the ascending aorta just proximal to the origin of the brachiocephalic arteries
(2) It is the second most common blunt injury to the great vessels
(3) About 20 percent of patients survive the original injury
(4) Common clinical manifestations include hypertension of the upper and lower extremities and superior vena cava syndrome

DIRECTIONS: Each question below contains five suggested responses. For **each** of the **five** responses listed with every question you are to respond either YES (Y) or NO (N). In a given item **all, some, or none of the alternatives may be correct.**

557. Correct statements regarding malignancies of the heart include which of the following?

  (A) Pulmonary embolism is most likely responsible for the distended neck veins in a patient who has undergone pericardial effusion

  (B) Atrial arrhythmias secondary to metastatic disease to the heart do not respond to conventional therapy

  (C) Patients who have received mediastinal irradiation are at increased risk for the development of coronary artery disease

  (D) Effective therapy for malignant pericardial effusion may include instillation of steroids into the pericardial space

  (E) Renal cell carcinoma extending into the inferior vena cava may mimic pericardial constriction

558. Correct statements regarding cardiac myxomas include which of the following?

  (A) Most cardiac myxomas are located in the left atrium

  (B) Myxomas usually originate from the atrioventricular (AV) groove

  (C) Children have a higher incidence of ventricular myxomas than adults

  (D) Constitutional symptoms and systemic illness with myxoma are rare

  (E) A "tumor plop" is a systolic sound that can resemble an ejection click

559. Correct statements regarding benign primary cardiac tumors include which of the following?

  (A) The most frequent cardiac tumor in children is a rhabdomyoma

  (B) Sudden death can occur in patients with intracardiac fibromas, primarily because of arrhythmias, outflow obstruction, or conduction system involvement

  (C) Papillary fibroelastoma most commonly occurs on the mitral valve

  (D) Mesothelioma of the atrioventricular (AV) node can cause sudden death and is more common in women

  (E) Rhabdomyomas are usually solitary and most often involve the atrial endocardium

XIV. Miscellaneous Causes of Heart Disease

Answers

545. The answer is A. *(pp 2021–2023)* Primary ileal carcinoids frequently metastasize to the liver and produce the carcinoid syndrome. The metastatic tumor releases products that create a distinctive endocardial and valvular pathological pattern. 5-Hydroxytryptamine (5-HT) secreted by the carcinoid tumor and bradykinin have been implicated in the pathogenesis of the cardiac lesions. Glistening white-yellow deposits are found on the pulmonary and tricuspid valves and to varying degrees on the right atrial and ventricular endocardium. Contraction of these deposits leads predominantly to pulmonary stenosis and tricuspid insufficiency and occasionally produces a restrictive type of myopathy. A harsh holosystolic murmur at the lower left sternal border that increases with inspiration is often heard, connoting tricuspid regurgitation. When the tricuspid regurgitation is significant, a diastolic flow rumble may be heard. Distended neck veins with a *v* wave that increases with inspiration also may be seen due to the tricuspid regurgitation. An upper left sternal systolic ejection murmur may be heard due to relative pulmonic stenosis. A parasternal heave is common, reflecting right ventricular volume overload, and a multinodular liver may be indicative of hepatic metastases. Echocardiography reveals right ventricular volume overload. The tricuspid valve is typically thickened, retracted, and fixed in a semiopen position; thus, regurgitation is common.

546. The answer is C. *(p 2010)* The clinical features of left atrial myxoma may mimic the features of mitral stenosis. Left atrial myxomas may obstruct either the mitral valve orifice or the pulmonary venous orifice, causing pulmonary hypertension and right-sided heart failure. Dyspnea on exertion, paroxysmal nocturnal dyspnea, and acute pulmonary edema may occur. Syncope or sudden death may be caused by prolapse of the tumor across the mitral valve with a profound decrease in cardiac output. Recumbancy may relieve dyspnea by changing the position of the myxoma. The "tumor plop" is an early diastolic low-pitched sound that occurs later than an opening snap but earlier than a third heart sound (S_3) and occurs when the tumor prolapses into the left ventricle. It may be distinguished from an opening snap because of its low frequency. The first heart sound (S_1) is generally loud and frequently split. The second component of S_1 corresponds with the expulsion of the tumor from the mitral orifice. Additionally, the pulmonic component of S_2 is increased when pulmonary hypertension exists. An apical systolic murmur may be heard when mitral regurgitation occurs with systolic expulsion of the tumor mass from the left ventricle to left atrium. A diastolic flow rumble may be heard because the tumor mass obstructs normal flow from the left atrium to the left ventricle in diastole. A rapid *y* descent may be noted in the pulmonary capillary wedge tracing due to the sudden decrease in left atrial volume when the tumor prolapses into the left ventricle. A large *v* wave may also be noted in the pulmonary capillary wedge tracing even in the absence of mitral regurgitation. This reflects the inability of the left atrium to accommodate the normal reflux of pulmonary venous blood due to the space-occupying effect of the myxoma.

547. The answer is B. *(pp 1991–1992)* Doxorubicin is a very common chemotherapeutic agent. Though electrocardiographic (ECG) changes may occur during the course of therapy, an increase in QRS voltage has not been reliably described. If anything, a reduction in QRS voltage has been used as a predictor of cardiomyopathy, but this too is unreliable. Cardiomyopathy is a very serious cardiotoxic effect. With doses of 430 mg/m^2, there is a 14 percent incidence of clinical congestive heart failure (CHF). A total dose of over 550 mg/m^2 is associated with an incidence of left ventricular dysfunction of up to 30 percent. Factors that may increase the chance of cardiomyopathy, even with lower doses, include prior radiation therapy, preexisting heart disease, hypertension, and associated use of other chemotherapeutic agents. A higher incidence is also noted in young children and other adults. The clinical presentation of doxorubicin cardiomyopathy is similar to that of idiopathic dilated cardiomyopathy. The clinical course is variable, but only a few patients improve and regress with medical therapy. The value of radionuclide determination of left ventricular ejection fraction at rest and with exercise has been reported. Serial determinations of ejection fraction may allow for higher doses without additional risk of CHF.

548. The answer is C. *(pp 1997–1999)* The path of electrical current through the body (entry to exit sites) is very important in determining the cardiac and central nervous system (CNS) effects of electricity. A current path from arm to arm or arm to leg is more likely to cause direct cardiac effects. Extensive body surface burns are also a predictor of myocardial damage. Electrocardiographic (ECG) changes, cardiac arrhythmias, and myocardial damage are common findings. Sinus tachycardia and nonspecific ST-segment and T-wave changes are also common findings. The catecholamine release often produces hypertension and tachycardia and can be successfully managed with intravenous beta-blocking drugs. Despite this, patients may develop significant left ventricular dysfunction. A number may return to near normal myocardial function with successful recovery. An alternating current, regardless of the voltage, is more hazardous than a direct current because tetanic muscle contractions prevent the "let-go" phenomenon.

549. The answer is C. *(pp 2031–2033)* Over 50 percent of victims with penetrating cardiac trauma succumb shortly after injury. The treatment of missiles to the heart depends on the clinical situation. Symptomatic missiles should be removed. Missiles that are free or partially protruding in a left cardiac chamber should be removed because they could embolize to the systemic circulation. Missiles in the right side of the heart may either be removed or left to embolize in the pulmonary vascular bed from which they can be easily retrieved. Intramyocardial or intrapericardial bullets or pellets are generally tolerated well and may be left in place. A missile that has embolized to the systemic circulation should be surgically removed without delay unless it has resulted in a significant neurologic deficit. Delayed sequelae may include ventricular or atrial septal defect; ventricular aneurysms; injury to valve cup, leaflets, or chordae tendineae; and recurrent post-traumatic pericarditis, which can occur in about 20 percent of penetrating cardiac injuries. Traumatic arteriovenous fistulas can be complicated by a bacterial endarteritis and endocarditis. They should be repaired as soon as possible after detection.

550. The answer is B. *(pp 2031–2032)* Most commonly, a single, free cardiac wall penetrating wound involves the right ventricle. In general, the relative frequency of such wounds is related to the area of exposure of the cardiac wall to the anterior chest wall. In decreasing order of frequency, the structures affected are the right ventricle, left ventricle, right atrium, and left atrium.

551. The answer is A (1, 2, 3). *(pp 1989–1990)* There are several cardiac side effects of the tricyclic antidepressants; despite these, however, they can often be used safely in patients with cardiovascular disease. A slight increase in heart rate is common and may persist even after discontinuation of therapy. This is usually a mild increase in heart rate and rarely exceeds 100 beats per minute. Orthostatic hypotension is a very common side effect. Several electrocardiographic (ECG) changes can be seen. These include prolongation of the QT interval, the PR interval, the QRS duration, and nonspecific ST-segment and T-wave changes. Depression of left ventricular function is very mild. Despite this, in patients with underlying ventricular dysfunction, these drugs should be used cautiously.

552. The answer is E (all). *(pp 1992–1993)* The incidence of myocardial infarction in premenopausal women is rare, but this risk is reportedly three to four times greater in patients on oral contraceptives. This risk appears to be greatest in women who are also cigarette smokers. Possible effects of oral contraceptives that might increase the risk of myocardial infarction include changes in lipid metabolism, decrease in glucose tolerance, relationship to hypertension, association with hypercoagulability, and possible implication in precipitating coronary spasm.

553. The answer is C (2, 4). *(pp 1993–1994)* Cocaine blocks the fast sodium (Na+) channel in the myocardium, producing a depression of depolarization and a slowing of conduction velocity; this causes a direct negative inotropic effect on the myocardium. Cocaine blocks the reuptake of catecholamines and increases the release of catecholamines. It also causes vasoconstriction of both nondiseased and diseased coronary artery segments. This is more pronounced in coronary segments already compromised by coronary atherosclerosis. It also produces significant constriction of smaller coronary microvessels. These effects on the coronary vessels may be inhibited by nitroglycerin or calcium blocking drugs. Electrocardiographic (ECG) effects of cocaine include prolongation of the PR, QRS, and QT intervals.

554. The answer is A (1, 2, 3). *(p 1995)* Caffeine has a sympathomimetic amine effect on the cardiovascular system. Acute administration causes an increase in blood pressure and heart rate. Caffeine is thought to have an arrhythmogenic effect on the heart. The relationship between caffeine use and coronary artery disease remains controversial. Caffeine toxicity causes marked catecholamine release and may be associated with tachyarrhythmias.

555. The answer is C (2, 4). *(pp 2033–2034)* Patients with contusion of the heart from nonpenetrating injuries are frequently asymptomatic, but they may complain of pain that is similar to that experienced with myocardial ischemia or infarction. Coronary thrombosis may result from nonpenetrating trauma, but this is a rare occurrence. Hemopericardium, with or without signs or symptoms of cardiac tamponade, may be associated with myocardial contusion. Creatine phosphokinase (CPK) elevation associated with electrocardiographic (ECG) manifestations of ST-segment or Q-wave changes is a diagnostic aid in patients with cardiac contusion. However, other causes must be excluded before these changes are attributed to cardiac contusion.

556. The answer is B (1, 3). *(p 2035)* Rupture of the aorta is the most common blunt injury of the great vessels. The most common sites of rupture of the aorta from blunt injury are the descending aorta just distal to the origin of the left subclavian artery (aortic isthmus) and the ascending aorta just proximal to the origin of the brachiocephalic artery. Only about 20 percent of patients with aortic rupture survive the original injury. False aneurysm is formed in these patients at the site of rupture. Common clinical manifestations of traumatic rupture of the aorta are chest pain, a new murmur, increased pulse amplitude, and hypertension of the upper extremities. Hoarseness, evidence of superior vena cava syndrome, and paraplegia are rare manifestations.

557. The answers are: A-N, B-Y, C-Y, D-N, E-Y. *(pp 2019–2021)* Pericardial effusion and tamponade may be the first manifestations of cardiac involvement by a malignancy. The persistence of neck vein distention after withdrawal of pericardial fluid is most often the result of constrictive physiology from a tumor mass encroaching on the heart. Atrial arrhythmias are common with metastatic cardiac disease with invasion of the atrium; the atrial flutter or fibrillation that results from this process are usually resistant to medical therapy. Ventricular arrhythmias or conduction disturbances may result from myocardial tumor invasion. In patients with malignant disease, angina or myocardial infarction may result from tumor embolization or compression of a coronary artery by tumor. Additionally, patients who have received radiation to the mediastinum may develop coronary fibrosis or accelerated atherogenesis leading to myocardial infarction. Malignant pericardial effusion usually recurs rapidly after pericardiocentesis. Radiation of the cardiac area may be effective if the tumor is radiosensitive. Malignant effusions may be drained, and intrapericardial administrations of 5-fluorouracil, radioactive gold, nitrogen mustard, or tetracycline have all been effective in temporarily diminishing the reaccumulation of fluid. Extension of tumors, such as renal cell carcinoma, along the inferior vena cava and into the right atrium can present as intracavitary obstructive masses. Right atrial and tricuspid obstruction may mimic constriction from tumor invasion or previous radiation to the mediastinum.

558. The answers are: A-Y, B-N, C-Y, D-N, E-N. *(pp 2007–2011)*   Primary tumors of the heart are less common than metastatic tumors, but myxomas are the most common of all primary tumors of the heart. Approximately 75 percent are located in the left atrium, although rarely (4 percent) myxoma can involve the right or left ventricle. Typically they originate from the fossa ovalis but can, on rare occasions, arise from the mitral valve, inferior vena cava, or the mitral annulus. There seems to be a higher incidence of women with myxomas in most series, and children have a higher incidence of ventricular myxomas than adults. Most patients present with a group of constitutional, embolic, or obstructive symptoms. Most affected patients present with weight loss, fever, fatigue, an elevated sedimentation rate, and increased serum immunoglobulins. Occasionally a hemolytic anemia can occur. Physical examination can reveal a loud first heart sound (S_1). An early diastolic sound called a "tumor plop" is heard just after the aortic closure sound and can be confused with a mitral valve opening snap or a third heart sound (S_3).

559. The answers are: A-Y, B-Y, C-N, D-Y, E-N. *(pp 2014–2016)*   Rhabdomyoma is the most frequent benign cardiac tumor in children and probably represents a hamartoma rather than a true neoplasm. They typically are multiple and more commonly involve the ventricular myocardium. Tuberous sclerosis is present in one-third of patients. Fibromas also occur more commonly in the ventricle and frequently are calcified. Sudden death occurs in one-third of patients, presumably because of conduction system involvement, arrhythmias, or outflow obstruction. Papillary fibroelastomas are usually found on the valves; however, there is a predilection for the aortic valve. Coronary ostial occlusion by the tumor can cause angina and sudden cardiac death. The high sensitivity of transesophageal echocardiogram (TEE) has led to an increased frequency in the diagnosis of papillary fibroelastomas. Mesothelioma is the smallest tumor capable of producing sudden death, usually by complete heart block or ventricular fibrillation. Although the tumor can occur in all ages, there seems to be a strong preponderance among women. Most patients with mesothelioma of the atrioventricular (AV) node demonstrate complete heart block and have recurrent Stokes-Adams attacks. This tumor should be suspected in all cases of sudden death without apparent cause, especially in children and young adults.

XV. Special Physiological Conditions and the Cardiovascular System

DIRECTIONS: Each question below contains five suggested responses. Select the **one best** response to each question.

560. In a pregnant woman, an in-depth search for underlying heart disease should be undertaken if on physical examination there is

(A) pedal edema
(B) a third heart sound (S_3)
(C) a grade 2/6 systolic murmur
(D) a grade 2/6 diastolic murmur
(E) a mammary soufflé

561. In view of the markedly increased incidence of mortality and morbidity, pregnancy should be absolutely contraindicated in patients with

(A) atrial septal defect, secundum variety
(B) atrial septal defect, primum variety
(C) mitral valve prolapse syndrome
(D) pulmonary hypertension
(E) coarctation of the aorta

562. Cardiovascular agents that do not cross the placental barrier include

(A) digitoxin
(B) acebutolol
(C) verapamil
(D) hydralazine
(E) heparin

563. If pregnancy occurs in a woman who has a mechanical prosthetic valve and requires full anticoagulation, the most appropriate regimen throughout the pregnancy would be to

(A) stop warfarin and treat with low-dose subcutaneous heparin
(B) stop warfarin and treat with full-dose subcutaneous heparin
(C) stop warfarin and treat with full-dose subcutaneous heparin during the first two trimesters, then stop heparin and resume warfarin in the last trimester
(D) stop warfarin and place on aspirin 325 mg/day and dipyridamole 75 mg three times a day
(E) reduce warfarin to 2 mg/day (mini-dose regimen) and add aspirin, 80 mg/day

564. In the cardiac evaluation of an athletically trained person, all the following findings are considered normal variants of the "athlete's heart" EXCEPT for

    (A) a first-degree atrioventricular (AV) block
    (B) periods of Möbitz I second-degree AV block
    (C) an early grade 1/6 diastolic murmur
    (D) a midgrade 2/6 systolic murmur
    (E) a third heart sound (S_3) gallop

565. During sustained static or isometric exercise, the cardiovascular physiological response in a conditioned, healthy heart may adapt by a decrease in

    (A) heart rate
    (B) cardiac output
    (C) systemic vascular resistance
    (D) stroke volume
    (E) mean arterial pressure

566. Correct statements concerning the assessment of hypertension in the elderly include which of the following?

    (A) Isolated systolic hypertension at rest may be considered abnormal
    (B) Isolated systolic hypertension during vigorous exercise may be considered abnormal
    (C) A resting and consistent diastolic blood pressure of greater than 90 mmHg but less than 100 mmHg may be considered a normal variant
    (D) Sympathetic hyperfunction is the underlying etiology of most hypertension
    (E) Beta-blockade therapy is the treatment of choice when significant hypertension is present

567. As part of a progressive age-related cardiovascular adaptation, exercise in normal elderly individuals will cause an increase in

    (A) use of the Frank-Starling mechanism
    (B) arterial vasodilatation
    (C) inotropic response
    (D) chronotropic response
    (E) response to catecholamines

568. To maintain cardiac output during exercise in the elderly, there is a decrease in

    (A) heart rate
    (B) use of the Frank-Starling mechanism
    (C) end-diastolic volume
    (D) end-systolic volume
    (E) contractility

569. In aged cardiac muscle, there is still preservation of the inotropic response to

    (A) digoxin
    (B) digitoxin
    (C) calcium
    (D) epinephrine
    (E) isoproterenol

DIRECTIONS: Each question below contains four suggested responses of which **one or more** is correct. Select

A	if	**1, 2, and 3**	are correct
B	if	**1 and 3**	are correct
C	if	**2 and 4**	are correct
D	if	**4**	is correct
E	if	**1, 2, 3, and 4**	are correct

570. The age-associated decrease in exercise capacity and the decrease in maximum rate of oxygen consumption during exercise in the normal geriatric population may be due to a

(1) direct limitation of the capability to increase cardiac output due to a geriatric myocardium
(2) decreased blood flow to skeletal muscles
(3) marked reduction of overall cardiac function
(4) variety of psychological factors

571. As a result of the aging process, the peripheral vasculature in elderly people manifests

(1) an increased compliance
(2) a preserved vasodilator response to nitrates and nitrites
(3) less tendency toward chronic structural dilatation of vessel walls
(4) a decreased vasodilator response to beta-sympathetic stimulation

572. Which of the following cardiovascular changes can occur as part of the normal process of aging?

(1) An increase in the beta-sympathetic response
(2) An increase in left ventricular mass and wall thickness
(3) A decrease in resting left ventricular function
(4) A slowed early diastolic left ventricular filling

573. During sustained or isotonic exercise, the cardiovascular physiological state adapts by an increase in

(1) heart rate
(2) systemic vascular resistance
(3) stroke volume
(4) end-systolic volume

574. Normal compensatory cardiovascular adjustments that may occur at various stages of pregnancy include

(1) an increase of plasma volume, which approaches its maximum in the second trimester
(2) a selective increase of uterine blood flow during exercise in the third trimester
(3) a fall in systemic vascular resistance in the first trimester
(4) a drop in cardiac output immediately after vaginal delivery

575. Peripartum cardiomyopathy has which of the following characteristics?

(1) It has an increased incidence among multiparous, older mothers
(2) It occurs almost exclusively in the middle of the second trimester
(3) It tends to occur in pregnancies complicated by hypertension
(4) It is an absolute contraindication for subsequent pregnancies

576. Diagnostic cardiovascular procedures that may be safely performed with minimal risk during pregnancy include

(1) a thallium exercise test
(2) a resting multigated acquisition (MUGA) scan
(3) a coronary angiography
(4) a two-dimensional echocardiogram

577. A physiological etiology for the reduced maximal aerobic capacity in women relative to men may be explained by a

(1) lower hemoglobin concentration
(2) higher blood volume
(3) higher percentage of body fat
(4) larger cross-sectional muscle mass

XV. Special Physiological Conditions and the Cardiovascular System

Answers

560. The answer is D. *(p 2044)* A variety of relatively normal physiological signs and symptoms may occur with pregnancy. Peripheral edema is found in as many as 80 percent of normal pregnant women. Pulmonary rales, visible neck vein pulsation, a third heart sound (S_3), and a systolic murmur less than grade 3/6 in intensity are not uncommon. These findings do not generally indicate significant cardiovascular disease that require an extensive cardiovascular workup. Although atrioventricular (AV) valve functional murmurs may occur with the increased cardiac output of pregnancy, a diastolic murmur is so unusual that it warrants the diagnosis of heart disease until proven otherwise. The mammary soufflé is an internal mammary flow sound that may have a diastolic component. Both the mammary soufflé and a venous hum are common in normal pregnancy and should be ruled out when a diastolic murmur is suspected.

561. The answer is D. *(p 2041, Table 113-1; pp 2045–2050, Table 113-3)* Mitral regurgitation from any cause and atrial septal defects, including both primum and secundum varieties, are generally well tolerated during pregnancy. Unless extremely unstable, pregnancy is not contraindicated in patients with these cardiovascular disorders, but they should be followed carefully throughout all trimesters and in the postpartum state. There is a relative risk during pregnancy in patients with coarctation of the aorta if blood pressure is not well controlled, but under usual circumstances, this is not an absolute contraindication for conception. Extremely elevated mortality and morbidity with pregnancy have been associated with right-to-left shunts, such as Eisenmenger's syndrome and tetralogy of Fallot, and Marfan's syndrome in association with a dilated aortic root. Pregnancy is absolutely contraindicated with these cardiovascular disease states. Pulmonary hypertension is an absolute contraindication to pregnancy regardless of the etiology and whether it is primary or secondary. The maternal mortality rate approaches 50 percent in patients with primary pulmonary hypertension and 30 to 70 percent when due to Eisenmenger's syndrome.

562. The answer is E. *(pp 2051–2052)* A great variety of cardiovascular agents cross the placental barrier. Long-term effects on the fetus and potential complications must be weighed against the necessity for therapy. Initial concerns about the theoretical possibility of beta blockers decreasing umbilical blood flow, initiating premature labor, and resulting in a small infarcted placenta have been counterbalanced by clinical experience with beta blockers in a large number of pregnant women without major adverse effects. In particular, the beta$_1$-selective agents such as acebutolol have been associated with successful, uncomplicated pregnancies. All of the calcium channel blocking agents cross the placental barrier, but verapamil is effective in managing supraventricular arrhythmias when such treatment is necessary. Vasodilator agents, such as hydralazine and the nitrate preparations, cross the placenta, but fetal tolerance appears to be high. Antiplatelet agents cross the placental barrier and may increase the incidence of bleeding. Heparin is a large molecule that does not cross the placental barrier and is the treatment of choice for patients who require full anticoagulation during pregnancy.

563. The answer is B. *(p 2051)* Warfarin derivatives cross the placental barrier and expose the fetus both to potential bleeding complications and teratogenic risk throughout pregnancy. Fetal exposure during the first 2 months of pregnancy results in a 15 to 25 percent incidence of the warfarin embryopathy syndrome, which consists of facial abnormalities, optic atrophy, digital malformations, epithelial changes, and mental impairment. The teratogenic effects of warfarin are reduced by the third trimester, but the risk of bleeding continues throughout pregnancy and during labor and delivery. In view of these significant complications, warfarin derivatives should be avoided if possible throughout pregnancy. Since heparin is a large molecule and does not cross the placental barrier, intravenous or subcutaneous heparin is the preferred alternative. Low-dose subcutaneous heparin does not adequately prevent embolic events; therefore, full-dose subcutaneous heparin is the anticoagulant of choice for home therapy during pregnancy. This generally is a subcutaneous dose every 12 hours, adjusting the doses to maintain a partial thromboplastin time (PTT) of 1.5 to 2 times normal. Placing a patient on a low-dose regimen of warfarin and aspirin is not appropriate. This still exposes the fetus to teratogenic effects and bleeding complications, and effective anticoagulation would not be achieved. Stopping warfarin and placing the patient on aspirin and dipyridamole also creates an ineffective anticoagulant regimen and still exposes the developing fetus to antiplatelet agents, which cross the placental barrier and may increase bleeding.

564. The answer is C. *(pp 2063–2064)* A third heart sound (S_3) and a fourth heart sound (S_4) may be heard in approximately 50 percent of trained athletes. A systolic heart murmur may be heard in approximately 40 percent of endurance athletes and is usually an ejection type heard best over the pulmonic or aortic area. Short, quiet ejection murmurs in midsystole are quite common, presumably reflecting a large stroke volume. Diastolic murmurs are rarely, if ever, caused by exercise training and warrant further study as they indicate underlying cardiac disease until proven otherwise. A variety of electrocardiographic (ECG) findings may be evident in athletes. First degree atrioventricular (AV) block may be found in approximately 20 percent of athletes, and even periods of Möbitz I second-degree AV block may be observed. The abnormalities are presumably vagally mediated, as these conduction variations disappear with exercise or atropine administration.

565. The answer is D. *(pp 2059–2060)* The normal cardiovascular physiological response to isometric or static exercise is to increase systemic vascular resistance. This is mediated by a local pressor response and is exacerbated by mechanical compression of resistance vessels due to sustained muscle contraction. Thus, mean arterial pressure increases, venous return may decrease, and stroke volume will actually fall. As a response to this, the heart adapts by increasing the heart rate to increase cardiac output. Static or isometric exercise may be thought of as a pressure or systolic load in contradistinction to dynamic or isotonic exercise, which is a volume or diastolic load.

566. The answer is A. *(p 2072)* Although aging is associated with an increase in arterial stiffness and a decrease in sympathetic arterial vasodilatory response, significant systolic hypertension at rest should be considered abnormal and an indication for treatment. Isolated systolic hypertension during exercise may be considered a normal adaptation. Any diastolic pressure consistently greater than 90 mmHg is abnormal and should be treated. Sympathetic hyperfunction is more often associated with hypertension in the young, and for that matter, beta-blockade therapy is the treatment of choice in the young age-group. In the elderly, on the other hand, because of a decrease in beta-sympathetic responsiveness, beta-blockade therapy is less effective, and vasodilator agents should be considered first.

567. The answer is A. *(p 2068)* The ability of the cardiac muscle to develop tension is well maintained in elderly people as is the inotropic response of the muscle to direct stimulation of the myofibrils with calcium (Ca^{2+}). However, with beta-sympathetic stimulation as with exercise, there is a decreased inotropic response, decreased arterial vasodilating response, and decreased chronotropic response. With left ventricular loading induced by exercise and other causes, there is enhanced use of the Frank-Starling mechanism to compensate for the increased work load and lower inotropic state.

568. The answer is D. *(p 2072)*   The basic factors used to maintain cardiac output in the face of stepwise increases in exercise are the same for both young adult and early age-groups. The difference is in the degree to which each factor is used. An increase in heart rate, an increase in inotropic response, and a reduction in impedance are all used in the elderly during exercise, but to a lesser extent than in the young adult. Proportionately, the Frank-Starling mechanism is used to a greater extent as a compensatory device in the elderly. This is reflected by a progressive increase in end-diastolic volume with stress and a decrease in end-systolic volume. Because of these balanced compensatory factors in all age-groups, cardiac output response to exercise is unchanged at any given level of work load in human beings from 20 to 80 years of age.

569. The answer is C. *(p 2069)*   In animal models of aging, studies on isolated cardiac muscle show a striking decrease in the response of tissues to inotropic factors such as catecholamines or digitalis glycosides. The inotropic response of cardiac muscle to calcium and the response of myofibrils upon direct exposure to calcium following chemical removal of the cell membrane are well maintained with age.

570. The answer is C (2, 4). *(p 2071)*   Although no study to date has clearly identified the factors that limit exercise capability in normal aging human beings, the age-associated reduction is not due to a straightforward limitation of the ability to increase cardiac output as a result of a marked reduction of overall cardiac function. Other possible mechanisms that may explain this decrease are increased work of breathing or overall decrease in pulmonary function; decreased blood flow to skeletal muscles; alterations in metabolism of skeletal muscle or a sensation of fatigue; psychological factors; and indirect mechanisms whereby the physiological alterations of geriatric cardiac function lead to an increased sense of fatigue or increased respiratory demands.

571. The answer is C (2, 4). *(p 2070)*   The arterial wall has increased intrinsic stiffness with age and, thus, has less compliance. Age-associated dilatation, particularly of the aorta, occurs. There is a distinct age-related decrease in the vasodilator response to beta-sympathetic stimulation. On the other hand, the response to other vasodilator agents, such as nitrates or nitrites, is relatively well maintained with age.

572. The answer is C (2, 4). *(pp 2068–2069)*   Age-related cardiovascular changes are numerous and include a marked decrease in the response to stimulation of beta-sympathetic receptors of cardiovascular tissues. This results in a decreased inotropic response of the cardiac muscle, a decreased arterial vasodilating response, and a decreased heart rate. There is, however, an enhanced use of the Frank-Sarling mechanism to compensate for the increased work load and lower inotropic state. Overall, noninvasive studies have shown a preservation of the resting left ventricular function. Left ventricular mass and wall thickness increase and diastolic volume is maintained. However, there is evidence of prolonged relaxation during diastole and therefore slowed early diastolic left ventricular filling.

573. The answer is B (1, 3). *(pp 2057–2059)*   The earliest hemodynamic response to acute isotonic or dynamic exercise is a marked vasodilation of the resistance vessels in the exercising muscles, which eventually results in a fall in systemic vascular resistance. Afterload falls, and the cardiac output is redistributed to the working muscles. The most striking factor in isotonic exercise is an increase in heart rate mediated by sympathetic stimulation. Overall, there is an increase in venous return, leading to an increase in end-diastolic volume and stroke volume. In addition, with acute exercise, most researchers have reported an independent increase in inotropism, manifested by a decrease in end-systolic volume, an increase in maximum dP/dt and an increase in fractional shortening. In its pure state, dynamic or isotonic exercise may be thought of as a volume or diastolic load, whereas static or isometric exercise is a pressure or systolic load. Dynamic exercise, thus, stresses the entire cardiovascular system as a result of increases in cardiac output or V_{O_2} in contradistinction to static exercise.

574. The answer is B (1, 3). *(pp 2042–2044)*   During pregnancy, plasma volume begins to increase as early as 6 weeks after conception, approaches its maximum in the second trimester, and increases overall by approximately 1.5 times normal by the time of delivery. Cardiac output increases early in pregnancy mainly due to an increase in stroke volume. This increase in cardiac output is accompanied by a fall in systemic vascular resistance, which occurs early in pregnancy and is associated with a slight fall in mean arterial blood pressure, which returns to the level of the nonpregnant state before delivery. Uterine blood flow increases by 50 to 100 mL/min over baseline by the end of the first trimester and peaks at 200 mL/min at term. However, during pregnancy, when redistribution of flow is required to serve the mother during periods of excitement, heat, exercise, or decrease in venous return, uterine blood flow preferentially decreases. It is not apparent that this transient diveresion during exercise has any permanent detrimental effect on the baby and should not deter a pregnant woman from participation in a reasonable exercise program. Immediately after vaginal delivery, cardiac output may increase as much as 60 to 80 percent. With a cesarean section, there may be an initial transient decrease in cardiac output.

575. The answer is B (1, 3). *(p 2050)* The specific etiology of peripartum cardiomyopathy is unknown. It occurs almost exclusively in the third trimester or in the first 6 postpartum weeks. This timing suggests some aspect of pregnancy as an etiologic or initiating agent. In the United States, peripartum cardiomyopathy is more common in black women, especially those who are multiparous, older, or pregnant with twins, and whose pregnancy is complicated by hypertension. The prognosis is good if heart size returns to normal within 6 months. If ventricular function returns to normal after pregnancy, a subsequent safe pregnancy is possible but mortality and morbidity still approach 10 percent and should be considered relative contraindications. In women whose ventricular function does not return to normal, subsequent pregnancies are associated with an exacerbation of disease and a maternal mortality rate approaching 50 percent.

576. The answer is D (4). *(p 2053)* All roentgenographic procedures, including radionuclide studies, should be avoided during pregnancy, particularly in the early phases. Even though many radioisotopes theoretically bind to albumin and do not cross the placental barrier, separation may occur and fetal exposure is possible. Cardiac ultrasound is of no known risk to the fetus and may be safely performed during pregnancy. Nevertheless, it should be reserved for clinical indications.

577. The answer is B (1, 3). *(p 2063)* In general, the physiological responses and adaptations of women to exercise are qualitatively similar to those seen in men. However, women may have up to 50 percent reduced maximal aerobic capacity compared to men. Part of this difference is secondary to the higher percentage of body fat in women. When V_{O_2max} is adjusted to lean body mass, this maximal aerobic capacity difference is reduced to approximately 10 to 15 percent. This is a reflection of true gender-specific differences in oxygen transport and delivery since women have a lower hemoglobin concentration and a smaller blood volume than men in addition to a smaller cross-sectional muscle mass. Ironically, the capacity to perform isotonic exercise as measured by time to muscle fatigue is probably greater in women than in men. This may be due to the possibility that estrogen results in preferential use of fatty acids as substrate during exercise with a relative sparing of glycogen stores.

XVI. Emotions and the Cardiovascular System

DIRECTIONS: Each question below contains four suggested responses of which **one or more** is correct. Select

A	if	**1, 2, and 3**	are correct
B	if	**1 and 3**	are correct
C	if	**2 and 4**	are correct
D	if	**4**	is correct
E	if	**1, 2, 3, and 4**	are correct

578. Stress has been proved to be associated with

(1) acute rise in blood pressure
(2) silent ischemia
(3) elevated lipids
(4) sustained hypertension

579. Examples of iatrogenic cardiac problems and disability include which of the following?

(1) Recognized side effects of a prescribed drug
(2) Misinterpretation of the electrocardiogram (ECG)
(3) Constrictive pericarditis secondary to radiation treatment
(4) Conversion of a sedentary cardiac patient into an exercise fanatic

580. Correct statements regarding panic attacks include which of the following?

(1) The age of onset of panic disorder is uniform and unimodal with a peak in the twenties
(2) Of the victims of panic disorder, 75 to 80 percent are women
(3) Symptoms of panic attack include chest pain, nausea, numbness, dizziness, shortness of breath, and a fear of dying
(4) Classes of medications that may be effective for treating panic disorder include benzodiazepines, tricyclic antidepressants, and monoamine oxidase (MAO) inhibitors

XVI. Emotions and the Cardiovascular System

Answers

578. The answer is A (1, 2, 3). *(pp 2087–2089)* Animal and human data conclude that stress can acutely elevate blood pressure, but it has not yet been proved to be related to sustained hypertension. Cholesterol levels rise in medical students taking examinations, in soldiers during training, and in patients anticipating surgery. A stress interview can raise lipid levels by 159 percent. The effect of stress, even mathematical calculation, is well established in the literature of silent ischemia. Vulnerability to ventricular fibrillation is increased experimentally by catecholamine infusion as well as by placing dogs in cages in which they were previously shocked.

579. The answer is E (all). *(pp 2109–2111)* Iatrogenic heart disease is usually defined as physician-induced heart disease. The term is generally accepted when referring to a complication of a procedure or a drug, recognizing that an "error" may not have always occurred. Thus, the expanded definition now includes unwanted side effects of drugs or procedures, misinterpretation of clinical data, patients' reactions to comments by physicians or other members of the health team, or patient fanaticism induced by well-intentioned rehabilitation efforts.

580. The answer is E (all). *(pp 2100–2104)* Panic attacks have been described as early as the 1800s. Since then, many different terms have been used to describe this syndrome including "irritable heart" syndrome, neurasthenia, anxiety neurosis, and "hyperdynamic β-adrenergic circulatory state." The age of onset of panic disorder is distributed uniformly and unimodally with a peak incidence in the twenties. It rarely starts before the age of 15 or after the age of 40. Most (75 to 80 percent) of the victims are women. Panic attacks occur regardless of educational status, ethnic background, or social status. Symptoms include nausea, dizziness, numbness, dyspnea, chest pain, and a fear of dying. Appropriate treatment includes the benzodiazepines, tricyclic antidepressants, and monoamine oxidase (MAO) inhibitors.

XVII. Environmental Factors and the Cardiovascular System

DIRECTIONS: Each question below contains five suggested responses. Select the **one best** response to each question.

581. High-altitude pulmonary edema (HAPE) is best characterized by which of the following statements?

(A) People with normal cardiopulmonary systems do not develop HAPE

(B) HAPE may develop at altitudes between 2000 and 8000 ft above sea level

(C) HAPE occurs in 100 to 1000 per 10,000 persons ascending rapidly to above 8000 ft

(D) HAPE is a form of noncardiac pulmonary edema

(E) Most people ascending to high altitudes develop some degree of pulmonary problems

582. The cardiac response to heat and cold stress is best characterized by which of the following statements?

(A) Angina occurs at similar work loads in cold and more temperate environments

(B) In patients with coronary artery disease, the cold presser test produces an increase in coronary blood flow

(C) Sweating is an important response that regulates thermal balance to excessive cold

(D) During heat stress, the skin may receive over 50 percent of the cardiac output

(E) At rest, cardiac output mildly decreases during periods of heat stress

DIRECTIONS: Each question below contains four suggested responses of which **one or more** is correct. Select

A	if	**1, 2, and 3**	are correct
B	if	**1 and 3**	are correct
C	if	**2 and 4**	are correct
D	if	**4**	is correct
E	if	**1, 2, 3, and 4**	are correct

583. Adjustments of cardiovascular performance to altitude include

(1)   an immediate increase in resting heart rate

(2)   a 25 percent decrease in stroke volume during the first week

(3)   unchanged myocardial contractility

(4)   increased end-diastolic volume

584. The decrease in stroke volume at high altitudes is due to a

(1)   decrease in myocardial contractility

(2)   decrease in plasma volume

(3)   increase in afterload of the left ventricle

(4)   decrease in venous return

585. Diving leads to which of the following physiological responses?

(1)   Increased central blood volume

(2)   Natriuresis

(3)   Aldosterone suppression

(4)   Increased atrial natriuretic peptide

586. Decompression sickness is most likely to occur

(1)   with severe exercise

(2)   after prolonged hyperbaric exposure

(3)   in obese people

(4)   with preexisting vascular disease

DIRECTIONS: The group of questions below consists of lettered headings followed by a set of numbered items. For each numbered item select the **one** lettered heading with which it is **most** closely associated. Each lettered heading may be used **once, more than once, or not at all.**

Questions 587–590

For each occupational exposure listed below, select the cardiovascular risk most likely to be associated with it.

(A)   Rebound vasospasm, leading to myocardial ischemia and death
(B)   Increased blood levels of carboxyhemoglobin
(C)   Hypersensitivity reactions
(D)   Cholinesterase inhibition
(E)   Increased left ventricular ejection fraction

587. Glyceric nitrol esters

588. Hand-held vibrating tools

589. Chronic carbon monoxide exposure

590. Phosphorous insecticides

XVII. Environmental Factors and the Cardiovascular System

Answers

581. The answer is D. *(pp 2121–2122)* Most people ascending to high altitudes experience no pulmonary problems. Occasionally, certain people develop acute high-altitude pulmonary edema (HAPE). The incidence is between 1 and 10 per 10,000 people ascending rapidly to altitudes above 8000 ft. Symptoms almost always appear during the first 2 to 7 days at such altitudes. The symptoms include undue shortness of breath and sinus tachycardia. Physical examination reveals moist rales, and the patient notes fatigue. Untreated, HAPE tends to be progressive and fatal; however, recovery is prompt on descent to lower altitudes. HAPE is a form of noncardiac pulmonary edema and may occur in healthy individuals with no underlying cardiovascular or pulmonary disease. The etiology of HAPE remains a mystery. Respiratory stimulation as by metolazone (Zaroxolyn) is both a rational and effective mode of prophylaxis for HAPE.

582. The answer is D. *(pp 2122–2125)* In a cold environment ($-10°C$), patients with effort angina are more likely to develop angina at a lower work load as compared to room temperatures of $+20°C$. In addition, in a cold environment, systolic blood pressure, heart rate, and rate pressure product are significantly higher during exercise testing under cold stress. The cold presser test normally produces an increase in coronary blood flow; however, in patients with coronary artery disease, there is a paradoxical decrease in coronary blood flow. Thermal balance is modified by the responses of sweating and shivering. Sweating is the response to heat stress. The skin is very important in regulating thermal control. Normally, the skin receives 5 to 10 percent of the cardiac output; however, in periods of heat stress, the skin may receive from 50 to 70 percent of the cardiac output. Cardiac output increases during periods of heat stress.

583. The answer is A (1, 2, 3). *(pp 2117–2121)* In high altitudes, there are some immediate changes in circulatory function. Initially, with the decreased P_{O_2}, there is a hypoxic stimulation of the sympathetic nervous system, leading to an increase in heart rate. This offsets the hypoxemia and preserves oxygen transport (oxygen transport = arterial content $\times$ cardiac output). Because of the contraction of the plasma volume, end-diastolic volume and stroke volume decrease during the initial weeks of exposure to high altitude; however, myocardial contractility remains unchanged. As a result of these circulatory adjustments, cardiac output both at rest and during exercise plateaus at levels about 20 percent below the values at sea level.

584. The answer is C (2, 4). *(pp 2117–2121)* During exposure to high altitude, there is a hemoconcentration and contraction of the plasma volume, which increase the hematocrit. With this compensation, there is a diminished venous return and diminished plasma volume, which decrease the stroke volume. Intrinsic myocardial contractility is not depressed. The decreased stroke volume is not due to increases in afterload. The baseline ejection fraction remains fairly constant in patients at high altitudes.

585. The answer is E (all). *(pp 2126–2131)* Diving elicits a number of physiological changes due to factors such as increased barometric pressure and loss of body heat to the surrounding water. The most characteristic cardiovascular response to these physical forces is bradycardia. Hydrostatic pressure from immersion increases the pressure gradient across the diaphragm and decreases venous compliance in the lower extremities, a combination that increases intrathoracic blood volume. This centralization of blood distends the atria and activates mechanoreceptors, initiating the immersion response, which includes both diuretic and natriuretic components. Diuresis is prompted by suppression of antidiuretic hormone (ADH). The natriuretic mechanism is due to renin-angiotensin activity, increased release of atrial natriuretic factor, and increased release of renal prostaglandins. The central hypervolemia distends the atria and elicits the release of atrial natriuretic factor.

586. The answer is A (1, 2, 3). *(pp 2128–2129)* Decompression is defined as the elimination of nitrogen or other inert gas from the body following a decrease in ambient pressure, as with return from a deep dive or rapid ascent to a high altitude. Decompression sickness occurs primarily during rapid decompression when nitrogen dissolves in body tissues and is no longer in equilibrium with the falling barometric pressure, undergoing a change in physical state. Bubbles form within tissues and venous blood, producing diverse clinical manifestations. It appears to occur in association with severe exercise, after prolonged hyperbaric exposures, and with excessive body fat. These associations are thought to be related to increased uptake of inert gas by body tissues. Other aggravating factors include increasing age, fatigue and preexisting vascular disease, presumably related to impaired gas transport from tissues to the external environment. The clinical manifestations of decompression sickness are most likely to involve ischemia in a limb or organ. In severe cases, central nervous system (CNS) dysfunction (i.e., loss of consciousness, coma, or vertigo) cardiorespiratory distress, and asphyxia may be seen. Management of decompression sickness requires prompt recompression in a hyperbaric chamber and breathing 100 percent oxygen with short breaths. Relief occurs within a few minutes in most cases.

587–590. The answers are: 587-A, 588-E, 589-B, 590-D. *(pp 2133–2134)* Patients who work with nitroglycol can experience angina during the weekend that disappears when they return to work; sudden death has also been reported to occur during the weekend. These workers frequently have headaches on Monday and Tuesday but not during the rest of the week. Nitroglycol, which is easily absorbed through the lungs and skin, appears to cause a vasodilatory effect on the heart. During the weekend when workers are no longer exposed to nitroglycol, rebound vasospasm occurs.

Severe ischemia of the digits has occurred in machinists, welders, steel workers, miners, and lumberjacks who repeatedly use high-frequency vibratory devices such as pneumatic hammers. Changes in the industrial design of these tools has decreased the prevalence of this problem. Cardiovascular changes in these workers include increased left ventricular ejection fraction due to an increase in left ventricular end-diastolic dimension and a decreased resting heart rate.

Carboxyhemoglobin levels are known to be higher in fire fighters and steel and foundry workers, who have chronic exposure to carbon monoxide; although this exposure does not appear to cause atherosclerotic heart disease, it does increase symptoms in workers with known coronary disease.

Chemical agents enter the body by skin absorption, inhalation, and ingestion and may produce cardiovascular toxicity by impairing the oxygen-carrying capacity of blood, directly affecting the myocardium, or by cholinesterase inhibition (as with organic phosphorous insecticides) that is evidenced by parasympathetic stimulation.

XVIII. Diseases of the Great Vessels and Peripheral Vessels

DIRECTIONS: Each questi below contains five suggested responses. Select the **one best** response to each question.

591. Regarding embolic stroke, all the following are true EXCEPT

   (A) mitral annular calcification is a risk factor for developing cerebral embolic events
   (B) there are probably more patients who have cardiac embolic events than are clinically recognized
   (C) patients with myxomatous mitral valves and mitral valve prolapse are at increased risk for embolic events
   (D) approximately 5 percent of all strokes can be attributed to cardiac embolic events
   (E) atrial fibrillation is the most common cardiac cause of embolic phenomena

592. A 75-year-old man with sick sinus syndrome and recurrent atrial fibrillation presents with the sudden onset of a right hemianopia, a right hemisensory loss, and the inability to read or name colors. He is still able to write and spell. The most likely diagnosis is

   (A) embolus to the upper division of the middle cerebral artery
   (B) embolus to the lower division of the middle cerebral artery
   (C) embolus to the posterior inferior cerebellar artery
   (D) embolus to the posterior cerebral artery
   (E) digitalis toxicity

593. Neurologic complications of cardiac surgery can be devastating to patients and their families. All the following statements about this clinical problem are true EXCEPT

   (A) most strokes that occur during CABG surgery are due to the brain hypoperfusion that is common with this operation
   (B) rates of neurologic complications, including alteration of behavioral and intellectual functions, are high after cardiac surgery
   (C) stroke rates are higher for those patients undergoing CABG surgery who have high-grade carotid artery disease
   (D) severe atheromatous aortic disease, or "trash aorta," is a common source of embolic stroke in patients undergoing CABG surgery
   (E) most alterations of behavioral and intellectual function resolve completely soon after surgery is completed

594. According to the NINDS Stroke Data Bank, cardiac conditions with a strong predilection to embolization include all the following EXCEPT

   (A) valvular surgery
   (B) atrial fibrillation
   (C) mitral valve prolapse
   (D) sick sinus syndrome
   (E) cardiomyopathy

595. The characteristic pathological aortic lesion in Marfan's syndrome is

    (A) Takayasu's arteritis
    (B) Reiter's arteritis
    (C) cystic medial necrosis
    (D) annuloaortic ectasia
    (E) diffuse atherosclerosis

596. One of the most common major complications of Takayasu's disease is

    (A) a myocardial infarction
    (B) a cerebrovascular accident
    (C) an aortic rupture
    (D) an aortic dissection
    (E) congestive heart failure (CHF)

597. The most common etiology of thoracic aortic aneurysm is

    (A) Marfan's syndrome
    (B) syphilitic aortitis
    (C) systemic arterial hypertension
    (D) atherosclerosis
    (E) cystic medial necrosis

598. A patient with a single focal occlusion in the right lower extremity experiences claudication of the entire calf with exercise. The lesion is located in the

    (A) pedal vessels
    (B) tibioperoneal trunk
    (C) popliteal artery
    (D) superficial femoral
    (E) common femoral

599. The most common major complications following percutaneous transluminal angioplasty (PTA) of a peripheral or renal artery is

    (A) arteriovenous fistula
    (B) limb and kidney loss
    (C) acute tubular necrosis
    (D) thrombus and embolism formation
    (E) arterial rupture and perforation

600. A 72-year-old man whose arteriogram is shown below is likely to have all the following signs and symptoms EXCEPT

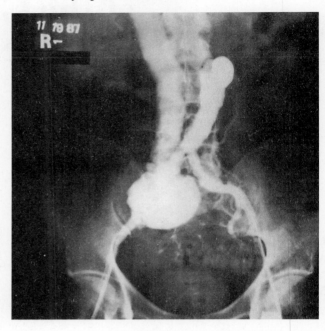

    (A) a continuous bruit in the right lower quadrant
    (B) high-output congestive heart failure (CHF)
    (C) resting claudication of both lower extremities
    (D) progressive fatigue and dyspnea
    (E) evidence of atherosclerosis elsewhere such as carotid bruits or coronary artery disease

601. Percutaneous transluminal renal angioplasty (PTRA) is generally successful in all the following clinical situations EXCEPT

    (A) unilateral fibromuscular dysplasia
    (B) bilateral fibromuscular dysplasia
    (C) ostial atherosclerotic disease
    (D) nonostial atherosclerotic disease
    (E) transplant arterial stenosis

602. Desirable pathological findings in a successful peripheral angioplasty would include all the following EXCEPT

    (A) fracture of the atheromatous plaque
    (B) dehiscence of the intima from the media
    (C) stretching of the media
    (D) adventitial deformation
    (E) incomplete tears and disruption of the media

603. The 73-year-old man in the photographs below presented with cyanotic toe pads, livoid plantar skin, and secondary livedo reticularis below the waist. The most likely diagnosis is

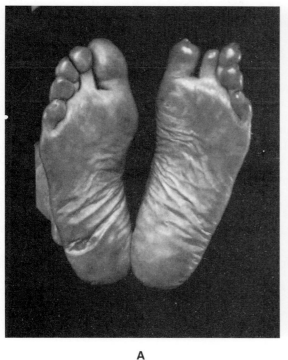 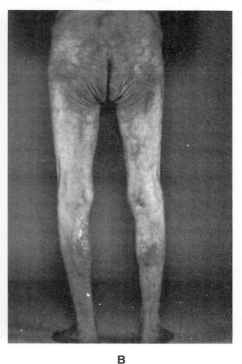

A   B

(A) ergot toxicity
(B) systemic lupus erythematosus with a circulating anticoagulant
(C) atherothrombotic microemboli
(D) thrombotic thrombocytopenia purpura
(E) heparin-induced thrombocytopenia

604. All the following statements concerning Doppler evaluation of the arterial and venous system are true EXCEPT

(A) a Doppler study ankle-arm index of less than 0.5 implies severe stenosis of a lower extremity vessel
(B) although the presence of stenosis can be determined using Doppler techniques, precise localization of obstructions is not possible by this method
(C) Doppler studies of extracranial vessels easily distinguish total occlusion from tight stenosis
(D) Doppler studies are useful in distinguishing myointimal hyperplasia from recurrent atherosclerotic plaque in patients who have undergone carotid endarterectomy
(E) Doppler ultrasound and plethysmography are sufficiently sensitive and specific for deep venous thrombosis that anticoagulant therapy may be begun or withheld on the basis of these tests

DIRECTIONS: Each question below contains four suggested responses of which **one or more** is correct. Select

A	if	**1, 2, and 3**	are correct
B	if	**1 and 3**	are correct
C	if	**2 and 4**	are correct
D	if	**4**	is correct
E	if	**1, 2, 3, and 4**	are correct

605. Surgical correction of an abdominal aortic aneurysm is indicated in

(1) asymptomatic patients with an aneurysm diameter less than 4 cm but with eggshell calcification

(2) asymptomatic patients with an aneurysm diameter of 5 cm or greater

(3) asymptomatic patients with an aneurysm diameter of less than 4 cm but affecting the renal arteries

(4) symptomatic patients with an aneurysm diameter of less than 5 cm

606. DeBakey type III aortic dissection is characterized by which of the following statements?

(1) The origin point occurs proximally to the right brachiocephalic artery

(2) Reentry channels may occur in the distal descending aorta

(3) Aortic insufficiency is a frequently related occurrence

(4) Medical therapy is the treatment of choice as long as no vascular compromise is present

607. Appropriate medical therapy in significantly hypertensive patients with acute aortic dissection may include the prompt intravenous use of

(1) hydralazine

(2) labetolol

(3) diazoxide

(4) propranolol and sodium nitroprusside

608. Mycotic aneurysms of the aortic wall may form as a result of

(1) bacterial septicemia without endocarditis

(2) infective bacterial endocarditis

(3) tuberculous infection

(4) fungal endocarditis

609. Severe atherosclerosis seems to center in the abdominal aorta and spare the ascending region with the exception of patients who have

(1) diabetes mellitus

(2) syphilitic aortitis

(3) type II hyperlipidemia

(4) type IV hyperlipidemia

610. Medical therapy of proven benefit in claudication includes

(1) vasodilator therapy

(2) nitroglycerin

(3) anticoagulation with warfarin

(4) a regular walking program

DIRECTIONS: Each question below contains five suggested responses. For **each** of the **five** responses listed with every question you are to respond either YES (Y) or NO (N). In a given item **all, some, or none of the alternatives may be correct.**

611. Correct statements concerning the surgical treatment of peripheral vascular disease include which of the following?

   (A) Symptomatic patients with carotid stenosis of 70 to 99 percent occlusion benefit from surgery
   (B) Symptomatic patients with carotid stenosis of 30 to 69 percent occlusion benefit from surgery
   (C) Asymptomatic patients with 75 to 80 percent carotid stenosis can be closely observed until symptoms occur without significant morbidity
   (D) Patients with lower extremity ischemia have an excellent prognosis and require only aspirin for long-term care
   (E) Patients requiring mesenteric revascularization are in a high-risk subgroup both for morbidity and mortality

612. Complications of phlebography include

   (A) pulmonary edema
   (B) deep venous thrombosis
   (C) renal failure
   (D) death
   (E) gangrene requiring amputation

613. The clinical application of impedance plethysmography is accurately characterized by which of the following?

   (A) It is useful for the diagnosis of below-the-knee thrombus
   (B) It is useful in patients with the nephrotic syndrome
   (C) It is accurate in the detection of proximal deep venous thrombosis
   (D) Detection of a proximal deep venous thrombosis by impedance plethysmography increases the likelihood of the subsequent development of pulmonary emboli
   (E) If impedance plethysmography does not detect a proximal deep venous thrombosis, the development of pulmonary emboli is unlikely

XVIII. Diseases of the Great Vessels and Peripheral Vessels

Answers

591. The answer is D. *(pp 2141–2162)*   Prior to the advent of echocardiography, the diagnosis of cardiac embolic disease was presumptive at best. Most careful studies of patients with strokes now attribute approximately 15 to 25 percent of all strokes to cardiac embolic phenomena. The cardiac sources can be divided into three groups: cardiac wall abnormalities (e.g., wall motion abnormalities, patent foramen ovale, tumors), valve disorders, and arrhythmias. Clearly, atrial fibrillation is the most common etiology of cardiac emboli. With the routine use of CT scans in patients with strokes, it has become obvious that many patients have subclinical embolic events. Mitral valve prolapse that is *not* associated with myxomatous valve leaflets probably does not increase a patient's risk of stroke. Mitral annular calcification has been associated with an increased risk of stroke, probably by ulceration and extrusion of calcium or thrombi from the overlapping cusps seen at autopsy.

592. The answer is D. *(pp 2142–2143)*   About 80 percent of emboli involve the anterior circulation. Occlusion of the upper division of the middle cerebral artery (MCA) leads to contralateral hemiparesis, hemisensory loss, aphasia (left hemisphere), and left side neglect with motor impersistence (right hemisphere). Occlusion of the inferior MCA branch leads to a Wernicke's aphasia, agitation, right upper quadrant anopia (right hemisphere) or agitation, neglect, and poor drawing (left hemisphere). MCA mainstream infarcts have features of both syndromes.

Posterior circulation sites are the recipient of emboli in but 20 percent of cases. The hallmark of a posterior cerebral artery (PCA) occlusion is hemianopia and hemisensory loss contralateral to the infarct. Patients with left PCA infarcts retain the ability to write and spell but cannot read or name colors. Amnesia lasting up to 6 months is common. Right PCA infarction is occasionally accompanied by left visual neglect. Occlusion of the posterior inferior cerebellar artery leads to ataxia, vomiting, and occipital headache.

593. The answer is A. *(pp 2141–2162)*   The rate of neurologic complications following CABG surgery has been reported as high as 60 percent if alterations of cognitive functions of intellect and personality are included in the analysis. Fortunately, these almost all completely resolve and are often quite subtle, except in elderly patients. The incidence of severe debilitating stroke is, however, quite low in programs with considerable experience. Most strokes that occur during CABG surgery are embolic in nature. The source of these emboli include atheroma from carotid artery disease, atheromatous aortic disease, air embolus, fat emboli, and embolization of particulate matter. In patients with coronary disease, the cardiologist and cardiovascular surgeon must look carefully for hemodynamically significant carotid artery disease. The risk of serious stroke following bypass rises to 5 to 6 percent if a carotid stenosis of greater than 90 percent occlusion is found. This degree of stenosis necessitates concomitant carotid artery surgery or carotid artery surgery under local anesthesia before CABG surgery. It is very rare for hypoperfusion to cause serious strokes in patients undergoing CABG surgery.

594. The answer is C. *(pp 2141–2142)* The NINDS Stroke Data Bank lists the following conditions as having a *strong* predilection to embolization: valvular surgery, atrial fibrillation, sick sinus syndrome, ventricular aneurysm, akinetic segments, mural thrombi, cardiomyopathy, and diffuse ventricular hypokinesis. Mitral valve prolapse is considered to have a weak embolic potential. The rate of recurrence in patients with mitral prolapse and stroke is low. The incidence of stroke, considering the number of patients with mitral prolapse, is very low. Coumadin is not recommended in patients with prolapse who have had an initial stroke; aspirin is felt to be sufficient therapy.

595. The answer is D. *(p 2164)* Cystic medial necrosis was for many years considered to be the hallmark histological lesion of medial degeneration. However, recent observations suggest that this light microscopy lesion is neither specific nor accurately named. A better descriptive terminology of "annuloaortic ectasia" has been applied to reflect the anatomical findings. The defect of disease in the medial aorta lies at a biochemical and subcellular level. Annuloaortic ectasia is the characteristic aortic lesion of Marfan's syndrome. There is a prototypical "Florence flask" or "onion bulb" appearance that reflects the severity of the medial degeneration in the aortic root. Rupture of these aneurysms or aortic regurgitation secondary to root dilatation is responsible for most of the premature deaths of Marfan's syndrome. Takayasu's arteritis refers to a nonspecific aortitis. Reiter's arteritis is a diffuse poorly understood inflammatory response. Diffuse atherosclerosis is not a usual complication of Marfan's syndrome.

596. The answer is B. *(p 2165)* Takayasu's disease is named for the Japanese ophthalmologist who first called attention to the funduscopic findings of this problem. The disease involves a nonspecific aortitis and has been labeled "pulseless" disease and aortic arch syndrome because of its predilection for brachiocephalic vessels. Cardiac manifestations may resolve from aortic regurgitation, coronary artery narrowing, or severe hypertension. Dilatation of the aortic root commonly accompanies the aortic valve incompetence. Angina pectoris, heart failure, and myocardial infarction are reported. However, cerebrovascular accidents and blindness are the most common major events. Congestive heart failure (CHF) and aortic rupture or dissection are less frequent.

597. The answer is D. *(p 2167)* Aneurysms develop at sites of medial weakness. Atherosclerosis is by far the most frequent cause of aortic disease and, thus, is the etiology of most thoracic and abdominal aortic aneurysms. However, the thoracic region may be subdivided into the ascending and descending regions. Syphilis and cystic medial necrosis rather than pure atherosclerosis have a predilection for the ascending aorta.

598. The answer is D. *(p 2182)* The site of claudication indicates the level of the occlusive process if there is a single, focal lesion. Claudication in the foot results from obstruction in the pedal and lower calf vessels. Calf and foot pain results from tibioperoneal occlusive disease. Lower calf discomfort results from popliteal occlusive disease. Superficial femoral occlusive disease causes claudication of the entire calf. Common femoral disease and external iliac occlusive disease lead to thigh and calf claudication. Aortoiliac occlusive disease can produce calf, thigh, buttock, and occasionally low back pain.

599. The answer is D. *(p 2213; Becker, Radiology 170:921–940, 1989)* Becker and colleagues reported the major complications of peripheral and renal artery angioplasty in 4662 patients. Thrombus and embolism occurred most commonly (4.8 percent), followed by arterial rupture and perforation (0.26 percent), death (0.23 percent), limb and kidney loss (0.21 percent) and arteriovenous fistula (0.09 percent). Minor complications included hematoma, pseudoaneurysm, and local injury (3.7 percent), while acute tubular necrosis occurred in 0.88 percent of the patients.

600. The answer is C. *(p 2182)* The patient described in the question has diffuse atherosclerosis in the aorta and a large iliac artery aneurysm that has ruptured into the adjacent iliac vein. Thus, signs and symptoms of high-output cardiac failure and a continuous bruit in the right lower quadrant are likely. Since atherosclerosis is a diffuse process, evidence of atherosclerosis elsewhere would be likely. Resting claudication is unlikely since flow would have to be impeded at rest. There is no obstruction to that degree, and flow is seen in both lower extremities on the arteriogram.

601. The answer is C. *(pp 2211–2213)* In general, fibromuscular disease responds better to renal angioplasty than does atherosclerotic disease. Both unilateral and bilateral fibromuscular diseases respond well. Most patients are cured or improved (93 percent) initially, while 5-year patency rates approach 90 percent. Atherosclerotic obstruction responds initially (89 percent) and remains patent 80 percent of the time. A notable exception is ostial renal atherosclerotic disease in which failure rates of 50 to 100 percent are reported. In this group of patients, plaques are frequently displaced not fractured, leading to poor results. Initial success in renal transplant arteries is likely in 80 percent of cases. Restenosis occurs in 20 percent but redilatation is again successful in 80 to 90 percent of cases.

602. The answer is D. *(p 2207)* Controlled injury is required for successful percutaneous transluminal angioplasty (PTA). Balloon dilatation fractures the atheromatous plaque and disrupts the intima from the media. Injury to the media varies from stretching and incomplete tears to disruption and rupture. Dilatation to the point of adventitial deformation can lead to aneurysm formation and arterial rupture. Thus, injury must be controlled, not extensive, to be effective.

603. The answer is C. *(pp 2188–2190)* Primary livedo reticularis is characterized by a bluish mesh like discoloration of the extremities and trunk, which is stimulated by cold and emotion and is relieved by warmth and exercise. Presumably spasm of cutaneous arterioles with secondary dilatation of the capillaries and venules creates the pattern. Treatment is rarely needed. Secondary livedo reticularis is patchy, focal, or asymmetric. The lesions are tender, elevated, and may be complicated by local infarction or ulcerations. Causes include atherothrombotic emboli, vasculitides, beta blockers, and reflux sympathetic dystrophy. The lesions of the patient pictured in the photographs that accompany the question are confined to below the waist, which localize them to a "nonsystemic process." This patient had a 7 cm abdominal aneurysm as the cause of his symptoms.

604. The answer is B. *(pp 2215–2217)* Systolic blood pressure recorded at the ankle is normally greater than that recorded in the arm. This so-called ankle-arm index is therefore usually greater than 1.0. With an occlusion in the peripheral vasculature of the lower extremity, systolic blood pressure of the lower extremity drops as blood must now course through high-resistance collateral channels. Continuous wave Doppler may be used to indirectly measure systolic blood pressure from the pedal arteries. The magnitude of the fall of pedal systolic blood pressure, and hence the ratio of ankle-to-arm blood pressure, is a reflection of vascular occlusion, and when the ankle-arm ratio is less than 0.5, the occlusion is severe. It is possible to examine the arterial system from the level of the aorta to below the knee. An area of stenosis can be localized by an increase in flow velocity through a narrowed segment and a total occlusion located by absence of flow in a lesion. Thus, obstruction can be relatively well localized. Estimates of degree of stenosis can be made fairly accurately in the extracranial system. Velocity of flow through a stenosis increases as the stenosis worsens. Flow becomes turbulent with changes in lumen diameter and the normal narrow band of frequencies demonstrated in systole becomes widened. Using this information for examining the carotid bifurcation, the sensitivity of Doppler is 98 percent and the specificity is 92 percent. Stenosis is easily distinguished from total occlusion. Doppler is useful for following patients after they have had carotid endarterectomy. About 10 to 20 percent of these patients may demonstrate high-grade restenosis from hyperplasia. Importantly, these smooth lesions are not associated with development of transient ischemic attacks. Doppler can distinguish this lesion from the recurrence of atherosclerotic restenosis, which carries a worse prognosis. The accuracy of Doppler ultrasound and plethysmography permits detection of deep venous thrombosis. Venous flow loses its phasic quality and becomes continuous distal to venous occlusion. Venous hypertension occurs below sites of venous thrombosis, and impedance plethysmography can measure the rate of venous emptying and define venous thrombosis in this way. The sensitivity and specificity of Doppler for diagnosis of deep venous thrombosis are sufficient to base treatment on the results of these tests.

605. The answer is C (2, 4). *(p 2170)*   Rupture of an abdominal aortic aneurysm is a frequent cause of death. The risk of rupture appears greatest for larger aneurysms, particularly those greater than 5 cm in diameter. There is general agreement that patients with aneurysms greater than 5 cm, even if asymptomatic, should undergo operative treatment. Aneurysms smaller than 4 cm appear rarely to rupture and do not ordinarily require surgery unless they become larger. Aneurysms between 4 cm and 5 cm fall into a gray zone in which there is controversy regarding the surgical intervention. Symptomatic aneurysms require urgent surgical treatments since early rupture can be confidently predicted.

606. The answer is C (2, 4). *(pp 2170–2171, 2175)*   According to the widely used DeBakey nomenclature, a proximal dissection is classified as type I and a distal dissection is classified as type III. Type II includes dissection limited to the ascending aorta. Type III dissection initiates distal to the left subclavian takeoff. Reentry channels may occur in the distal descending aorta in both type I and III dissections. Aortic insufficiency may be found in type I and type II dissections due to dilatation of the ascending aorta, but it is not part of the pathophysiological process of a type III dissection. Surgical therapy is generally indicated in cases of type I dissection. Medical therapy is the best course of action in type III dissection as long as there is no impairment of the distal aortic circulation.

607. The answer is C (2, 4). *(p 2175)*   The goal of pharmacological therapy in acute and subacute aortic dissection is to reduce the overall hydraulic stress by lowering aortic pressure and reducing contractility. Hydralazine, minoxidil, and diazoxide are contraindicated since they produce reflex inotropic stimulation of the left ventricle and may propagate the dissection. Although sodium nitroprusside used alone has this theoretical fault, when combined with propranolol, there is an appropriate balance of effects, which makes this regimen appropriate. Intravenous labetolol is also a useful alternative to the combination of nitroprusside and a β-adrenergic blocking agent.

608. The answer is E (all). *(p 2164)*   The term "mycotic" aneurysm is a misnomer. Invasion of the aortic wall in this entity is not exclusively by a fungal infection but by any potential organism, particularly a bacterial invasion. These invading organisms are blood-borne and enter the aortic wall via the lumen or from the vasa vasorum. Since the intact endothelium is resistant to invasion, a previously damaged area usually provides the nidus point for infection. The invasion may occur as a result of septicemia with or without endocarditis. Tuberculous infection may spread into the aortic wall from adjacent lymph nodes. On occasion, fungal endocarditis may cause mycotic aneurysms.

609. The answer is A (1, 2, 3). *(pp 2163–2164)*   Atherosclerosis characteristically tends to spare the ascending aorta in most concomitant states. The major exceptions are in patients with diabetes mellitus and in patients with type II familial hyperlipidemia. Both of these processes may result in the development of severe atherosclerotic plaque throughout the entire aorta. Syphilis is another exception, but in this setting, atherosclerosis may overlay regions of aortitis that have a predilection for the ascending aorta.

610. The answer is D (4). *(p 2186)*   Vasodilators improve cutaneous flow but do not improve claudication or arterial flow. Anticoagulants do not change the course of atherosclerotic obstructive disease but are used in cases of embolic phenomena or clotting disorders. Pentoxifylline can increase the distance until exercise-induced claudication occurs by 30 to 60 percent. A regular walking program of 30 to 45 minutes at least 4 days per week can improve walking distance by 200 percent or more.

611. The answers are: A-Y, B-N, C-N, D-N, E-Y. *(pp 2197–2201; NASCET, Stroke 22:711–720, 1991; ECST, Lancet 337:1235–1243, 1991; Roederer, Stroke 15:605–613, 1984)* The North American Symptomatic Carotid Endarterectomy Trial (NASCET) and the European Carotid Surgery Trialists' Collaborative Study (ECST) both concluded that symptomatic patients with 70 to 99 percent occlusion would benefit from carotid endarterectomy. Groups with more moderate occlusion are still under investigation. In data provided by Seattle researchers, 35 percent of asymptomatic patients with 80 percent or greater stenosis had a stroke, transient ischemic attack (TIA), or carotid occlusion within 6 months of discovery of the lesion, and 45 percent had similar events within a year. Peripheral lower extremity surgery has a 1 to 4 percent operative mortality rate, but a 50 percent 5-year mortality is expected in the subgroup of patients with severe ischemia. An ankle-brachial index less than or equal to 0.30 is associated with a 64 percent mortality in the ensuing 6 years. Operative mortality for celiac or mesenteric bypass approaches 5 to 9 percent. There is a high (about 50 percent) frequency of complications including myocardial ischemia, pulmonary insufficiency, sepsis, and local wound complications.

612. The answers are: A-Y, B-Y, C-Y, D-Y, E-Y. *(pp 2219–2222)* Phlebography remains the more accurate test compared to radionuclide and noninvasive techniques in the diagnosis of venous thrombosis of the lower extremity. The technique is, however, far from totally benign. Adverse reactions, ranging from nausea to hemodynamic collapse, occur in about 12.7 percent of patients receiving ionic contrast agents and in 3.1 percent of patients receiving nonionic contrast agents. Death occurs in every several hundred cases. Pulmonary edema can occur as a result of volume overload. Renal failure can result from nephrotoxic effects of the dye. Endothelial injury due to irritant effects of the dye can lead to thrombosis or thrombophlebitis (wide variability from 0 to 48 percent). Contrast extravasation can lead to ulceration, necrosis, and even amputation of a gangerous extremity.

613. The answers are: A-N, B-N, C-Y, D-Y, E-Y. *(pp 2223–2225)* Plethysmography is useful for the detection of proximal deep venous thrombosis. If a proximal deep venous thrombosis is not detected, there is a low likelihood for the subsequent development of pulmonary embolization. Impedance plethysmography is of limited use in the detection of a thrombus below the knee or in patients with morbid obesity or peripheral edema as seen in patients with nephrotic syndrome. Positive impedance plethysmography for the detection of proximal deep venous thrombosis is correlated with an increased risk of the development of subsequent pulmonary embolization, though such development is not inevitable.

XIX. Special Diagnostic Ultrasound Techniques Used in the Evaluation of the Cardiovascular System

DIRECTIONS: Each question below contains five suggested responses. Select the **one best** response to each question.

614. Nonexercise stress echocardiography is best described by which of the following statements?

(A) Dipyridamole echocardiography has a high sensitivity but a low specificity for coronary disease

(B) Dobutamine stress echocardiography is contraindicated in patients with diastolic blood pressures greater than 95 mmHg

(C) Echocardiography has a sensitivity and specificity of 85 to 90 percent in detecting dobutamine-induced wall motion abnormalities

(D) Significant side effects from high-dose dobutamine infusion are common and necessitate termination of the test in roughly one-third of patients

(E) Dobutamine stress echocardiography has a distinct advantage over exercise echocardiography because only one parasternal view is necessary with dobutamine stress testing

615. An absolute contraindication to transesophageal echocardiography (TEE) is

(A) a grade I esophageal varix

(B) a recently successfully dilated esophageal stricture

(C) cervical spine instability

(D) an active gastric ulcer

(E) an indwelling nasogastric tube

DIRECTIONS: Each question below contains four suggested responses of which **one or more** is correct. Select

A	if	**1, 2, and 3**	are correct
B	if	**1 and 3**	are correct
C	if	**2 and 4**	are correct
D	if	**4**	is correct
E	if	**1, 2, 3, and 4**	are correct

616. The evaluation of aortic regurgitation by the Doppler deceleration slope and velocity half-time technique can be influenced by

 (1) the presence of mixed aortic stenosis and regurgitation
 (2) associated ischemic ventricular damage
 (3) the presence of a poorly compliant left ventricle
 (4) a very high systolic blood pressure

617. Correct statements regarding the evaluation of ventricular septal defects by Doppler echocardiography include which of the following?

 (1) Large ventricular septal defects usually produce a low shunt flow velocity
 (2) Multiple defects are most easily demonstrated by using pulsed Doppler
 (3) Compared with angiographic findings, Doppler can detect ventricular septal defects with a sensitivity of 95 to 100 percent
 (4) The ratio between the pulmonary and systemic flow volumes do not correlate well with the $\dot{Q}_p/\dot{Q}_s$ measured at cardiac catheterization

618. In the evaluation of mitral stenosis, the mitral valve area obtained by the Doppler pressure half-time technique is relatively unaffected by

 (1) mitral volumetric flow
 (2) presence of coexisting mitral regurgitation
 (3) heart rate
 (4) associated significant aortic regurgitation

619. Transesophageal echocardiography (TEE) is superior to transthoracic echocardiography (TTE) in the assessment of

 (1) an intracardiac tumor
 (2) an atrial septal defect
 (3) a flail mitral leaflet
 (4) aortic stenosis

620. Exercise echocardiography provides a distinct advantage to exercise electrocardiography (ECG) because

 (1) the exercise ECG is often abnormal in patients on digoxin even in the absence of coronary artery disease
 (2) exercise echocardiography is more sensitive than exercise ECG without sacrificing specificity
 (3) left ventricular hypertrophy is unlikely to cause a false-positive echocardiographic response, whereas it can cause a false-positive exercise ECG response
 (4) exercise-induced changes in aortic flow velocity and estimated cardiac outputs as seen on Doppler exercise echocardiography are indicative of global left ventricular function

DIRECTIONS: Each question below contains five suggested responses. For **each** of the **five** responses listed with every question you are to respond either YES (Y) or NO (N). In a given item **all, some, or none of the alternatives may be correct.**

621. Evaluation of prosthetic valve function by transthoracic Doppler echocardiography is accurately described by which of the following statements?

(A) Aortic valve functional orifice area can be calculated by using the continuity equation

(B) The pressure half-time should not be used to calculate the mitral valve functional orifice areas

(C) Mitral regurgitation is adequately evaluated by color Doppler

(D) The velocity of antegrade flow across a prosthesis varies with cardiac output

(E) Many bioprostheses as well as mechanical prostheses normally do permit some regurgitation

622. Intracoronary ultrasound can be used to

(A) detect thrombus

(B) differentiate between therapeutic and pathological dissection after percutaneous transluminal coronary angioplasty

(C) provide luminal characteristics for lesion-specific therapy with coronary angioplasty

(D) detect the presence of coronary artery disease with more sensitivity than coronary angiography

(E) quantify luminal measurements with more accuracy than coronary angiography

XIX. Special Diagnostic Ultrasound Techniques Used in the Evaluation of the Cardiovascular System

Answers

614. The answer is C. *(p 2270)* Intravenous dipyridamole in high doses can cause a coronary steal phenomenon. Over 50 percent of patients who receive these high doses have side effects; therefore, in the United States, dobutamine stress echocardiography is the more popular modality. Nonetheless, studies by Italian investigators reveal a very high specificity for the detection of coronary disease but a sensitivity of only 60 to 74 percent. Dobutamine stress echocardiography is both sensitive and specific, and side effects are relatively infrequent. Premature ventricular contractions (PVCs), paroxysmal atrial fibrillation, nausea, and jitteriness are not uncommon, but few side effects are severe enough to terminate the test. Standard dobutamine stress echocardiography requires multiple echocardiographic views to visualize all segments of the myocardium. Mild hypertension is not a contraindication to dobutamine stress echocardiography; however, in patients with significant hypertension at rest, it is usually recommended that the blood pressure be controlled prior to initiation of any stress testing.

615. The answer is C. *(p 2254, Table 131-2)* A transesophageal echocardiography (TEE) is generally well tolerated. There are no contraindications if a patient has a nasogastric tube, a hiatal hernia, a duodenal ulcer, a tracheostomy; or is critically ill or elderly. Relative contraindications include grade I varices, a meal within 4 hours, an esophageal stricture successfully dilated, mild esophagitis, an oropharyngeal deformity, or a gastric ulcer. TEE in a patient with cervical spine instability may cause major neurological trauma and, therefore, is an absolute contraindication. Other absolute contraindications include large esophageal varices or a recent bleed, carcinoma of the esophagus or a tumor invading the esophagus, Zenker's esophageal diverticulum, a ruptured esophagus, a tracheoesophageal fistula, a nondilated esophageal stricture, a Mallory-Weiss tear, or dysphagia of unknown etiology.

616. The answer is E (all). *(pp 2243–2245)* Quantification of the severity of aortic regurgitation can be performed by measuring deceleration slopes and velocity half-times obtained by continuous wave Doppler. It is important to remember, however, that the time course of the aortic regurgitant velocity curve reflects the time course of the corresponding gradient and is, therefore, affected by factors that are associated with poor left ventricular compliance, such as coexisting aortic stenosis, ischemic ventricular damage, or markedly elevated aortic systolic pressure.

617. The answer is B (1, 3). *(p 2247)* Multiple ventricular septal defects are usually best visualized by using color flow images. Doppler techniques are quite sensitive for the detection of ventricular septal defects (95 to 100 percent). In general, there is a good correlation between the $\dot{Q}_p/\dot{Q}_s$ ratio obtained by Doppler echocardiography and that measured from cardiac catheterization. Large ventricular septal defects are nonrestrictive and, thus, produce low shunt flow velocity.

618. The answer is A (1, 2, 3). *(pp 2241–2242)* In the evaluation of mitral stenosis, the Doppler pressure half-time can be determined directly from the transmitral diastolic flow velocity curve. The Doppler pressure half-time is the time required for the pressure to drop to half of its initial value or it is the time required for the initial maximum velocity to decline to a level of 70 percent of the maximum initial velocity. The mitral orifice can be calculated by dividing 220 ms/cm² square by the Doppler half-time measured in milliseconds. Mitral valve areas derived by this technique are relatively unaffected by mitral volumetric flow, heart rate, or the presence or absence of coexisting mitral regurgitation. On the other hand, the accuracy of the pressure half-time technique has been questioned in patients with mitral stenosis and associated moderate-to-severe aortic regurgitation.

619. The answer is A (1, 2, 3). *(pp 2258–2260)* With the retrocardiac orientation, transesophageal echocardiography (TEE) is better able to interrogate the mitral valve. Intracardiac tumors and atrial septal defects are seen much better than with transthoracic echocardiography (TTE). The aortic valve is not as well analyzed due to the retrocardiac orientation of TEE; thus, TTE is probably still the best way of assessing pathology in this region. Aortic dissections are more effectively analyzed by TEE as quite commonly the intimal flap, entry site, and true and false lumens may be evaluated.

620. The answer is E (all). *(pp 2267–2269)* There are many potential causes of false-positive responses to exercise electrocardiography (ECG), including the use of digoxin, intraventricular conduction delays, left bundle branch block (LBBB), left ventricular hypertrophy, Wolff-Parkinson-White syndrome, and electrolyte abnormalities. Exercise echocardiography, however, provides a visualization of left ventricular function at rest and with exercise. The development of a new regional wall motion abnormality or a worsening of an existing wall motion abnormality is highly suggestive of coronary disease. Exercise echocardiography increases the sensitivity for single-vessel disease to 75 percent and to 90 to 95 percent for multivessel disease. This is a distinct advantage over exercise ECG. The specificity is high and is comparable to that of exercise ECG. Doppler interrogation of aortic flow velocity can be used to calculate stroke volume and cardiac output. The peak velocity achieved during exercise and the time to peak velocity are additional measures of exercise ventricular systolic function. In normal subjects, these exercise-induced changes in aortic flow velocity and the derived cardiac outputs correlate well with changes in cardiac output determinations by the traditional methods of Fick oximetry and thermodilution.

621. The answers are: A-Y, B-N, C-N, D-Y, E-Y. *(pp 2246–2247)* In the evaluation of prosthetic valve function by Doppler transthoracic echocardiography (TTE), it is important to remember that the prosthetic valve may conceal Doppler evidence of mitral regurgitation because of acoustic masking of the left atrium. For this reason, when the severity of mitral regurgitation across a prosthetic valve needs to be evaluated, transesophageal echocardiography (TEE) is valuable. Mitral valve functional orifice area can be determined from pressure half-time measures for bioprosthetic and tilting disk mechanical valves. The continuity equation can be used to determine the functional orifice area of an aortic valve prosthesis. Although the amount of regurgitation may be negligible, many bioprostheses and mechanical prostheses have a limited amount of valvular regurgitation.

622. The answers are: A-N, B-N, C-N, D-Y, E-Y. *(pp 2275–2276)* Intracoronary ultrasound has potential exciting applications. At present, it is generally accepted that ultrasound is more sensitive in the detection of coronary artery disease and in the quantification of luminal measurements than coronary angiography. Future potential applications include the ability to differentiate therapeutic from pathological dissections and to guide lesion-specific therapy. At present, the density of thrombus and blood is similar and cannot be differentiated with intracoronary ultrasound.

XX. Diagnostic Radionuclide and Nuclear Techniques Used in the Evaluation of the Cardiovascular System

DIRECTIONS: Each question below contains five suggested responses. Select the **one best** response to each question.

623. The extent of myocardial salvage following thrombolytic therapy administered during an acute myocardial infarction is best assessed with

- (A) technetium-99m methoxy isobutyl isonitrile [^{99m}Tc-MIBI (sestamibi)]
- (B) technetium-99m teboroxime (^{99m}Tc-teboroxime)
- (C) planar imaging with thallium-201 (^{201}Tl)
- (D) dobutamine stress echocardiography
- (E) left ventriculography

624. All the following statements regarding ultrafast computed tomography (CT) are true EXCEPT

- (A) it is a promising diagnostic technology for the detection of coronary artery disease in asymptomatic patients
- (B) it is a better diagnostic tool for evaluating native heart valves than echocardiography
- (C) it is one of the diagnostic procedures of choice for the rapid diagnosis of dissecting aneurysms of the thoracic aorta
- (D) it is one of the diagnostic methods of choice for evaluating the pericardium
- (E) it has been shown to predict accurately patency of bypass grafts

625. The gated blood pool scans below at end-diastole (*top*) and end-systole (*bottom*) represent an example of

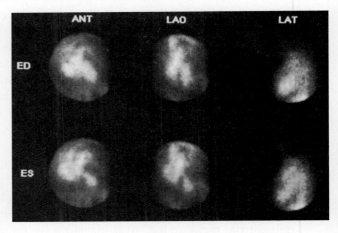

- (A) a normal study
- (B) a dilated cardiomyopathy
- (C) right ventricular dysfunction in a patient with cor pulmonale
- (D) a left ventricular aneurysm
- (E) a left ventricular pseudoaneurysm

626. All the following statements regarding ultrafast CT are true EXCEPT

(A) the speed of acquisition of ultrafast CT images depends on how fast the gantry moves around the patient

(B) one mode of ultrafast CT allows for real-time cross sections of the beating heart

(C) another imaging acquisition mode for ultrafast CT allows for evaluation of myocardial blood flow

(D) ultrafast CT is probably the best modality for determining the volumes of the cardiac chambers and cardiac mass

(E) ultrafast CT is a diagnostic modality that has no moving parts but uses roentgenograms to image the heart

627. All the following statements regarding ultrafast computed tomography (ultrafast CT) and coronary calcification are true EXCEPT

(A) coronary calcification is present in most patients with significant coronary disease

(B) sensitivity of ultrafast CT for predicting obstructive coronary disease is very high

(C) young patients with acute myocardial infarction frequently have no calcification present in the coronary artery

(D) the degree of coronary calcification is not related to age

(E) patients with symptomatic coronary disease have a more rapid progression of coronary artery calcification than asymptomatic patients

628. Correct statements regarding technetium-99m–teboroxime (^{99m}Tc-teboroxime) tracer include which of the following?

(1)   It is chemically similar to the cationic complexes, which include technetium-99m methoxy isobutyl isonitrile [^{99m}Tc-MIBI (sestamibi)]

(2)   It exhibits high myocardial extraction

(3)   It washes out slowly from the myocardium

(4)   Regional washout rates are related to regional myocardial blood flow

629. In a thallium-201 (^{201}Tl) study, increased lung thallium activity can be seen in patients with

(1)   aortic stenosis and left-sided heart failure

(2)   dilated cardiomyopathy

(3)   left-sided heart failure from mitral regurgitation

(4)   severe coronary artery disease

630. Exercise radionuclide cineangiography is correctly characterized by which of the following statements?

(1)   The test can be performed using gated equilibrium imaging but not the "first-pass" technique

(2)   An abnormal response of the left ventricular ejection fraction to exercise is sensitive but not specific for coronary artery disease

(3)   The widely accepted normal response of left ventricular ejection fraction to exercise is to increase by 15 percent or more

(4)   Resting left ventricular ejection fraction and exercise duration are helpful in determining the optimal time for valve replacement in aortic regurgitation

DIRECTIONS: Each question below contains five suggested responses. For **each** of the **five** responses listed with every question you are to respond either YES (Y) or NO (N). In a given item **all, some, or none of the alternatives may be correct.**

631. In the evaluation of coronary artery bypass grafts, ultrafast computed tomography (ultrafast CT)

    (A) has difficulty differentiating fully patent grafts from partially or distally obstructed grafts

    (B) has a high sensitivity and specificity in evaluating graft patency

    (C) is ineffective for evaluating internal mammary artery grafts

    (D) uses intravenous contrast

    (E) easily visualizes proximally occluded saphenous vein grafts

632. Which of the following positron-emitting tracers are used to evaluate myocardial tissue?

    (A) ^{15}O water is used to measure myocardial blood flow

    (B) ^{18}F 2-fluoro-2-deoxyglucose is used to measure exogenous glucose use

    (C) ^{11}C CGP 12177 is used to measure the activity of beta adrenoreceptors

    (D) ^{18}F mizonidazole is used to measure hypoxic-ischemic myocardium

    (E) ^{11}C-labeled methiodide salt of quinuclidinyl benzylate (^{11}C MQNB) is used to measure muscarinic receptors

DIRECTIONS: The group of questions below consists of lettered headings followed by a set of numbered items. For each numbered item select the **one** lettered heading with which it is **most** closely associated. Each lettered heading may be used **once, more than once, or not at all.**

Questions 633–635

For each clinical pathology listed below, select the findings on positron emission tomography (PET) that are most likely to be associated with it.

(A) Normal blood flow and normal glucose metabolism
(B) Decreased blood flow and normal glucose metabolism
(C) Decreased blood flow and decreased glucose metabolism
(D) Normal blood flow and decreased glucose metabolism

633. Myocardial scar

634. Hibernating myocardium, acute

635. Hibernating myocardium, chronic

XX. Diagnostic Radionuclide and Nuclear Techniques Used in the Evaluation of the Cardiovascular System

Answers

623. The answer is A. *(pp 2286–2287)* Technetium-99m isobutyl methoxy isonitrile [^{99m}Tc-MIBI (sestamibi)] has relatively stable myocardial concentration with little washout over a 3- to 4-hour period. Therefore, it does not demonstrate redistribution phenomenon. To assess the extent of myocardial salvage following thrombolytic therapy, one dose of the tracer is injected prior to the administration of thrombolytic therapy, and imaging is performed several hours later because of the very slow washout. The patient is then reinjected and reimaged 24 hours later. The difference between the two defects represents the salvaged myocardium.

624. The answer is B. *(pp 2325–2338)* Ultrafast computed tomography (ultrafast CT) has primarily been a research tool; however, recent technical advances have brought this technology into the forefront of cardiac diagnoses for several disease entities. Ultrafast CT is an excellent diagnostic tool for visualizing the heart and great vessels. Because the scan times are in the millisecond range, cardiac motion can be stopped, allowing for good resolution of cardiac structures. Ultrafast CT has been shown to predict accurately patency of coronary artery bypass grafts when compared to conventional angiography. It is also one of the diagnostic modalities of choice for evaluating the pericardium. One of the most promising applications for ultrafast CT may be the early diagnosis of coronary artery disease in asymptomatic patients. Diagnosis of coronary artery disease by ultrafast CT is made by visualizing calcification in the coronary arteries. The amount of calcium (Ca^{2+}) in the coronary arteries can be graded and correlated to the severity of disease. This is very useful to clinicians who can diagnose coronary artery disease in asymptomatic patients and then focus on risk-factor modification. Currently, a number of studies are designed to evaluate the long-term incidence and prevalence of asymptomatic coronary disease as well as the effects of risk-factor modification on the long-term prognosis of these patients. Ultrafast CT is one of the diagnostic modalities of choice in evaluating patients with suspected dissecting aortic aneurysms. Relative to magnetic resonance imaging (MRI), the ultrafast CT has a much more open architecture that allows continued medical treatment of patients with suspected dissecting aortic aneurysms. Thus, ultrafast CT and transesophageal echocardiography (TEE) are the diagnostic tests of choice for making the diagnosis of dissecting aneurysms. Echocardiography continues to be the diagnostic standard for evaluating native leaflet structure and motion.

625. The answer is D. *(p 2308)* Left ventricular aneurysm and pseudoaneurysm are both easily detected by three-view multigated blood pool imaging. An aneurysm is suggested by an akinetic or dyskinetic segment most commonly seen at the apex as shown in the figure that accompanies the question. A pseudoaneurysm is suggested by a large aneurysmal dilatation with a narrow neck connecting it to the main body of the ventricle.

626. The answer is A. *(pp 2325–2338, Figures 135-1 and 135-3)* Ultrafast computed tomography (ultrafast CT) is a diagnostic modality that images the heart with x-radiation. This technology has no moving parts. The electron gun is positioned at a distance from the gantry, which holds the tungsten target that encircles the thorax. The electron beam is deflected by a powerful magnetic coil, and when the electron beam strikes the tungsten targets, x-radiation is generated and then passes through the patient to a detector located 180° from the tungsten target. By sweeping the electron beam in a circular fashion, a 360° arc can be made around the patient in as little as 50 ms. There are a number of modes of operation for ultrafast CT. The most common is a cine mode. This mode creates a cross-sectional view of a beating heart that can be played on a television screen in realtime. Another mode is the flow mode. In this imaging protocol, images are acquired at different times throughout the cardiac cycle and timed on the electrocardiogram (ECG), following intravenous injection of a iodinated contrast material. This allows the construction of time activity curves or time density curves that have been validated in animals against the gold standard of radioactive microspheres. Because image acquisition with ultrafast CT is quick, frame-by-frame analysis can be used to determine accurate measures of cardiac chamber size and wall thickness; thus, it is not difficult to then calculate myocardial mass. Ultrafast CT has now become the gold standard for measuring cardiac mass.

627. The answer is D. *(pp 2329–2331)* Ultrafast computed tomography (ultrafast CT) has a very high resolution and scanning frequency. This technology is seen as a potential tool for evaluating and diagnosing coronary artery disease. Ultrafast CT can be used to determine regional left ventricular function and volumes and to detect coronary calcification. In general, the higher the amount of calcification present, the more severe the coronary disease; however, coronary calcification is an age-related phenomenon. Even normal elderly patients without angiographically significant coronary disease have a higher level of coronary calcification as determined by ultrafast CT than younger patients. The absence of any calcification on ultrafast CT in an older man has a very high specificity for ruling out hemodynamically obstructive coronary disease. Younger patients with acute myocardial infarction frequently do not have significant calcification on ultrafast CT scanning. The presumed reason is that the acute infarction is caused by rupture of a soft plaque, platelet aggregation, and thrombosis and not to a chronic high-grade stenosis within the coronary artery. One small study has actually shown a decrease in the severity of coronary calcification in patients who are aggressively treated with risk-factor modification. The current generation of scanners are not adequate to permit clinically diagnostic coronary angiography, although future developments in spatial resolution may make it feasible to perform diagnostic coronary angiography with this device.

628. The answer is C (2, 4). *(pp 2287–2288)* Technetium-99m–teboroxime (^{99m}Tc-teboroxime) is similar to thallium in that it exhibits high myocardial extraction, and it distributes proportionately to regional myocardial perfusion. Teboroxime clears rapidly from the myocardium and has a half-life for myocardial clearance of about 6 to 10 min. For this reason, images must be acquired rapidly. ^{99m}Tc-teboroxime is a member of a class that is chemically different from the cationic complexes, which include technetium-99m methoxy isobutyl isonitrile [^{99m}Tc-MIBI (sestamibi)].

629. The answer is E (all). *(pp 2290–2291)* Increased lung thallium activity can be seen in patients with conditions leading to left-sided heart failure. These include valvular heart disease, dilated cardiomyopathy, or severe ischemic heart disease. Patients with cardiomyopathy or left ventricular volume overload can demonstrate transient left ventricular dilatation on thallium studies following exercise.

630. The answer is C (2, 4). *(pp 2309–2311)* Ejection fraction and wall motion can be assessed during exercise stress using either "first-pass" or gated-equilibrium blood pool imaging. Both techniques can be applied using upright bicycle exercise. The widely accepted normal response of left ventricular ejection fraction to exercise is to increase by 5 percent or more. This response can be normally blunted in elderly patients. The value of ejection fraction at peak exercise in determining the time for aortic valve replacement in patients with aortic regurgitation is not clear. However, two parameters are helpful in this regard: resting left ventricular ejection fraction and exercise duration.

631. The answers are: A-Y, B-Y, C-N, D-Y, E-N. *(p 2329)* Conventional computed tomography (CT) can assess coronary artery bypass graft patency, but ultrafast computed tomography (ultrafast CT) is much more accurate. A multicenter prospective study suggested an overall predictive accuracy exceeding 92 percent. A disadvantage of ultrafast CT is that it requires intravenous contrast with the associated risks. This technique appears to work well for both arterial and venous conduits. While ultrafast CT is good at determining flow down the proximal portion of a graft, visualization of the more distal portions is difficult. Scan artifacts secondary to surgical clips can interfere with the resolution in the more distal portion of the vein graft. Therefore, a vein graft with a 90 percent distal stenosis may appear patent by ultrafast CT when in fact hemodynamically obstructive narrowing exists. Further studies involving graft flow velocity and graft time-density curves have been suggested as potential solutions.

632. The answers are: A-Y, B-Y, C-Y, D-Y, E-Y. *(p 2362)* The metabolic aspects of myocardial tissue function can now be measured with positron emission tomography (PET). The various aspects that can be measured include myocardial blood flow, myocardial metabolism of glucose and fatty acids, neuronal control, and other specified functions. Myocardial blood can be measured with ^{15}O water. This tracer is retained in the myocardium in proportion to blood flow. Aspects of myocardial metabolism can be measured, including glucose use with ^{18}F 2-fluoro-2-deoxyglucose and fatty acid metabolism with ^{11}C acetate. An emerging application of PET scanning includes the evaluation of neuronal control of the heart. Beta adrenoreceptors can be measured with ^{11}C CGP 12177, an experimental compound, and muscarinic receptors can be measured with ^{11}C-labeled methiodide salt of quinuclidinyl benzylate (^{11}C MQNB). Hypoxic-ischemic myocardium can be evaluated with ^{18}F mizonidazole to demonstrate ischemic but salvageable myocardium.

633–635. The answers are: 633-C, 634-A, 635-B. *(pp 2368–2370)* Assessment of myocardial viability is an important clinical application of positron emission tomography (PET). Blood flow–metabolism mismatch indicates potential areas of salvageable myocardium. This can be identified by normal glucose metabolism with decreased blood flow (myocardial hibernation, chronic). The identification of decreased blood flow and decreased glucose metabolism indicates myocardial scar. Viable myocardium is characterized by normal blood flow and normal glucose metabolism (pure stunning).

XXI. Diagnostic Techniques of Cardiac Catheterization and Vascular Angiography

DIRECTIONS: Each question below contains five suggested responses. Select the **one best** response to each question.

636. The left ventriculogram shown below confirms the diagnosis of

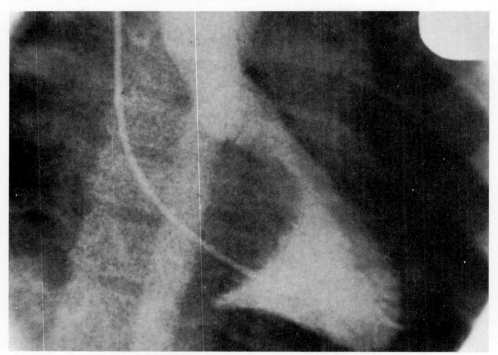

(A) isolated congenitally corrected transposition
(B) isolated transposition of the great vessels
(C) atrioventricular (AV) canal defect
(D) Ebstein's anomaly
(E) right atrial myxoma

637. The arteriogram in the right anterior oblique projection that follows shows

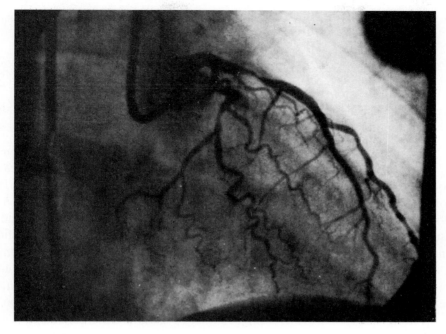

(A) significant occlusion of the left main artery
(B) significant occlusion of the left anterior descending artery
(C) significant occlusion of the circumflex artery
(D) dissection in the left coronary artery
(E) diffuse coronary arteritis

---

638. Indicator-dilution injection into the right atrium and sampling a peripheral arterial site reveals which of the following indicator-dilution curves?

(A) A normal recirculation curve
(B) An early recirculation curve
(C) No recirculation curve
(D) A very late recirculation curve
(E) Unintelligible results since the recirculation prevents dye from being detected by the catheter

639. The most frequently expected complication following cardiac catheterization is

(A) death
(B) myocardial infarction
(C) cerebral emboli
(D) a local arterial complication
(E) ventricular fibrillation

DIRECTIONS: Each question below contains four suggested responses of which **one or more** is correct. Select

A	if	**1, 2, and 3**	are correct
B	if	**1 and 3**	are correct
C	if	**2 and 4**	are correct
D	if	**4**	is correct
E	if	**1, 2, 3, and 4**	are correct

640. Patients who require supervision after catheterization and who are, therefore, not candidates for ambulatory cardiac catheterization include those with

(1)   morbid obesity
(2)   uncontrolled blood pressure
(3)   severe chronic lung disease, hypoxia, and pulmonary hypertension
(4)   brittle insulin-dependent diabetes mellitus

641. Clues to catheterization of the coronary sinus include

(1)   acute catheter angle in the right atrium in the right anterior oblique position
(2)   catheter blood samples that reveal marked oxygen desaturation
(3)   posterior position of the catheter in the lateral view
(4)   a course near the right atrioventricular (AV) groove since it removes venous drainage of the right coronary artery distribution

642. Right atrial angiography is useful in defining

(1)   the severity of tricuspid regurgitation
(2)   the position of the tricuspid valve in Ebstein's anomaly
(3)   cor triatriatum
(4)   right atrial myxoma

643. In detecting a left-to-right shunt, which of the following oxygen stepups is significant?

(1)   A 9 percent saturation increase between the superior vena cava and the right atrium indicates an atrial shunt
(2)   A 3 percent saturation increase between the right atrium and the right ventricle indicates a ventricular shunt
(3)   A 3 percent saturation increase between the right ventricle and the pulmonary artery indicates a pulmonary artery shunt
(4)   A 3 percent saturation increase between the inferior vena cava and right atrium indicates an atrial shunt

644. Correct cardiac catheterization laboratory determinations include

(1)   a spurious gradient caused by left ventricular cavity obliteration with catheter entrapment
(2)   a mean pulmonary artery pressure with exercise no higher than 25 mmHg in a normal patient
(3)   left ventricular femoral artery pressures to calculate the gradient in patients with aortic stenosis
(4)   rapid atrial pacing, leading to a decrease in left ventricular end-diastolic pressure, in patients with significant coronary artery disease

XXI. Diagnostic Techniques of Cardiac Catheterization and Vascular Angiography

Answers

636. The answer is C. *(p 2400)* The catheter used in the ventriculogram that accompanies the question arises in the venous system not in the aorta. Since an anatomic left ventricle is injected, an intracardiac defect was crossed. Injection into the left ventricle reveals a typical "swan's neck" deformity of the left ventricular outflow tract followed by ejection of dye into the aorta. In either isolated congenitally corrected transposition or transposition of the great arteries without other defects, there would be no connection to the systemic side of the heart. In transposition of the great arteries, the right atrium leads to the right ventricle, which leads to the pulmonary artery. Likewise, in corrected transposition, the right atrium leads to the anatomic left ventricle, which leads to the pulmonary artery. In either Ebstein's anomaly or right atrial myxoma, an intracardiac defect must exist to see a left ventriculogram and aorta, and injection into the left ventricle would not demonstrate pathology on the right side.

637. The answer is B. *(p 2409)* The coronary arteriogram in the right anterior oblique projection that accompanies the question shows a high-grade occlusion of the left anterior descending artery proximal to the first septal perforator secondary to coronary atherosclerosis.

638. The answer is B. *(p 2392)* One may quantitate left-to-right shunts and estimate right-to-left shunts by indicator-dilution techniques in the cardiac catheterization laboratory. By injecting an indicator into the right atrium and sampling either a peripheral arterial site or other sites in the heart, the presence of a left-to-right shunt is possible. In a normal heart, injection of an indicator-dilution dye into the right atrium reveals an initial curve with a very large peak and falloff reflecting the initial pass through the circulation and its detection in a peripheral arterial site.

639. The answer is D. *(p 2412)* The frequency of any complication following cardiac catheterization is low. Arterial complications, such as hematomas, arterial occlusion or stenosis, false aneurysm, and infection, occur more frequently than the thromboembolic events, such as death, myocardial infarction, cerebral emboli, or ventricular fibrillation.

640. The answer is E (all). *(p 2382, Table 138-1; Pepine, J Am Coll Cardiol 18:1149–1182, 1991)* The American College of Cardiology and American Heart Association have published criteria specifying clinical characteristics of patients who are not candidates for ambulatory cardiac catheterization because they need postcatheterization supervision. These include patients with mechanical prosthetic valves, general debility, low ejection fraction, uncontrolled hypertension, pulmonary hypertension, severe lung disease, morbid obesity, uncontrolled diabetes, and a history of allergies to contrast materials. In addition, patients under 21 years of age and those who have had a stroke or extreme ischemia during stress testing are not candidates for ambulatory cardiac catheterization. However, as pressures mount to increase savings, more patients with the above criteria are allowed to go home after catheterization so long as they tolerate the procedure well.

641. The answer is A (1, 2, 3). *(p 2383)* Catheterization of the coronary sinus is often performed to obtain measurement of coronary sinus lactate. Coronary sinus lactate reflects the myocardial oxygen supply and demand balance, and measures of coronary sinus blood flow reflect left anterior descending coronary blood flow. Consequently, coronary sinus blood flow may be used as a measure of coronary flow reserve under conditions of maximal coronary vasodilation from drug intervention or rapid atrial pacing. It is, therefore, important to be able to localize specifically the tip of the catheter in the right atrium or in the coronary sinus. Because the coronary sinus has a fairly posterior location, an acute angle of the catheter must be formed in the right anterior oblique position to sample the coronary sinus. Because the coronary sinus is the venous drainage of the myocardial bed, the blood is markedly desaturated; therefore, a blood sample for oxygen saturation can localize the position of the catheter in the coronary sinus.

642. The answer is C (2, 4). *(p 2398)* Right atrial angiography is useful in evaluating patients with Ebstein's anomaly in that the attachment of the inferiorly displaced septal tricuspid valve leaflet may be seen. With right atrial angiography, masses in the right atrium, particularly prolapsing tumors like right atrial myxomas, may be seen quite clearly. In cor triatriatum, the left atrium is bisected by an intra-atrial membrane, and right atrial injection usually allows inadequate visualization of the left atrium to be of diagnostic value. There is great difficulty judging the severity of tricuspid regurgitation with right heart angiography. The right ventricle is typically catheterized and contrast injected into the right ventricle to estimate the severity of tricuspid regurgitation. However, the catheter itself produces some degree of regurgitation in crossing the tricuspid valve. Grading the degree of tricuspid regurgitation on right atrial angiography is extraordinarily difficult in that the blood does not reach the right ventricle in severe tricuspid regurgitation and will, therefore, not allow the degree of the regurgitant stream back into the right atrium into the inferior vena cava and superior vena cava to be determined. Consequently, Doppler echocardiography is one of the current standards for judging the severity of tricuspid regurgitation.

643. The answer is B (1, 3). *(p 2389)* Oxygen saturation stepups on the right side of the heart are used to detect left-to-right shunts in the cardiac catheterization laboratory. As the catheter is advanced from the inferior vena cava into the right atrium, samples are taken as the oxygen run is performed from the inferior vena cava to the superior vena cava and back into the pulmonary artery. With shunting, more complete mixing occurs further downstream or distal to the actual shunt lesion. Therefore, in an atrial septal defect, better mixing occurs in the pulmonary artery than occurs in the right atrium. Consequently, it takes less of an oxygen stepup to make the diagnosis of a left-to-right shunt in the more distal parts of the right heart circuit. A 9 precent saturation increase between the superior vena cava and the right atrium indicates an atrial shunt; a 5 percent saturation increase between the right atrium and the right ventricle indicates a ventricular shunt; and a 3 percent saturation increase between the right ventricle and the pulmonary artery indicates a pulmomary artery shunt.

644. The answer is A (1, 2, 3). *(p 2388)* Many hemodynamic measurements are made in the cardiac catheterization laboratory of pressures in various cardiac chambers. Spurious data may be obtained if the appropriate placement of the catheters is not understood. A spurious left ventricular outflow tract gradient can be created with a single catheter advanced in the left ventricular apex that becomes entrapped during a transaortic pullback. This may lead to an incorrect diagnosis of idiopathic hypertrophic subaortic stenosis (IHSS) in some cases of hyperdynamic left ventricle. Measurement of the mean pulmonary artery during exercise in the catheterization laboratory can be used to determine pulmonary vascular reactivity in patients with a tendency toward primary hypertension and to estimate the severity of mitral stenosis. In patients with significant mitral stenosis, there is a marked elevation in the mean pulmonary artery pressure to more than 25 mmHg. When using the left ventricular and femoral artery pressures to calculate the pressure gradient across the aortic valve, proper alignment of these pressures is important because there is a natural temporal delay in the wave form generation between the left ventricle and the femoral artery. The occurrence of myocardial ischemia may be assessed through the technique of rapid atrial pacing. In normal patients, the left ventricular end-diastolic pressure falls as the heart rate increases. Patients with coronary artery disease who are unable to meet the increased myocardial oxygen demand experience an increase in left ventricular end-diastolic pressure.

XXII. The Heart, Anesthesia, and Surgery

DIRECTIONS: Each question below contains five suggested responses. Select the **one best** response to each question.

645. Used as a sole agent, which of the following has the LEAST cardiovascular effect?

(A) Benzodiazepines
(B) Barbiturates
(C) Opioids
(D) Meperidine
(E) Propofol

646. All the following patients require pulmonary catheter monitoring in the intraoperative period EXCEPT those

(A) requiring high levels of positive end-expiratory pressure
(B) with recent myocardial infarction
(C) with left ventricular dysfunction and mitral regurgitation
(D) who undergo tricuspid valve replacement
(E) with pericardial tamponade

DIRECTIONS: Each question below contains four suggested responses of which **one or more** is correct. Select

A	if	**1, 2, and 3**	are correct
B	if	**1 and 3**	are correct
C	if	**2 and 4**	are correct
D	if	**4**	is correct
E	if	**1, 2, 3, and 4**	are correct

647. Administration of which of the following agents is often associated with tachycardia and hypertension?

    (1) Doxacurium
    (2) Pancuronium
    (3) Vecuronium
    (4) Succinylcholine

648. Spinal anesthesia is relatively contraindicated in patients with

    (1) significant valvular heart disease
    (2) hypertrophic obstructive cardiomyopathy
    (3) tetralogy of Fallot
    (4) coronary artery disease

649. Indications for central venous line placement for intraoperative monitoring include

    (1) major trauma
    (2) patients who require frequent blood sampling but do not require an arterial line
    (3) intravascular volume assessment in the setting of renal failure
    (4) major operations involving larger fluid shifts in patients with good left ventricular function

650. Indications for intra-atrial monitoring in the operative period include patients

    (1) undergoing aortic surgery that requires cross-clamping
    (2) requiring inotropes or an intra-aortic balloon pump
    (3) with massive ascites
    (4) who are morbidly obese, making accurate blood pressure measurements difficult

651. Hematologic abnormalities associated with cardiopulmonary bypass include

    (1) platelet dysfunction
    (2) fibrinolysis
    (3) protamine reactions
    (4) antithrombin III deficiency

652. Recognized gastrointestinal complications following bypass include

    (1) pancreatitis
    (2) bowel infarction
    (3) gastrointestinal bleeding
    (4) cholecystitis

XXII. The Heart, Anesthesia, and Surgery

Answers

645. The answer is A. *(pp 2437–2438)* When used as sole agents, benzodiazepines have minimal cardiovascular effects. When used in combination with opiates and potent volatile anesthetics, benzodiazepines produce hypotension that may be due to myocardial depression or decreased systemic vascular resistance. Opioids, though important anesthetic agents for patients with cardiovascular disease, are associated with "breakthrough" hypertension and tachycardia. Meperidine causes tachycardia and histamine release and is a direct myocardial depressant. Barbiturates and propofol have dose-dependent myocardial depressant effects.

646. The answer is D. *(p 2435, Table 140-3)* Widely accepted indications for pulmonary artery catheter monitoring in the intraoperative period include patients with recent myocardial infarctions, pericardial tamponade, left ventricular dysfunction, and mitral regurgitation; patients requiring high levels of positive end-expiratory pressure; and patients undergoing aortic surgery, procedures involving large fluid shifts, or hepatic transplantation. Surgeons should avoid placing a pulmonary artery catheter during tricuspid valve surgery for fear of clotting, valve trauma, or sewing the balloon into the operative area.

647. The answer is C (2, 4). *(pp 2439–2440)* Doxacurium is a new benzylisoquinoline, nondepolarizing, neuromuscular blocker with minimal cardiovascular effect. Pancuronium is a steroidal, nondepolarizing, neuromuscular blocking drug, which can lead to hypertension, tachycardia, and myocardial ischemia during surgery. Vecuronium is a new steroidal, neuromuscular blocker with minimal cardiovascular effects at usual dosages. Succinylcholine is a depolarizing, short-acting, neuromuscular blocker with which either nicotinic (tachycardia and hypertension) or muscarinic (bradycardia and hypotension) effects may occur.

648. The answer is A (1, 2, 3). *(p 2436)* Spinal anesthesia is relatively contraindicated in patients whose hemodynamic stability depends on preservation of high preload and afterload, such as patients with significant valvular heart disease, hypertrophic myopathy, or tetralogy of Fallot. Patients with coronary artery disease tolerate spinal anesthesia well as long as diastolic arterial pressure maintains adequate coronary perfusion.

649. The answer is E (all). *(p 2434, Table 140-2)* Widely accepted indications for central venous line placement include operative procedures that involve large fluid shifts, that have a high risk of air embolism, and that involve major trauma; and for patients who require intravascular volume assessment, frequent blood sampling, and rapid infusion of intravenous fluid. In addition, central venous line placement is used for patients with tricuspid stenosis and for chronic drug administration.

650. The answer is E (all). *(p 2434, Table 140-1; Cheney, Clinical Anesthesia, pp 35–44, 1989)* Basic intra-operative monitoring standards were established in 1986 by the American Society of Anesthesiologists. Digital pulse oximetry is now almost universal. Specific indications for intra-arterial monitoring include surgical procedures involving large fluid shifts, requiring cardiopulmonary bypass, involving the aorta, and for massive trauma; and for patients with pulmonary disease, recent myocardial infarctions, coronary artery disease, massive ascites, congestive heart failure (CHF), electrolyte disturbances, and right-sided heart failure. In addition, patients requiring inotropes or an intra-aortic balloon pump or in whom blood pressure is not able to be measured also need intra-arterial monitoring.

651. The answer is A (1, 2, 3). *(pp 2448–2449)* Prolonged heparinization prior to the bypass procedure (e.g., for the treatment of an intracoronary clot or myocardial infarction) can produce a significant antithrombin III deficiency, which makes the patient difficult to anticoagulate and requires large doses of heparin during bypass. After weaning the patient from cardiopulmonary bypass, protamine is infused to reverse the heparin effect. Infused too rapidly, protamine may cause hypotension and deterioration of myocardial function. Severe anaphylactic reactions may occur in patients previously exposed to protamine, protamine-zinc insulin, or possibly postvasectomy. Marked peripheral vasodilation, massive histamine release, capillary leak, pulmonary vasoconstriction, and right ventricular failure have all been reported in this setting. Coagulopathy after bypass is characterized by platelet dysfunction and fibrinolysis. Severe bleeding occurs in approximately 5 percent of patients with 1 to 3 percent requiring reoperation to control the bleeding.

652. The answer is E (all). *(p 2448)* Severe gastrointestinal complications may occur in 0.5 to 2.0 percent of patients undergoing bypass procedures. Gastrointestinal bleeding occurs as a result of increased stress with gastritis and bleeding ulcers most common. Pancreatitis and cholecystitis can occur acutely or following a prolonged difficult course with multiple drugs and prolonged nutritional support. The exact cause of these complications is often obscure. Bowel infarction usually follows distal embolization of cholesterol-laden debris or clots from inside the heart. The result is often catastrophic.

XXIII. Insurance and Legal Problems

DIRECTIONS: Each question below contains four suggested responses of which **one or more** is correct. Select

A	if	**1, 2, and 3**	are correct
B	if	**1 and 3**	are correct
C	if	**2 and 4**	are correct
D	if	**4**	is correct
E	if	**1, 2, 3, and 4**	are correct

653. Factors that may indicate a high insurance risk in patients following a myocardial infarction include

(1) poor left ventricular systolic function (less than 30 percent)

(2) persistent ventricular ectopy

(3) a positive postinfarction exercise electrocardiogram (ECG)

(4) the extent and severity of coronary artery obstructive disease

654. The medical assessment of cardiac disease for legal purposes is impaired by

(1) the subjective nature of medical complaints

(2) the frequent discrepancy between subjective complaints and objective findings

(3) the dynamic state of cardiac impairments and secondary variability in day-to-day performance

(4) the influence of psychological factors in objective performance

655. In medical malpractice cases, issues that are important in proving a patient's allegation of professional negligence include which of the following?

(1) The physician owed a duty that is implied in the physician-patient relationship

(2) The physician breached the standard of care owed

(3) The patient suffered injury or harm

(4) The physician's negligence was the cause of the patient's harm

XXIII. Insurance and Legal Problems

Answers

653. The answer is E (all). *(p 2455)* There are several factors involved in the risk assessment of the postinfarction patient with regard to insurability. Patients often have problems obtaining insurance after a myocardial infarction. They are either denied insurance or forced to pay very high premiums. Factors considered by insurance underwriters include left ventricular systolic function, extent and severity of coronary artery disease, ventricular arrhythmias, and postinfarction angina. In addition, a positive postinfarction exercise electrocardiogram (ECG) indicates a poor risk. Associated risk factors for coronary artery disease (e.g., diabetes, hypertension, hyperlipidemia, or cigarette smoking) also result in high premiums or denial of insurance.

654. The answer is E (all). *(pp 2472–2473)* Medical assessments of cardiac performance and impairment for legal purposes are difficult due to a variety of reasons. Objective measurements of functional status often do not correlate with subjective complaints. The variability of objective performance varies such that performance may not be constant over a given period of time. In addition, motivation of the patient is an important key factor. Patients who have a lack of motivation and a lack of desire to return to activity often will not perform as well despite similarities in objective functional status.

655. The answer is E (all). *(pp 2473–2474)* There are several issues that are important in medical malpractice cases. In general, the physician must be identified as responsible by virtue of the physician-patient relationship. The physician must adhere to the standard of care owed the patient as a result of this relationship. As a result of negligence on the part of the physician, some injury or harm must have occurred because the standard of care was not followed. In some jurisdictions the patient's conduct may or may not be important as a contributing factor to the harm that resulted (the doctrine of contributory negligence). The fact that a patient suffered an injurious result of a treatment or procedure by itself does not raise the presumption of negligence; the physician is not legally responsible (necessarily) for all adverse outcomes.

Bibliography

Ad Hoc Task Force, Pepine CJ (chairman): ACC/AHA Guidelines for cardiac catheterization and cardiac catheterization laboratories. *J Am Coll Cardiol* 18:1149–1182, 1991.

Aretz HT, et al: Myocarditis. *Am J Cardiovasc Pathol* 1:3–14, 1986.

Becker GJ, et al: Noncoronary angioplasty. *Radiology* 170:921–940, 1989.

Bradbury S, Eggleston C: Postural hypotension: A report of three cases. *Am Heart J* 1:73–86, 1925.

Brensike JF, et al: Effects of therapy with cholestyramine on progression of coronary arteriosclerosis. Results of the NHLBI Type II Coronary Intervention Study. *Circulation* 69:313–324, 1984.

Brown G, et al: Regression of coronary artery disease as a result of interior lipid-lowering therapy in men with high levels of apolipoprotein B. *N Engl J Med* 323:1289–1298, 1990.

Burack B, Furman S: Transesophageal atrial pacing. *Am J Cardiol* 23:469–472, 1969.

Canner PL, et al: Fifteen year mortality in Coronary Drug Project patients: Long-term benefit with niacin. *J Am Coll Cardiol* 8:1245–1255, 1986.

Cardiac Arrhythmia Suppression Trial (CAST) Investigators: Preliminary Report: Effect of encainide and flecainide on mortality in a randomized trial of arrhythmia suppression after myocardial infarction. *N Engl J Med* 321:406–412, 1989.

Cheney FW, et al: Medicolegal aspects of anesthetic practice. In *Clinical Anesthesia,* edited by Barash PG, et al. Philadelphia, Lippincott, pp 35–44, 1989.

Cobb LA, et al: Clinical predictors and characteristics of the sudden cardiac death syndrome. In *Proceedings of the First US-USSR Symposium on Sudden Death,* Yalta, October 3–5, 1977. Washington, DC, US Department of Health, Education, and Welfare, Public Health Service, National Institutes of Health (DHEW publication no NIH 78-1470, 1978).

Cox JL, et al: The surgical treatment of atrial fibrillation: 4. Surgical technique. *J Thorac Cardiovasc Surg* 101:584–592, 1991.

D'Alonzo GE, et al: Survival in patients with primary pulmonary hypertension. *Ann Intern Med* 115:343–349, 1991.

European Carotid Surgery Trialists' Collaborative Group: MRC European Carotid Surgery Trial: Interim results for symptomatic patients with severe (90–99%) or with mild (0–29%) carotid stenosis. *Lancet* 337:1235–1243, 1991.

Expert Panel: Summary of the second Report of the National Education Program (NCEP) Expert Panel on detection, evaluation, and treatment of high blood cholesterol in adults (Adult Treatment Panel II). *JAMA* 269:3015–3023, 1993.

Forrester JS, et al: Medical therapy of acute myocardial infarction by application of hemodynamic subsets (second of two parts). *N Engl J Med* 295:1404–1413, 1976.

Frick MH, et al: Helsinki Heart Study: Primary-prevention trial with gemfibrozil in middle-aged men with dyslipidemia. Safety of treatment, changes in risk factors, and incidence of coronary heart disease. *N Engl J Med* 317:1237–1245, 1987.

Furchgott RF, Bawadzki JV: The obligatory role of endothelial cells in the relaxation of arterial smooth muscle by aceytlcholine. *Nature* 288:373–376, 1980.

Guiraudon GM, et al: Combined sinoatrial node atrioventricular node isolation: A surgical alternative to His bundle ablation in patients with atrial fibrillation (abstract). *Circulation* 72 (Suppl 3):220, 1985.

Hancock EW: Subacute effusive-constrictive pericarditis. *Circulation* 43:183–192, 1971.

Huxley HE, Hanson J: Changes in the cross-striatums of muscle during contraction and stretch and their structural interpretation. *Nature* 173:973–976, 1954.

Jones EL, et al: Clinical, anatomic, and functional descriptors influencing morbidity, survival and adequacy of revascularization following coronary bypass. *Ann Surg* 192(3):390–392, 1980.

Lubell DL: Cardiac pacing from the esophagus. *Am J Cardiol* 27:641–644, 1971.

Lipid Research Clinics Program: The Lipid Research Clinics Coronary Prevention Trial results. I. Reduction in incidence of coronary heart disease. *JAMA* 251:351–364, 1984.

Lipid Research Clinics Program: The Lipid Research Clinics Coronary Prevention Trial results. II. The relationship of reduction in incidence of coronary heart disease to cholesterol lowering. *JAMA* 251:365–374, 1984.

Multiple Risk Factor Intervention Trial Research Group: Multiple Risk Factor Intervention Trial. Risk factor changes and mortality results. *JAMA* 248:1465–1477, 1982.

North American Symptomatic Carotid Endarterectomy (NASCET) Steering Committee: North American Symptomatic Carotid Endarterectomy Trial: Methods, patient characteristics, and progress. *Stroke* 22:711–720, 1991.

Rodbard S: Blood velocity and endocarditis. *Circulation* 27:18–28, 1963.

Roederer GO, et al: The natural history of carotid arterial disease in asymptomatic patients with cervical bruits. *Stroke* 15:605–613, 1984.

Shy GM, Drager GA: A neurologic syndrome associated with orthostatic hypotension. *Ann Intern Med* 82:336–341, 1975.

von Reyn CF, et al: Infective endocarditis. An analysis based on strict case definitions. *Ann Intern Med* 94:505–518, 1981.

Wiggers CJ: Studies on the consecutive phases of the cardiac cycle: I. The duration of the consecutive phases of the cardiac cycle and the criteria for their precise determination. *Am J Physiol* 56:415–438, 1921.

Working Group on Hypertension in the Elderly: Statement on hypertension in the elderly. *JAMA* 256:70–74, 1986.

ISBN 0-07-052011-9

9 780070 520110

90000>